PEDIATRICS - LABORATORY AND CLINICAL RESEARCH

PRETERM INFANTS

DEVELOPMENT, PROGNOSIS AND POTENTIAL COMPLICATIONS

Pediatrics - Laboratory and Clinical Research

Additional books in this series can be found on Nova's website under the Series tab.

Additional e-books in this series can be found on Nova's website under the e-book tab.

Pregnancy and Infants: Medical, Psychological and Social Issues

Additional books in this series can be found on Nova's website under the Series tab.

Additional e-books in this series can be found on Nova's website under the e-book tab.

PEDIATRICS - LABORATORY AND CLINICAL RESEARCH

PRETERM INFANTS

DEVELOPMENT, PROGNOSIS AND POTENTIAL COMPLICATIONS

DIOGO CONTREIRAS
AND
JOHANN SAMPAIO
EDITORS

Nova Science Publishers, Inc.
New York

Library of Congress Cataloging-in-Publication Data

Library of Congress Control Number: 2012937530
ISBN: 978-1-62081-819-0

Published by Nova Science Publishers, Inc. † New York

CONTENTS

PREFACE

In this book, the authors present current research from across the globe in the study of the development, prognosis and potential complications of preterm infants. Topics discussed in this compilation include the cognitive and behavioral problems in moderately preterm children at preschool age; the socio-emotional development and early intervention of preterm infants; later preterm birth and the developing brainstem; readiness of preterm infants to start breastfeeding; hormonal dysregulation of the HPT and HPA axes in preterm infants; effect of additional weight in proximal and distal adjustments of reaching behavior in preterm infants; language and literacy in preterm children; and cognitive, motor and communicative-linguistic developmental trajectories of extremely low gestational age preterms.

Chapter 1 - The social and emotional development of the infant emerges within the context of the first relationships with primary care-givers, most often his mother and father. For the baby, in a state of 'absolute dependency', these relationships will support the baby's physical and physiological integrity and homeostasis. They will provide an environment within which the baby's experiences, internal and external may be gradually processed and become meaningful and where his changing emotional and behavioural states are regulated. These relationships also are the setting within which the baby's innate propensity to relate to others takes place. They also provide the scaffolding for the baby's motor, cognitive and language development and emergent sense of self. Infant mental health has been defined as "the young child's capacity to experience, regulate and express emotions, form close and secure relationships and explore the environment and learn". The care-giving environment which supports the development of these capacities is integral to the existence of infant mental health, namely the family, their community and the culture within which the child is born. Attachment, the unique emotional bond between the infant and his caregivers that develops in the first years of life, has been found to play a crucial role in the subsequesnt social and emotional health of the child..

When the baby is born preterm,, parents and infant must adapt to the dramatic change in each of their lives. The baby's prematurity may necessitate neonatal intensive care; there may be medical complications and separation from the parents. The parents may experience emotional upheaval, anxiety and stress. These experiences may impact on the developing relationship, which is vital for the infant's social and emotional development.

The following chapter aims to review current knowledge on the attachment and social emotional development of preterm infants.

The chapter will begin with a review of the literature on the parent's experiences and psychological adjustment to preterm birth. The neurobehavioural and psychological sequealaefor the infant will then be considered.. A review the literature on preterm infant-parent interaction and attachment will be followed by outcome findings on preterm infant mental health and development. The chapter will conclude with a review of existing interventions to support the developing infant-parent relationship and the social-emotional development of the preterm infant.

Chapter 2 - Carefully monitoring the neurologic status and development in early life is important for preterm infants. A decrease in gestational age is often associated with an increased incidence of neurodevelopmental abnormalities or deficits such as cerebral palsy, even for those infants born at late pregnancy or late preterm. Of all preterm births, late preterm birth comprises about 70%. Therefore, late preterm infants are an important population in preterm infants. Numerous previous studies have shown that infants who are born at very or extremely preterm are predisposed to brain damage and neurological impairment. By comparison, there is relatively limited information available for brain function and neurodevelopment in late preterm infants. Over the last decade, there is an increased interest in studying neurodevelopment in these infants.

Recently, there are investigators who studied brainstem auditory evoked response (BAER) in late preterm infants using the maximum length sequence technique (MLS). In those who had no major perinatal conditions or problems, MLS BAER was basically normal, except for a moderate abnormality at high-rate click stimulation. This finding implies that low-risk late preterm infants have a mild delay in neural conduction in the brainstem and that late preterm birth has limited or no major effect on the immature brain. In late preterm infants who had major perinatal conditions or problems, there were some major abnormalities in those MLS BAER components that mainly reflect functional status of the more central or rostral brainstem. The abnormalities indicate that the functional integrity of the auditory brainstem, mainly in the central regions, is impaired in late preterm infants with perinatal problems. Since late preterm birth *per se* does not exert any significant effect on the immature auditory brainstem, the major MLS BAER abnormalities and, in turn, this functional impairment must be predominately caused by the perinatal problems that are associated with the late preterm birth. This is consistent with some clinical observation that perinatal problems associated with late preterm birth contribute to the overall risk of brain injury in late preterm infants. These findings shed some lights on functional integrity of the brain, specifically the auditory brainstem, in high-risk late preterm infants. Further research into brain development and injury in these infants will help develop focused plans to optimize their management and prevent adverse neurological outcomes.

Chapter 3 - An estimated 3.1 million neonatal deaths occur annually worldwide, accounting for more than 40% of all deaths in children younger than five years of age Complications of preterm birth (before 37 weeks of gestation) are the leading direct cause and major risk factor for neonatal deaths, accounting for 27% or approximately 1 million neonatal deaths annually. However, there is a marked regional difference in these rates, with 99% of the neonatal deaths occurring in low and middle-income countries.

There are approximately 13 million preterm infants born each year worldwide. Data from a systematic review conducted between 1997 to 2007 revealed a world preterm birth rate of 9.6%, with more developed countries having a rate of 7.5% compared to 8.8% in less-developed countries and 12.5% in least-developed countries.

Chapter 4 - Survival for infants born prematurely now exceeds 80%. These infants are at high risk of abnormal neurodevelopment with disabilities affecting 1 in 8 survivors Hormonal dysregulation is common in prematurity. In adaptation, maternal factors and the placenta control many aspects of the fetal endocrine milieu. After preterm birth, the infant suddenly has to cope and adapt to the external environment. Abnormal values of endocrine tests such as the thyroid and cortisol axes are commonly encountered in preterm infants and infants with more extreme endocrine disturbances are at increased risk of abnormal development.

The optimal way to manage endocrine problems in preterm infants is not clear. In part, this is because infants born at extreme prematurity have different physiology from term infants and older children. What constitutes a "normal" physiological hormone level of a preterm infant at different gestations remains unclear. Examples of delayed adaptation have been evident in the hypothalamic-pituitary-thyroid axis (HPT) and the hypothalamic-pituitary-adrenal (HPA) axes in preterm infants.

The developmental origins theory proposes that events and stress in fetal life provokes adaptive changes in endocrine and metabolic function which can be permanently programmed resulting in an adverse impact in late adult health. Reduced birth weight has been associated with risk for type 2 diabetes mellitus, hyperlipidaemia, hypertension and syndrome X in adulthood. Maternal exposure to exogenous glucocorticoids leads to increased fetal brain exposure to excess glucocorticoids which may result in permanent modification of hypothalamo-pituitary-adrenal (HPA) axis and can have life-long effects on later neuroendocrine function. [9] Maternal hypothyroxinaemia has been reported to be a serious risk factor for neurodevelopmental difficulties that can be identified in neonates as young as 3 weeks of age.

Chapter 5 - Prematurely born infants tend to be less alert, less attentive, less active and less responsive than infants born at full term, and their mothers tend to have greater difficulty knowing when and how to modulate their interactions. Although premature birth alone is not necessarily a risk factor for the parent-infant relationship or attachment, the prevalence of insecure attachment is higher in preterm infant-mother dyads. It does become a risk factor for attachment and parent-infant interactions in the presence of low socio-economic status, low maternal education, co-morbid infant health problems, or maternal depression. The primary focus of this chapter is the mother-infant relationship in the context of prematurity. We propose a literature review of three domains: a) mothers' experience and representations of premature delivery and infant development; b) mothers' interactions with preterm infants and c) the quality of mother-infant attachment. Since insecure attachment can be prevented, we include a brief review on practices promoting secure relationships and supporting mothers.

Chapter 6 - The use of additional weight on infant's voluntary motor skills has been a strategy used to examine how infants adjust their movements when submitted to context manipulations. The evaluation of these issues in a population at risk, such as premature infants, is extremely important since there are significant differences in their motor behavior when compared to full-term infants. Thus, the aim of this chapter was to assess the effects of additional weight on proximal and distal adjustments of the reaching behavior and whether additional weight can be use to facilitate manual reaching.

Chapter 7 - We tested the hypothesis that extremely low gestational age (ELGA) preterm birth without major cerebral damage impacts developmental outcomes and trajectories in the first year, expecting poorer developmental outcomes, a higher rate of impairments and different developmental trajectories in ELGA with respect to full term (FT) infants. Direct tools and a parental questionnaire with four assessments in the first year were employed.

Method. Seventeen monolingual Italian ELGA (≤28 weeks) preterms without major cerebral damage and 11 monolingual Italian full terms, comparable for biological and social characteristics, were evaluated at 3, 6, 9 and 12 months (corrected age for preterms) through the Griffiths Mental Development Scales (GMDS-R), providing a general developmental quotient (DQ) and five sub-quotients (SQ). The "Primo Vocabolario del Bambino" -PVB- (Italian form of the MB-CDI) was administered to the parents at 9 and 12 months.

Results. Use of repeated measure multivariate analyses of variance showed that, compared to FTs, ELGA infants exhibited significantly lower DQ and SQ scores (personal and social skills, eye and hand coordination, performance, tendency in locomotor and hearing and language) in the GMDS-R, with mild or moderate impairments in some ELGA at 6 (6%), 9 (12%) and 12 months (24%), while not in FT infants. ELGA compared to FT infants showed also significantly lower gesture/action production and word comprehension scores in the PVB. Differences between the two samples became larger toward the end of the first year of life.

Conclusions. Our findings highlight that several domains are impacted by ELGA preterm birth in the first year with poorer developmental outcomes, evidence of impairment in some infants and different developmental trajectories between ELGAs and FTs. Relevance of repeated assessments by employing both developmental scales assessing specific cognitive, motor, and linguistic competences and a parental questionnaire providing deeper information for communicative-linguistic competences observed in natural daily contexts was shown.

Chapter 8 - Several studies have highlighted how language and literacy can be affected by preterm birth. This review aims at analyzing the effects of preterm birth on specific language (lexicon, grammar and phonological awareness) and literacy competencies (reading and writing) from the first years of life to adolescence, through the description of studies carried out in the last two decades. The conclusions point out that difficulties found in preterms' language and literacy development do not depend on a slower rhythm of acquisition in all competencies, but on their atypical development. In fact, some competencies are more compromised than others and difficulties in specific competencies emerge at different ages during development. In particular, lexical difficulties become more evident at preschool age, while grammar and phonological awareness are affected by preterm birth since their emergence. With regard to literacy, both reading and writing are affected, but with a greater compromise in the area of writing. This review also highlights that preterm birth does not determine a single developmental trajectory, but several developmental trajectories that relate to the level of neonatal immaturity, the presence of neurological damage, and the biological and environmental risk factors associated to preterm birth. Preterms with a higher immaturity (gestational age <28 weeks and/or birthweight <1000 grams) show diffuse linguistic difficulties from the first years of life to adolescence, while preterms with a moderate neonatal immaturity have more specific difficulties particularly evident from preschool-age.

In conclusion, this review provides a useful contribution both for theoretical and clinical aims. At the theoretical level, following a neuroconstructivist approach, it points out how preterm birth is associated with atypical developmental trajectories, since preterms' development occurs in the context of multiple interacting constraints which differ from typical development. At the clinical level, this review highlights the importance to know which specific competencies are particularly affected by preterm birth and need well-timed interventions.

Chapter 9 - The chapter proposes a research study on the likely developmental outcomes of preterm birth and, in particular, on cognitive and behavioural problems in moderately preterm children at preschool age.

The objective of the study is to investigate the likely occurrence of precursors of ADHD, meant as a complex disorder, in moderately preterm children at preschool age, characterised by distraction, impulsiveness and hyperactivity, at school and home. Therefore, the study is aimed at broadening the knowledge on some specific features of the evolutional paths of moderately preterm children, in order to provide directions for the activation of the training, useful for improving their life quality.

The research has involved 55 moderately preterm children (M: 34,6-week gestational age, SD: 2) without any medical and/or neurological neonatal complications, and low birth weight (M:2100 g, SD: 350 g); a control group of 55 full term children without any pre- and perinatal complications (M: 40-week gestational age, SD: 2). Parents and reference teachers of children were administered specific questionnaires and Italian scales (IPDDAI - *Attention Deficit Hyperactivity Disorder Early Detection for Teachers;* IPDAG - *Attention Deficit Hyperactivity Disorder Early Detection for Parents*; IPDA- *Early Learning Deficit Detection Questionnaire*) to detect attention deficit and hyperactivity in the child's everyday and school life.

The results show a profile of moderately preterm children at risk of attention deficit and hyperactivity, and highlight statistically significant differences related to gender (IPDDAI [$F_{(2, 110)} = 2.9$, p=.04]), birth (IPDAG [$F_{(2, 110)} = 3$, p =.04]) and interaction (IPDDAI [$F_{(2, 110)} = 2$, p=.01]). The moderately preterm children show a deficit in self-regulation and self-control (IPDAG [$F_{(1)} = 3.6$, p=.04], and attention deficit in both everyday family (IPDAG [$F_{(1)} = 5.7$, p=.02]) and school life (IPDDAI [$F_{(1)} = 2.9$, p=.04]. In particular, preterm young girls show a higher risk of disattention, compared to young boys.

The outcomes would suggest assessment paths, aimed at monitoring the aspects of cognitive, motor and behavioural development of moderately preterm children, recognised as signs of problematic functioning profiles.

Therefore, the chapter suggests the activation of training for children showing precursors of ADHD at preschool age. The training would involve children in experiential activities, which are aimed at improving the management of their attention and self-regulation processes, in order to prevent ADHD syndrome from occurring.

In: Preterm Infants
Editors: Diogo Contreiras and Johann Sampaio
ISBN 978-1-62081-819-0

Chapter 1

PRETERM INFANT MENTAL HEALTH: THE ATTACHMENT AND SOCIAL-EMOTIONAL DEVELOPMENT OF PRETERM INFANTS

***Aoife Twohig**,1,2,3,4*,**
***Eleanor J. Molloy*[1,2,3,4]*, and Fiona McNicholas*[4]**
[1]Department of Paediatrics, National Maternity Hospital, Dublin, Ireland
[2]Department of Child Psychiatry, Our Lady's Children's Hospital, Dublin, Ireland
[3]The National Children's Research Centre, Dublin, Ireland
[4]University College Dublin, Ireland

ABSTRACT

The social and emotional development of the infant emerges within the context of the first relationships with primary care-givers, most often his mother and father (Stern, 1977 & 2002). For the baby, in a state of 'absolute dependency' (Winnicott, 1949), these relationships will support the baby's physical and physiological integrity and homeostasis. They will provide an environment within which the baby's experiences, internal and external may be gradually processed and become meaningful and where his changing emotional and behavioural states are regulated. These relationships also are the setting within which the baby's innate propensity to relate to others takes place. (Stern, 1985 Bruschweiler-Stern, 2009). They also provide the scaffolding for the baby's motor, cognitive and language development and emergent sense of self. Infant mental health has been defined as "the young child's capacity to experience, regulate and express emotions, form close and secure relationships and explore the environment and learn" (Zero to Three, 2001). The care-giving environment which supports the development of these capacities is integral to the existence of infant mental health, namely the family, their community and the culture within which the child is born. Attachment, the unique emotional bond between the infant and his caregivers that develops in the first years of life, has been found to play a crucial role in the subsequesnt social and emotional health of the child..

* Correspondence: Aoife Twohig, MD student, National Maternity Hospital, Holles St., Dublin 2, Ireland. Tel:00353-87-1215238; Fax:00353-1-6614623.Email: aoife.twohig@gmail.com.

When the baby is born preterm,, parents and infant must adapt to the dramatic change in each of their lives. The baby's prematurity may necessitate neonatal intensive care; there may be medical complications and separation from the parents. The parents may experience emotional upheaval, anxiety and stress. These experiences may impact on the developing relationship, which is vital for the infant's social and emotional development.

The following chapter aims to review current knowledge on the attachment and social emotional development of preterm infants.

The chapter will begin with a review of the literature on the parent's experiences and psychological adjustment to preterm birth. The neurobehavioural and psychological sequealaefor the infant will then be considered.. A review the literature on preterm infant-parent interaction and attachment will be followed by outcome findings on preterm infant mental health and development. The chapter will conclude with a review of existing interventions to support the developing infant-parent relationship and the social-emotional development of the preterm infant.

INTRODUCTION

The concept of mental health in infancy is increasingly becoming a focus of attention for many disciplines working with infants and their parents.. Over the past century clinicians and researchers such as Winnicott (1942), Bion (1962), , Bowlby (1969, 1980), Ainsworth (1979)and many others identified the salience of early experiences for the development of the infant and the richness of the internal world during the first years of life, however infant mental health may still be a relatively new phenomenon in many parts of the world. The work of Fraiberg (1980) was seminal in defining the realm of infant mental health. Fraiberg described her work with infants at risk, identifying the 'ghosts in the nursery', the unspoken parental experiences of childhood trauma, which came in the way of their relationship with their own babies. It was this movement to working with infants and parents who were struggling in their relationships that led to the growth and understanding of infant mental health

Infant mental health has been defined as "the young child's capacity to experience, regulate and express emotions, form close and secure relationships and explore the environment and learn" (Zero to Three, 2001), within the context of the care-giving environment which best supports the development of these capacities. This is namely the family, their community and the culture within which the child is born. The healthy social and emotional development of children depends upon the environmental facilitation of these emerging capacities. Central to the infant's mental health is the formation of selective attachments to his primary care-givers (Zeanah, 2009). It is in the milieu of these attachment relationships that emotional, social and cognitive development occurs.

Recognising the importance of early relationships to the social and emotional development of infants and the potential difficulties that can arise in paediatric populations, in particular when infants have been born prematurely or with medical problems requiring neonatal intensive care has led to a significant body of research in the hope of improving mental health for these infants and parents. The complex situation of preterm birth in particular constitutes a risk for later development.

For the infant, preterm birth results in the loss of the environment of the womb. The continuity or '*going along*' (Winnicott, 1949) of fetal development is disrupted at sensitive and critical periods in neurological development. The environment to which the fetus has adapted is suddenly and irrevocably changed. The birth may be physically traumatic and at earlier gestational ages there will be need for resuscitation and intensive care treatment. At a somatic and a neurobiological level this is a time of extreme stress for the neonate. In addition there is separation from the mother, who can act as protector and modulator of the infant's experiences.

The experience of preterm birth may be traumatic for the mother. She must cope with the loss of the pregnancy and also with the possibility of death of her infant. Separation from her infant, to be cared for by the medical team, may lead her to feel lack of confidence and competence in her mothering. Past feelings of loss and separation may be reactivated in the context of preterm birth. For the father there may be complex emotional reactions also as he tries to protect and support his wife and cope with his own emotional distress following the birth.

In the Neonatal Intensive Care Unit (NICU), the preterm infant recieves life sustaining treatment. While necessary, these interventions may be painful and unpredicatable. The NICU is also an environment of excessive stimulation.. These experiences may be physiologically dysregulating (Slevin, et al. 2000). Recurrent experiences of pain and invasive care procedures as well as the necessary handling of the babies can result in the premature infant becoming disorganised (Muller Nix et al., 2009).

The baby may require assisted ventilation and parenteral feeding. Establishing breast or bottle feeding maybe difficult, due to the immaturity of the infant sucking reflexes. The elements of early attachment relationship formation, namely infant behaviours and communication and maternal looking, holding and handling may be obscured by the surroundings of the incubator and the attachment process disrupted. Yet the preterm infant's communicative capacities and regulatory potential has also been observed (Trevarthen, 2010; Als, 1986) and his need for the presence of and contact with his parents is profound.

We will first consider how attachment and social-emotional development unfold normally in development and then consider how this may be impacted upon by preterm birth.

I. Relationships, Attachment and Social-Emotional Development

The social and emotional development of the infant emerges within the context of the first relationships with mother and father (Stern, 1977 & 2002). For the baby, in a state of 'absolute dependency' (Winnicott, 1949), these relationships will support the baby's physical and physiological integrity and homeostasis. They will provide an environment within which the baby's experiences, internal and external may be gradually processed and become meaningful and where his changing emotional and behavioural states are regulated. These relationships also are the setting within which the baby's innate propensity to relate to others takes place. (Stern, 1985; Bruschweiler-Stern, 2009). They also provide the scaffolding for the baby's motor, cognitive and language development and emergent sense of self (Stern, 1985).

Bowlby (1969) held that the quality of the relationship an infant forms with their caregiver over the first 12 months of life will influence the infant's social-emotional development and later mental health. Having observed and worked with children who had suffered separation from their mother, during the Second World War, Bowlby, a child psychiatrist and psychoanalyst became acutely aware of the significance of the earliest relationships, in particular the relationship with the mother, for the emotional development of infants.. His interest lay in the fundamental need of humans to seek, through specific attachments, or bonds, protection, comfort and support (Joyce, 2005), Bowlby integrated psychoanalytic theory with ethology and systems theory to elaborate a theory of infant-parent attachment (Bretherton, 1991; Bowlby, 1980). The quality of this "affectional tie" (Bowlby, 1969 & 1980) to the mother is displayed through the behavioural and affective responses of the infant to separations and reunions with the caregiver, particularly evident in the second half of the first year. The quality of these specific attachments was found to be related to the sensitivity and responsiveness of mothers as observed naturalistically in the home interacting with their 3 month old infants (Ainsworth et al., 1978). Sensitivity relates to the capacity of the mother to perceive in her infant a a range of states and emotions and to the timing, consistency and appropriateness of her responses to the infant's communications. The importance of maternal sensitivity arose out of Ainsworth's original Ganda studies, where infant's whose mothers were able to provide rich spontaneous detail about their infant's and sensitive to the infant's communications were found to have infants later to be called secure. The quality of the mother or other care-giver's responses, or responsiveness, to the infant and their contingency to the infant's needs at that time was also deemed important. Mothers vary individually in sensitivity and in responsiveness. Crittenden (2005) has also noted the dyadic nature of sensitivity, where the infant's temperament becomes integral to the adult's sensitivity to the particular needs of their infant.

Early patterns of mother-infant interaction have been the focus of attachment and developmental research over the past several decades (Stern, 1977 & 2002). The early 'dance' between mother and infant that unfolds over the weeks and months following the infant's birth is the basis of the infant's growing attachment relationship with his mother. This includes the early gazing, facial play and reciprocal vocalization, characteristic of early mother-infant interactions (Trevarthen, 1978). Both infant and mother play a part in this emerging rhythm which will, through repetition and over time become internalized or learned as a mental representation, or internal working model (Bowlby, 1980) of the relationship. A mental representation may be thought of as the internal component, or a 'map' of the relationship and recurrent patterns of the subjective experience of that relationship (Zeanah, 2007). For example, an infant who has repeated experiences of being responded to, cuddled and comforted by his care-giver when in distress, builds up an expectation that distress can be managed and will pass and a representation of his relationship with his care-giver as reliable and comforting. These representations are built upon, providing the child with a sense of self that is worthy of comfort and love and others as reliable. As Stern has described the infant builds his internal world of representations based upon the 'reality of lived experience', echoing in many ways Winnicott's thesis on the mother's role in 'holding and handling' her infant in helping him contruct his internal world (Winnicott,1971). Central to attachment formation are the infant's innate capacity for person-to person communication, also termed primary intersubjectivity (Trevarthen, 2010) and the emerging capacity of the infant for emotional regulation , which develops initially through mutual regulation (Tronick, 2008) within the relationship.

Ainsworth developed a classification of observed attachment behaviours in 12 month old infants following lengthy naturalistic observations of infants in their homes with their mothers, both in Baltimore and in Uganda (Ainsworth et al., 1978). In the strange situation procedure the infant is separated briefly from his caregiver and his behaviour is observed both on separation and reunion. Securely attached infants will be distressed and protest at separation but on reunion will approach and be comforted by the parent. Their distress is assuaged and they are free to begin exploration and play following the reunion. The parent forms a secure base from which the infant will explore the room and toys. There are two patterns of insecurity of attachment. Insecure ambivalent infants will be distressed on separation but not comforted by the parent's presence or holding on reunion and may even become more distressed. Insecure avoidant infants do not appear outwardly to be distressed, and tend to absorb themselves in play rather than seek comfort from their caregiver during the reunion. A further classification of disorganisation of attachment strategy was developed by Main et al (1986). Children with disorganised attachment lack a strategy for seeking comfort and exhibit unusual or chaotic behaviour, such as freezing, stereotypies or retreating from the caregiver.

Secure attachment may be seen as protective, conferring resilience, as has been described in several longitudinal studies (Sroufe et al., 2005). Insecure attachment may be a risk factor for later emotional and behavioral problems and problems with stress management (Bakermans-Kranenberg et al., 2009). Infant attachment is influenced by parents' behaviours and interactional styles, such as sensitivity, warmth and responsiveness, parental states of mind in relation to their own childhood experiences of attachment relationships, and parental mental health. Infant factors include infant communicative capacities, sensory and neurological integrity and temperament (Fuertes et al., 2006; Sroufe et al., 2005; Van Ijzendoorn et al, 1992).

Main and colleagues (Main et al.,1985) developed amethod of assessing parental characteristics that were strongly associated with infant security of attachment through their development of the Adult Attachment Interview. This method assesses narrative qualities of parents relating their relationships to primary caregivers to identify patterns of adult attachment representations. This linking of the narrative quality to internal representations is connected to Bowlby's construct of internal working models and those of cognitive psychology (Zeanah, 2007). Further developments in the area of parental representations of the child, was pursued by Zeanah and colleagues (Zeanah et al., 1986) with the design of the Working Model of the Child Interview. This interview elicits parent's descriptions of their infants and young children and focuses on the qualitative features of the parent's narrative. (Zeanah, 2007). The parental representation of the infant has been shown to predict infant attachment security (Zeanah et al., 1986; Benoit et al.,198)

Theearliest relationships and attachment formthe core of subsequent individual social-emotional development, optimally a sense of security and self worth. They will influence the child's experience of the world and how he will interact and with his environment. We have also seen how parental attachment experiences and representations may influence the developing relationship with their infant, the so called 'ghosts' and 'angels' in the nursery (Fraiberg et al.1975; Lieberman et al., 2005). How does preterm birth affect parent's emotionally? How do patterns of parent-infant interaction develop in the context of preterm birth? How will they influence the evolving attachment relationship and the preterm infant's development? Thefollowing sections of the chapter will review our current knowledge of this area.

Psychological Adjustment of Parents to Preterm Birth

The social-emotional development of preterm infants has stimulated researchers due to the increasing prevalence of preterm birth and the survival of the most premature infants. There is now awareness of the traumatic impact of preterm birth on parents and an understanding of the complex social and family influences on outcomes for preterm infants (Johnson et al., 2010; Milgrom et al., 2010).

Approximately 10% of all births are preterm, globally (Beck et al, 2010). Advances in maternal-fetal medicine, obstetrics and neonatology have led to the increasing survival of infants born as early as 23 weeks gestation and also to improved morbidity(Tucker et al., 2004; Tyson et al., 2008). These infants however are at significantly higher risk of medical and neurodevelopmental complications and may require extended periods of hospitalisation and intensive care. The loss of the adaptive environment of the womb and the stress experienced by the preterm infant in order toto maintain physiological homeostasis has been found to impact on the infant's development (Milgrom, 2010.) Milgrom et al.,(2010) have highlighted that the increased risk of neurobehavioural outcomes associated with medical and structural brain impairment do not fully explain the variance in these outcomes. The importance of environmental factors which influence the preterm infant's outcomes has been highlighted also (Rauh et al, 1990; Newnham et al 2009; Treyvaud et al 2009). Tronick (2008) has described how the infant's neurobehaviour can affect parental care-giving behaviour which further shapes the infant's behaviour, highlighting the complexity of the interaction between the infant and the environment.

We will look firstly at the parent's experience of preterm birth followed by the infant's experience, before considering the implications for the infant-parent relationship.

Pregnancy may be conceptualised as a time of great psychological changes in both the mother and father, these psychological changes mirroring the physical changes of the pregnancy. For expectant mothers there is a process of personal change. There is a growing awareness of the fetus during pregnancy, through the perception of fetal movements and the unfolding physical and emotional changes of pregnancy. These changes foster in health, the growing relationship with the baby both in fantasy and reality. Finally toward the end of the pregnancy there is a period described by Winnicott as "primary maternal preoccupation", a state of mind in the mother in the last weeks of pregnancy characterised by a deep inward preoccupation with the baby and herself to the exclusion of outside interests. This process in turn facilitates her identification with the baby during and following the birth (Winnicott, 1975). This identification is of great significance to her subsequent relationship with the infant and may last for some weeks following the birth, a period where the mother and baby are getting to know each other and the rhythms of feeding, sleeping and other regulatory processes are evolving.

For parent's who experience the sudden and potentially traumatic end of the pregnancy, when the baby is "sent before" his time (Cohen, 2003), these normal developmental processes may be disrupted. Birth may be viewed as a developmental crisis for parents, however when the baby is born very prematurely or critically ill, this normative developmental process is altered irrevocably (Zeanah et al., 1984). Preterm birth may begin spontaneously. and the unexpected labour may be frightening and a potentially overwhelming experience for the mother and father. The decision to deliver the infant early may be due to concern about the moher's health or the fetus' development or growth. The infant's appearance and condition at birth may be a source of worry or concern for the parents as they must adjust their image of the fantasised baby. The parents may feel helplessness and uncertainty facing the unknown future for their infant. Parents may feel dependent and become passive in the face of their child's care passing to the medical team. Guilt and grief are intensified by the separation from their infant. Grief following transfer of a critically ill infant to intensive care has been found to be comparable to a parent's grief experienced following the death of an infant (Zeanah, 1984). Anticipatory mourning may also be a reaction to the infant's birth, irrespective of the infant's actual viability. impact on the mother's sense of the developing bond with the baby (Muller-Nix, 2009). Those infants of very low birth weight are at ongoing risk of postnatal complications such as intraventricular haemorrhage, infection and respiratory problems. The perceived threat to the baby's survival may be a source of great anxiety and anger for new parents. Fear for the infant's survival may remain for a considerable time following the infant's discharge(Muller Nix et a., 20091). Lack of resolution of grief following the birth may impact on the mother-infant relationship and has been associated with more insecure attachment of the infant (Shah et al., 2011).

Parents experience a range of emotional reactions following the preterm birth of their infant, which include anxiety, depression and post traumatic stress (Brisch et al, 2003; Pianta et al, 1999, Muller Nix & Forcada-Guex, 2009; Muller Nix et al., 2004). The effects of the experience of a preterm birth may have acute and long term emotional consequences for both parents (Muller-Nix et al., 2009). Studies have reported chronic anxiety and depression (Minde, 1985; Miles et al', 2007; Padden & Glenn, 1997; Singer et al., 1999). Parents may experience the preterm birth differently. Mothers have been found to experience more stress compared with fathers and also have more difficulty adjusting(Hughes & McCollum; Miles et al., 2007). This may be related to the feelings of guilt often aroused in the mother following preterm birth.

Post traumatic stress experienced by parents following preterm birth has been described in several studies (DeMier et al., 2000; Jotzo & Poets, 2005; Holditch-Davis et al., 2003; Pierrehumbert et al., 2003; Binder et al., 2009). Maternal recollected traumatic experience has been linked to reduced sensitivity in interaction with their infants at 6 months and at 18 months preterm infants whose mothers experienced the birth as traumatic showed interactional differences, compared with full term infants (Muller-Nix et al., 2004).

Maternal anxiety has also been associated with preterm infants' interactional behaviour (Wijnroks, 1999). It has also been found that infants of depressed mothers display interactional differences and emotional and behavioural problems later in infancy and early childhood. Therefore the potential impact of preterm birth on the child's development through the effects on the parents' psychological wellbeing is complex.

The setting of the Neonatal Intensive Care Unit, physical separation from the baby and the observation of paradoxical distressing yet life saving interventions may preclude bonding and recognition of the infant by the mother. Maternal feelings of competence and adequacy as a mother may be affected, as the immediate care of the baby is dependent on highly technological equipment and expert medical and nursing staff (Zeanah et al, 1984). Therefore holding, familiarizing, first gazes, loving caresses and feeding may be postponed. These normative experiences are the basis for the growing relationship between infant and mother. While extremely preterm and low birth weight infants are most at risk of adverse neurodevelopmental and social-emotional outcomes, infants of greater gestational age and birth weight are also at risk of somatic and psychological complications (Pietrini et al.,2000). Parents of infants so deemed to be at lower risk have also been found to have disengaged representations of their infants. Parental emotional distress that is persistent can be deleterious for parental representations of the baby (Borghini et al., 2006), the parent-infant relationship and may impact on the formation of attachment (Minde et al, 1983).

Muller Nix et al., (2009) have described the importance also of qualitative approaches in elucidating the experience of preterm birth for parents and these approaches offer a deeper understanding of the experience of parents following the preterm birth of an infant.

II. Preterm Infant Development, Complications and Capacities

Preterm birth affects the infant's capacity to maintain homeostasis and to organize neurobehavioural states due to the infant's immaturity for life outside the womb (Tronick, 2008). Factors which may influence this are the gestational age and maturity of the infant, intrauterine conditions, such as infection, which may have a deleterious effect on the fetus during its development and also genetic processes. The preterm infant must face the challenges of birth and the environment outside the womb ill equipped. This variable level of need for support determines the subsequent course of the infant, who may require assistance with respiration, including mechanical ventilation, parenteral nutrition and other treatments to maintain his life. The infant's prematurity means that he is vulnerable to complications such as chronic respiratory disease, necrotising enterocolitis, retinopathy of prematurity among others. From a neurological perspective the immature brain is vulnerable to intraventricular haemorrhage and peri-ventricular white matter damage as well as a range of other insults. These are associated with longer term impairments such as Cerebral Palsy, but also with cognitive delay, learning disability and attentional problems such as attention deficit hyperactivity disorder (Johnson et al., 2010).

The impact on the preterm infant of the neonatal intensive care environment has been studied extensively in attempts to understand how this affects the preterm infant and how this can be ameliorated (Als et al., 1983). The preterm infant's experiences of pain and stress (Milgrom, 2010; Muller-Nix & Ansermet, 2009) may impact on pain processing, resulting in hyperalgesia. Chronic and recurrent pain can contribute to changes in brain structures and function and impact on neurodevelopmental outcomes (Smith et al., 2011). The pain pathways of the nervous system are functioning by 24 weeks gestation. Pain is most obviously experienced in relation to medical procedures which are life sustaining. Pain and stress are also associated with medical complications such as respiratory distress and environmental stimulation such as excessive noise and light. Positioning of the infant in the incubator contributes to the infant's overall organisation and state. Nesting of infants with soft blankets, provides the infant with a sense of containment and has been found to be regulating for extremely preterm infants (Als et al. 1986). Lying the infant prone and with their arms and legs flexed or on their side are also regulating physical positions, aiding the infant obtain more stable state organisation. In order to evaluate and assess infant pain and stress in the NICU there are several validated instruments, such as the Premature Infant Pain Profile (PIPP) (Holsti et al., 2008) and the Behavioural Indicators of Pain Profile (Stevens et al.) which may be used to evaluate painful experiences. The Observation Sheet of the Newborn Individualised Developmental Care Program (Als, 1986; Als et al., 2004) may be used during the hospitalisation to record physiological and neurobehavioural indicators of pain, stress and self-regulation. These observations can then inform the care and management of the infant to reduce stress and pain where possible. The use of the Neonatal Behavioural Assessment Scale (Brazelton, 1995) is particularly helpful prior to the infant's discharge, in helping parents observe the responses and self-regulatory capacities of their infants (Bruschweiler-Stern, 2009; Rauh et al., 1991). In addition the Assessment of the Preterm Infant's Behaviour (Als et al., 1982) and the NICU Network Neurobehavioural Scale are both specifically designed to assess the neurobehavioural integrity of the preterm and high risk neonate (Tronick, 2007). Naturalistic observations also inform the understanding of the infant's psychological experiences and how these may come to be meaningful for the infant. The Tavistock model of infant observation is one such model which has been used to observe the infant's experiences (Negri, 1994; Cohen 2003; Mendelsohn, 2005).

The Psychological Experience of the Preterm Infant

While we cannot ultimately 'know' the experience of the preterm infant, psychodynamic theory may illuminatethe infant's experiences of preterm birth. Winnicott has written eloquently on the impact of birth trauma on psychological development (Winnicott, 1949a). He hypothesised a rudiment of emotional development before birth. The fetus during the pregnancy is protected from excessive disturbances from the environment, so that there is continuity of fetal emotional development, which he termed 'going along'. In the uncomplicated pregnancy, *"the birth experience is an exaggerated sample of something already known to the infant"*. The unborn infant is prepared through the sensations and experiences during the pregnancy for the birth.. For Winnicott the continuity of the emerging self is essential, The 'soon to be born infant' must have opportunity to return to a state of "not having to react" in which the infant self can begin to come into being. Winnicott, described birth as a *"temporary ...interference with the personal 'going along', not so powerful or prolonged as to snap the thread of the infant's continuous personal progress"*. Winnicott has in this piece conveyed in a most sensitive way, the possible experiences of the fetus and infant during the journey from womb to the world. Traumatic birth, on the other hand, is a situation of "prolonged impingement" of the environment on the infant and the infant's loss of identity. The loss of identity gives an extreme sense of insecurity and lays the basis for expectation of further loss of continuity of self. Winnicott also postulated that a sense of hopelessness may develop.

The experience of the infant may also be linked to the experience of the mother during labour, during which the mother "has to be able to resign herself to a process almost exactly comparable to the infant's experience at the same time.' This "special state of sensitivity" in the mother Winnicott later called "primary maternal preoccupation" (Winnicott, 1956). During episodes of stress the infant has no sense of when this feeling will end and no way of being comforted by the knowledge that the experience will end, which makes this experience of helplessness so intolerable.. Following premature and traumatic birth, infants are exposed to an environment not ready to adapt in the way that in the normal course of events the mother would. One can postulate that Winnicott's 'thread of going along' may be subject to episodes of snapping, fraying and tangling in the postnatal period. Winnicott also believed that the development of the baby could be affected by the experience of traumatic birth as the immature ego endeavors to integrate in the face of considerable stress.

Winnicott (1956) considers "primary maternal preoccupation", as facilitating integration of the infant's experiences, that will promote the "going along" of the infant and the development of the mind. He believed that this was crucial to the infant's tendency toward integration or what may be termed organisation: "The tendency to integrate is helped by two sets of experience: the technique of infant care, whereby the infant is kept warm, handled and bathed and rocked and named, and also the acute instinctual experiences which tend to gather the experiences together from within". Thus the infant too brings his own personal contributions to the relationship and the environment and how these are integrated into his own subjective experience.

That the emotional relationship with the mother at the beginning was critical for the developing infant's mind was central also to Bion's thesis in 'Leanring from Experience' (1962) (b)..

Bion believed that in the very earliest stages of development the baby uses a means of primitive communication, projective identification, evoking in the mother the feelings the baby can himself not understand or tolerate. The mother in the early relationship has identified with her baby and through a process of "reverie", the mother's capacity to really understand her baby's experiences, is capable of receiving his communications (Bion, 1962 b). Bion called this maternal function the "container". The mother receives these primitive communications and allows the baby's state to be evoked in herself, as she sifts and ponders his experiences, processing them, tending to them, naming them and returning the experiences in a modified form to the baby, the baby then has the experience of being "contained". Britton (1992) has described this process as a transformation of a "near-sensory and somatic" experience for the infant to "something more mental" by the mother, which could be used for thinking or stored as memory. The mother performs this initial function, acting as container, a secure holding place, where meaning is made of the baby's primitive first experiences. These modified first experiences become the "schemas-of-being-with" or the mental representations of the earliest relationships described above. The human infant learns about his emotions as tolerated by the mother, and through the particular way in which they have been tolerated and handled (Likierman, 2001). This view of the containing process, according to Likierman, has played an important role in clarifying the nature of maternal emotional provision and highlighting the importance of the mother's "mental resilience". In this section we have seen how the parents, in particular the mother may be affected by the birth and also the impact of the birth, biologically, behaviourally and psychologically on the infant. The next section will review the areas of preterm infant interaction and attachment in considering the impact of preterm birth on the parent-infant relationship.

III. The Preterm Parent Relationship - Interaction, Communication, Representation

Infant-Parent Interactions

Following preterm birth, parents and infants have the task of forming their relationship under conditions of considerable stress. Does preterm birth hold particular risks for infant-parent interaction and the developing relationship? Studies of mother-infant interaction and attachment have attempted to answer this question...

The intimate moment to moment interactions between infants and their mothers have been the subject of an immense literature spanning several decades of research. This research initially began with the recognition of infants as individual persons with the capacity and desire for communication with other persons. Studies such as those of Trevarthen (1979) and Tronick (1977)_where mothers and their infants were filmed in face to face interactions and which were then subsequently analysed frame by frame, highlighted the complex behavioural repertoire of infants as early as one month of age in communicative interactions with their mothers. Just as these 'protoconversations', early preverbal communication patterns, (Trevarthen, 2010) are the product of the infant's "delicate and specifically human system for person to person communication", these interactions and communications are also the means with which the infant begins to develop in the first months of life the attachment relationship with his primary caregiver.

There are qualitative differences between how infants interact with the physical world and with persons. Infants use physical objects to discover their physical qualities and out of interest. Infants communicate with persons using expressive movement. A crucial feature of the subjectivity of infants is their repertoire of organized emotional expressions and movements, in relation to objects as well as to persons. These movements not only convey felt emotions but also personality or temperament to caregivers, who are emotionally moved by them. Communication occurs for a variety of reasons, to communicate state, needs, to share experiences and also for the pleasure of both self and the other (Stern, 2002). Communication consists of nonverbal as well as verbal means. Nonverbal means include the use of gaze; head movement, facial expression, hand gestures and body posture. Different patterns of communication differentiate feeding, defensive and distress behaviour and also communicative behaviour that is purely for social purposes (Trevarthen, 1979).

Maternal social behaviours are elicited by the newborn and are the mother's most valuable resources to regulate interaction with her infant. Maternal interaction with her infant comprises initiating, maintaining and terminating an interaction, and adjusting to the infant's level of attention, arousal and emotional tone (Stern, 1977 & 2002)). According to Stern the sequences and timing of maternal behaviours create "the tempo, theme and variation on themes which enhance her infant's experience of human interaction and communication". These early patterns of communication and interactive behaviours between infants and their mothers, fathers and caregivers have been shown to be strongly associated with the quality of the attachment relationship later in the first year. Ainsworth's (1978) studies have shown that maternal characteristics of sensitivity, responsiveness and warmth in interaction with her baby in the first three months of life, are associated with secure infant attachment at one year.

Preterm Infant-Parent Interaction

A significant body of research has grown in the area of preterm infant -mother interaction indicating that there are qualitative differences in the interactive behaviours and interactional quality of preterm infants and their parents. As noted above interaction may be described in terms of the behaviours of infant and mother during the interaction or by the quality of the interaction of the dyad. The findings of studies of preterm infant-mother interactions will be presented from these three perspectives.

In the neonatal period early studies found mothers of preterm infants to be less actively involved with their infant (DiVitto & Goldberg, 1979; Leifer et al 1972.) However at 4 months of age mothers of preterm infants have been found to be more stimulating as they may attempt to elicit responses from their infants who may be less active (Bakeman & Brown, 1980; Field, 1977). Mothers of preterm infants may be more controlling and less sensitive in interpreting their infant's affective communications (Crawford, 1982; Crnic, 1983, McGehee & Eckerman, 1983; Feldman & Eidelman, 2007; Malatesta et al 1986).

Crnic et al. (1983) found mothers of preterm infants, compared with full term controls, to be more active and express less positive affect in interaction across the first year with less frequency of smiles. Mothers of preterm babies held their babies more and tended to engage in more tactile kinesthetic stimulation of their babies.. Mothers of preterm infants vocalised more at 4 months. the preterm mothers faced their infants less than the term infants' mothers effectiveness and sensitivity.

Leiderman et al.,(1972) found that mothers of preterm infants smiled less towards their infant at 12 months. Brachfield et al., (1980) found that interactive differences, namely higher activity, at 8 months had resolved at 12 months. In a study of maternal play and caretaking of preterm infants, Minde et al., (1985) found that mothers of preterm infants differed from mothers of full-term infants in their interactions with their infants at 1, 2 and 3 months, corrected for gestational age. This was not related to past maternal experiences, however the degree of neonatal illness was related to behavioural disorganisation in the preterm infants. The authors conclude that behavioural disorganisation lead to differences in caretaking (Minde et al., 1985).

Muller Nix et al. studied the effect of prematurity, medical risk and maternal stress on mother-child interactions (Muller-Nix et al., 2004) Mothers of high risk preterm infants were found to be more controlling and less sensitive at 6 months. Mothers that had experienced post traumatic stress were also more controlling and less sensitive at 6 months during the dyadic play. This difference resolved at 18 months.

Early studies of preterm infant behaviour found that preterm infants may be less alert, less active and less responsive than full term infants during the first months of life (Bakeman & Brown, 1980; Di Vitto & Goldberg, 1979; Field 1977 & 1980). Preterm infants display more gaze aversion and inattention than full term infants which may be related to overstimulation and disorganisation in the face of external stimuli. Crnic (1983) et al., found preterm infants to smile less often and averted gaze from their mothers significantly more than full-term infants. Gaze aversion declined rapidly with age in the preterm group. Preterm infants averted their bodies from their mothers more frequently. displayed less positive affect , vocalised less frequently during a vocal elicitation episode, and their clarity of cues and responsiveness was lower.

Montirosso has shown that healthy preterm infants displayed more self regulatory behaviours in the form of distancing or turning away than full term infants during the face to face still face paradigm. In addition during the reunion episode of the paradigm, preterm infants showed greater social monitoring than full-term infants.

Infant interactional behaviour has been shown to differ from full-term infants at 18 months and is associated with parental post traumatic stress (Muller-Nix et al. 2004). The infant's behaviour differed at 18 months only for infants whose mothers experienced high stress following the birth. The infants of low stress preterm mothers had high levels of passivity, where as infants of high stress mothers have significantly higher compulsive compliance.

Dyadic Characteristics

Dyadic characteristics in social interaction with mothers include social signalling, vocalizing and regulatory processes. Synchrony is the ability to change affective or behavioural states in temporal coordination with each other. Bi-directionality is the capacity to share the lead in interaction. Matching describes the sharing of joint attentional, affective or behavioural states at the same moment in time (Beebe & Lachmann…; Cohn, Tronick, Feldman, Greenblum& Yirmiya, 1999; Jaffe, Beebe, Feldstein, Crown, & Jasnow, 2001 Tronick & Cohn, 1989). Mismatches occur when the infant and mother are in different behavioural states and are associated with interactive stress. Mothers and infants spend most of the time in mismatching states, which are corrected in the following interactive sequence (Tronick, 1989)

Crnic et al (1983) found that in preterm mother-infant dyads there were differences in the dyadic interactions compared to full term dyads, reflecting the individual social behaviour characteristics of preterm infants and their mothers outlined above. There was less reciprocity of signaling, with the interaction balanced on one member of the dyad ie: when the mother was active, the infant was not. Crnic et al. hypothesised that this pattern of dyadic interaction became circular with more infant unresponsiveness eliciting greater maternal activity, leading to gaze aversion and inattention. In their sample these interactive characteristics persisted over the first year, even while preterm infants gaze aversion lessened. The dyads appear to enjoy the interaction less as the less positive affective quality and tone of the interaction reveals.

Contrastingly several studies have found mothers of preterm infants to be particularly responsive to their infant's signals. Barrat et al.,(2006) studied the attentional, vocal and affective signals of preterm infants and their mothers during home observations. Preterm infants demonstrated heightened vocal and affective responsiveness. Shermann-Eizirik et al., (1997) found that preterm infants and mothers did not differ during observed interactions during changing and face to face interaction over the first six months compared to healthy full term infants.

In their sample, Montirosso et al., found that preterm dyads were comparable to full term dyads in coordination as measured by matching, reparation rate and synchrony following the still face paradigm. During the still-face paradigm the mother holds a still face during a play interation with the baby. The preterm infants hwoever were observed to use more self-regulatory behaviours and social monitoring than full term infants. For both groups of infants the still-faceparadigm and subsequent reunion was stressful, requiring a complex mutual dyadic adjustment for mothers and infants (Montirosso et al., 2010). The authors suggest that for preterm infants normal interactions can be experienced as more stressful and they have less capacity for self regulation compared to full term infants. Increased use of social monitoring may be a compensatory strategy used by preterm infants. They found healthy preterm infant-mother dyads were able to coordinate interactions comparably to full term dyads. levels of reparation following disruptions in the interactions were equal for both preterm and full term groups. Reparation according to Tronick (2007), is one of the "primary mechanisms underlying normal development, including the development of trust, attachment mastery. Having the experience that negative affect or stress can be transformed into positive affect and the elaboration of coping capacities (Tronick, 2007)" Such findings can reassure parents of typical interactive experience and developmental outcome. Tronick emphasises the normative nature of mismatching during interactions and, that reparation is possible. This potential for repair and reconstruction in the relationship is in fact advantageous to the infant's development. This awareness may help parents who search for the perfect, wished for interaction.

While some authors suggest that the differences in interaction may be adaptive qualities of parental interaction to the prematurity of the infant (Browne, 2009), others suggest that interactive differences may be considered to contribute to the dyadic vulnerability and may be related to later relationship difficulties (Muller-Nix et al., 2004; Stern , 2002).

Socio-cultural factors need also to be taken into account. Fuertes et al (2011) investigated the impact of socioeconomic status on mother-infant interaction. They found that lower socioeconomic status contributed more to the variance in sensitivity in interaction compared to birth status in their full term and preterm sample.

Korja et al., (2011), in their systematic review of 18 studies of mother-infant interaction note the variability in methods used to assess mother-infant interaction. These differences in methodology between studies make comparisons between the studies difficult. These authors conclude that although there are differences in interaction quality between preterm infants and their mothers these generally resolve in the second year. Patterns of interaction may transform as the infant moves into toddlerhood and early childhood. Further studies of parent-child interactions in the subsequent years may elucidate how these patterns evolve and may give further information on the evolving relational patterns.

IV. Studies of Preterm Infant Attachment

Preterm birth as a risk factor for attachment security has been a focus of research for several decades. The results of early studies (Bakeman & Browne 1980, Field et al 1981, Frodi et al 1983, Rode, 1981)suggested that preterm infants were as likely as term born infants to develop secure attachment relationships. These studiesincluded infants born at a wide range of gestational ages and birth weights, including infants born close to term. The studies also included infants who were relatively healthy, heavier birth weights and of families of generally middle class backgrounds. In addition methodological differences, in the assessment of attachment security, between the studies made the studies difficult to compare (Plunkett et al., 1986). Plunkett (1986) highlighted the need to focus research on attachment in preterm populations of specific conditions of high risk which may place these already vulnerable infants at risk of attachment disturbances.

Brown and Bakeman, (1980) studied attachment in 26 preterm infants and found no difference in distribution of attachment patterns to full term samplesAs discussed by Plunkett et al.(1986) these authors utilised recordings of sections of the Strange Situation Procedure (SSP) to make attachment classifications and so their results are not generalisable and difficult to compare with other studies. Field et al. (1981), studied 46 preterm neonates with Respiratory Distress Syndrome. This sample was also relatively healthy, with birth weights greater than 1660g, hospitalisations less than 32 days and gestational age 32 or more weeks. The results are difficult to evaluate as full term infants are compared with preterm and post-term infants, so that the distribution of attachment in the preterm group cannot be determined. Frodi 1983 studied 20 relatively healthy preterm infants, with a mean birth weight of 1990g and whose hospitalisations did not exceed 24 days also finding no differences in attachment patterns. Rode 1981 studied the impact of separation rather than preterm birth and included 4 term infants with 20 preterm infants in her sample. Goldberg et al. (1986) studied high risk very low birth weight infants, with birth weight's less than 1500g, singletons and twins and found that 75% of their sample secure in the Strange Situation procedure at one year. Higher medical risk was associated with greater security of attachmentEasterbrooks (1989) found the distribution of attachment among preterm infant's to be similar to term infants in a predominantly white, middle class sample. Attachment to mother and to father was similar to full term groups. The studies above examined relatively healthy preterm infants, of middle class backgrounds. Butcher et al (1993), posing a different question, examined maternal rigidity of attitudes in parenting and the relationship to attachment classifications of preterm infants and found that in their sample of 35 infants, 71% were securely attached, while there was an association between maternal rigidity and insecure attachment. Brisch, 2005, studied the relationship of maternal attachment representations in the Adult Attachment Interview at 6 months and infant neurological impairment with attachment security at 14 months corrected age, found that 64.7% of their 70 very low birth weight preterm infants were securely attached.

These studies indicate that for preterm infants across gestational ages, birth weights and with more favourable medical risk status, attachment security and insecurity is distributed in a similar way to full term infants.

Other researchers have however found differences in attachment patterns among preterm infants when neonatal medical risk was taken into account. Plunkett et al. (1986) studied the quality of the attachment relationship of preterm infants with respiratory illness and a length of hospitalisation greater than one month. These authors found that their high risk ill infants had significantly more insecure attachment than healthy preterm group who were similar to normative samples. Their preterm sample included a high number of infants classified as anxious-resistant. The authors hypothesise that the attachment relationship for these infants occurs in the context of the infant's experience of distress, difficulties being soothed and difficulties communicating and signaling to their care giver. The care giver is in turn anxious, may disengage emotionally from the infant, being overwhelmed by the infant's condition and distress. These early interactions and transactions lead to more stable but conflicting patterns of interaction into the second year. Parents who may have emotionally disengaged to cope with their infant's precarious hold of life, can find this too difficult to overcome, and become, as the authors quote Stern (1977), "unwilling victims of an involuntary inhibition of their caregiving".

Wille (1991) investigated the effects of preterm birth and perinatal medical risk on mother-infant interaction at 6 months and the quality of attachment at 1 year in a sample of infants from low socioeconomic backgrounds. In this sample, infants were of low birth weight, less than 2,500g and 30-36 weeks gestation. Infants were subdivided into those of high and lower medical risk according to their need for more than 48 hours oxygen at birth or the presence of intraventricular haemorrhage. The author found that preterm infants had higher risk of insecure attachment than full term infants, at 12 months, irrespective of medical risk status. With regard to mother-infant interaction in this study, mothers of full term infants used more positive affect in interaction, these infants were also more likely to come from marginally higher SES backgrounds. Attachment quality was related to level of maternal involvement and positive affect. A high level of involvement was related to lower synchrony. Birth status was found to predict quality of attachment but was not mediated by positive affect. Socioeconomic status may moderate the impact of preterm birth on the quality of the infant-mother attachment. Low SES is associated with a range of factors including single parent families, increased stress and low social support. Previous studies have shown that these factors associated with SES impact on the infant-parent attachment relationship and appear to compound the effect of preterm birth. The impact of preterm birth on maternal positive affect was also significant in this study however this was not found to mediate the effects of preterm birth on attachment. The authors suggest that the mother-infant interaction under more stressful circumstances may give more information as to the aspects of maternal behaviour in interaction which mediate attachment development.

Manglesdorf et al. (1996) further studied the effect of high medical risk and very low birth weight on attachment using naturalistic home observations of attachment and the strange situation procedure in a sample compared with a full term cohort. This study also investigated the stability of attachment from 14 to 19 months. Infants had birth weights < 1,250g and mean gestational age was 27.9 weeks. While there were no differences between preterm and full term groups in attachment classification in the strange situation procedure at 14 months, at 19 months high risk preterm infants were more likely to be insecurely attached. Insecure full term infants were more likely to move to secure over time, where as preterm infants were more likely to become insecure. Preterm infants were more likely to be insecure during the home observation at 14 months. The parents of infants in this study also reported in a separate study, that the impact of their child's prematurity had increased over time (Clafin et al.,1992). The 14 month strange situation procedure may not have allowed for the delay in development of the sample indicating a delay in attachment consolidation in the preterm group. Another reason for the difference may be the diminishing of ongoing support to parents during the second year which may stress the relationship.

A recent meta-analysis found that of the 8 studies of infant attachment as assessed in the strange situation which they included, only two studies reported higher levels of insecure attachment among preterm infants compared with full term populations (Korja et al., 2011). These authors conclude that preterm infants are not at higher risk of insecure attachment. Further review has identified several recent studies indicating that attachment is impacted on in specific ways.

Fuertes et al. (2007) studied the effect of infant temperament, infant regulatory behaviour and maternal sensitivity on attachment in a sample of 48 preterm infants, ranging from 30 to

36 weeks gestation. The study involved evaluation of mother's descriptions of their infant's behaviour at 1 and 3 months, the infant's capacity to regulate stress during Tronick's Face to Face Still face paradigm and maternal sensitivity during free play using the CARE-index. Infant attachment during the Strange situation procedure revealed that in this sample only one third were securely attached, with these infants being described by their mothers as less difficult and to display more positive behaviours during the still face paradigm. A further third of infants who were classified as insecure-avoidant tended to self sooth during the still face paradigm and their mothers were more controlling during free play. The remaining third of infants classified as insecure ambivalent tended to show more distress during the still face paradigm and mothers who were more unresponsive during free play. The authors conclude that multiple factors including temperament, coping behaviour and maternal sensitivity influence attachment in preterm infants.

Udry-Jorgensen et al (2011) studied mother-infant play interaction and attachment in 33 preterm infants born at less than 33 weeks gestational age and their mothers. Attachment was assessed using the Strange Situation Procedure (Ainsworth et al. 1978) at 12 months corrected age and the play interaction was scored using the CARE-index (Crittenden, 2003). The hypothesis of their study was that both medical risk status and mother infant interactions would predict attachment security, with preterm infants to show more insecure attachment compared to community samples. The results showed that 47% of infants of their high risk preterm infants were insecurely attached. In addition there was a significant correlation between the severity of perinatal medical problems as measured with the perinatal risk inventory and the risk of insecure attachment but not with SES, as has been previously found. The vulnerability to insecure attachment in this sample was not related to developmental delay. The authors conclude that the social and emotional difficulties may be mediated by factors such as temperament and self-regulation of preterm infants. With respect to care-giving quality and mother infant interaction, maternal controlling behaviour and infant compulsive compliance correlated with insecure attachment in this sample. Sensitive dyadic interaction was associated with secure attachment and therefore a protective factor. Limitations of the study include the small sample size and lack of a full term control group. The authors also acknowledge that their sample represents a healthy if high risk preterm group, exclusion criteria including infants without significant medical complications of preterm birth or impairments.

A recent study by Candelaria et al (2011) found that psychosocial and sociodemographic risk, but not the infant's medical condition influenced attachment outcomes. The impact on attachment security of these risk factors was mediated by maternal sensitivity. These authors used Attachment Q-sort measures to evaluate maternal sensitivity at 4 months and infant attachment at 12 months.

Less frequently is the concept of attachment disorganization, where the infant displays momentary or indeed prolonged breakdown in attachment behavior, following preterm birth. Previous research has shown that disorganisation is more prevalent in clinical samples and in certain populations (Van Ijzendoorn, 1992) and is associated with more stress in infancy (Hertsgaard et al., 1993; Spangler & Grossman, 1993), aggressive behavior in young children (Lyons-Ruth 1996) and dissociative and other emotional problems in adolescence and young adulthood (Hesse & Van IJzendoorn, 1998; Carlson, 1998). Cox et al., (2000), reported in their sample of 50 preterm infants, disorganised attachment was related both to high levels of maternal experiences of parental rejection and also to preterm infant's intraventricular haemorrhage. This may indicate that neurological factors may place vulnerable infants further at risk of disorganization and the emotional distress that is associated with this. In a further study by Brisch et al. (Brisch et al., 2005) neurological impairment was also associated with insecure attachment. In view of these findings and given the increasing prevalence of neurological sequelae for extremely preterm infants, thearea of attachment disorganisation and neurological impairment warrants further research. Cox found in her predominantly African American sample that insecure attachment was related to maternal representations and not to infant characteristics overall.

Maternal Representations of Attachment

That mothers' representations of their attachment histories, assessed using the Adult Attachment Interview (George et al, 1985), influences the attachment security of their infants has been shown and replicated in several studies (van IJzendoorn1995; Fonagyet al., 1991; Fonagy et al.,1995); Parent's internal representations of their infants, as assessed using the Working Model of the Child Interview (Zeanah et al 1995., Benoit et al., 1997) have also been shown to be predictive of infant attachment security, In the WMCI maternal represeantions are coded as balanced, disengaged or distorted, corresponding to secure, avoidant and ambivalent in the infant classification system based on the Strange Situation Paradigm. In relation to maternal representations in the event of preterm birth a number of studies have illustrated both similarities and differences in quality and patterns of distribution of attachment represenations in samples of mothers of preterm infants compared with normative sample.. Cox et al. (2000) found that in their sample of 50 high risk preterm infants at 19 months of age, 68% of mothers had balanced representations of their infants, 18% had disengaged representations and 14 % had distorted representations, a distribution similar to normative samples. Mothers' representations of their current relationship with their preterm infants predicted attachment security of the infants. Korja et al., (2009) found the distribution of maternal attachment representations in their sample of preterm infants was similar to full term samples, however they also noted qualitative differences between the preterm na dfull term samples. Distorted representations were associated with symptoms of depression. In a study of an early intervention programme for preterm infants, Meijssen et al., (2011) found 30% of their sample, total 78 mothers of preterm infants less than 32 weeks had non-balanced representations when assessed with the WMCI at 18 months. Expression of negative feelings on first seeing their infant and following discharge was found to be related to non-balanced representations. Borghini et al.,(2006), however found that in their sample of preterm infants there was ahigher proportion of insecure maternal representations, both disengaged and distorted when compared to full term infants. The severity of the infant's perinatal risk was associated with mother's attachment representations. Only 20% of the sample had balanced or secure representations at 6 months and 30% were balanced at 18 months. There were also qualitative differences in that mothers of higher risk infants had more distorted representations and mothers of lower risk infants had more disengaged representations. This sample was of lower socioeconomic status than in the previously described studies which may account for the higher rates of insecure or non-balanced representations.

Brisch et al., (2005) studied maternal attachment with the AAI in a sample of preterm infant-mother dyads, however they found no associations between maternal attachment representations in the AAI with infant attachment security at 14 months. These authors however found more insecure attachment in those infants with neurological impairment as noted above. Coppola et al (2007) have found an association between maternal attachment organisation and maternal sensitivity at 3 months of age in preterm infants, with an interaction between secure attachment and prematurity. Sensitivity was affected by medical risk and maternal trauma. Baldoni et al., (2010), report preliminary results that parental insecure attachment is predictive of parent-infant interaction and also with preterm infant development at at two years.

Other maternal experiences such as grief, trauma and depressionhave been explored in relation to infant attachment. Shah et al. (2011) found that maternal unresolved grief following the birth was related to a higher risk of attachment insecurity at 16 months. Symptoms of post traumatic stress and depression have both been found to correlate with maternal representations and infant attachment (Korja, 2009).

Attachment may be viewed as a risk or protective factor for later mental health (Sroufe et al., 2005; VanIJzendoorn et al., 1996). The next section will review the literature on preterm infant social, emotional and behavioural development.

Preterm Infant Social-emotional Development and Psychopathology in Infancy and Later Childhood

While many studies have been conducted on the neurodevelopmental, cognitive and language outcomes of preterm infants, increasingly attention is being paid to the social-emotional development of these infants and children. These areas of difficulties may be more subtle yet may be significantly impairing and distressing for both the child and the family.

Preterm infants may exhibit a variety or regulatory, social and emotional symptoms during the first years of life. Spittle et al.,(2009) found that very preterm infants < 30 weeks and with birth-weights less than 1250g, had significantly greater internalising and regulatory disturbances than their full term peers at age 24 months corrected age. The preterm born children also had lower social-emotional competency. These difficulties were associated with lower birth weight, female sex, white matter abnormalities and postnatal steroids. Treyvaud et al.(2009) have found that parent-child synchrony at age two and parental sensitivity, positive affect and facilitative behaviour was associated with positive cognitive development and social-emotional competence in preterm toddlers. Parents who described their children as more withdrawn, anxious and inhibited showed more negaitive affect during the interaction assessment. However negative affect also correlated with psychomotor development on the Bayley scales of infant development. These studies reveal both the importance of neurodevelopmental and medical factors and parental sensitivity to preterm infant development.

Many studies have focused on neurodevelopmental outcomes such as Attention Deficit Hyperactivity Disorder (ADHD). More recently social communication difficulties including autism spectrum disorders have been found in preterm populations. Extremely preterm infants are at three times higher risk of a range of mental health outcomes (Johnson et al., 2010) For example in a longitudinal study of extremely low birth weight, preterm infants born less than

26 weeks gestation, Johnson et al. (2010) have found of ADHD and autism spectrum disorders significantly higher than in the full term population. Anxiety disorders were also significantly higher and risk was associated with cognitive impairment. Previously several longitudinal and cross-sectional cohort studies have found higher rates of inattention, some reaching clinical diagnoses (Aarnoudse-Moens, 2009; McCormick, 1990 ; Szatmari, 1990 ; Whitaker et al., 2006 ; Botting et al., 1997; Saigal et al., 2000 ; Indredavik et a., 2005 ; Stevenson; Levy-Shiff, et al., 1994)

McCormick showed that children born at very low birth weights were significantly more likely than peers to have higher scores on the hyperactivity subscale of the Behavior Problem Index. Szatmari and colleagues diagnosed attention-deficit hyperactivity disorder (ADHD) in 16% of the children born with birth weights of less than 1,000 grams compared with 6.9% of the children in a matched control group. Aarnoudse-Moens and colleagues conducted a metanalysis of behavioural problems in very preterm and very low birth weight children. These authors found that attention problems were the most evident emotional or behavioural difficulties in their children, with teacher and parent ratings being 0.43 to 0.59 SD, respectively, higher than for controls. Whitaker found that 22% of their sample of 6 year old children, followed prospectively as part of the New Jersey Neonatal Brain Haemorrhage Study birth cohort (birthweight 501-2000g), had a psychiatric disorder; 15.6% of the cohort had a DSM-IIIR diagnosis of ADHD.

In the study by Levy-Shiff of 13 to 14-year-old VLBW children, these children reported a wide array of emotional problems, such as anxiety and depression. After controlling for IQ and visuomotor functioning, only the anxiety scale distinguished the groups. Both parents and teachers reported a higher prevalence of emotional and behavioural problems in VLBW teenagers (Stevenson et al., 1999). Saigal's comparison of 143 Canadian ELBW children of mean gestational age 27 weeks with normal birth weight peers at age 12-16 years demonstrated significantly higher depression subscale scores on the parent-reported Ontario Child Health Study-Revised (OCHS-R) questionnaire (Saigal et al., 2003). , While preterm or very low birth weight children and adolescents do not usually meet diagnostic criteria for depression in the studies, they are more likely to report depressive symptoms more frequently than their full term peers of normal birth weight. In addition 8% of children of very low birth weight met diagnostic criteria for generalised anxiety disorder, compared with 1% of the control grouo (Botting et al., 1997). Some studies however have found no differences (Rickards 1993; Dahl, 2006). There appear to be gender and developmental factors which influence outcomes. Patton (2004)found that adolescent very preterm females were at significantly higher risk of depression.

Several studies have investigated the socialization of preterm and very low birth weight children. These studies have found them to have more socialisation difficultes, more self-regulation difficulties, to be more socially withdrawn and to be described as sad or unhappy , playing alone and more lonely by their peers (Hoy & Sykes., 1997). Social problems have also been found in other studies of very preterm and extremely preterm children (Whittaker et al.1997; Hille et al. 2001; Elgen et al. 2004; Schothorst & van Engeland., 1996) These also have been found to persist into adolescence (Rickards et al., 1993; Saigal et al.,2003 ;)

The link has been made between attentional and socialisation difficulties of very preterm and very low birth weight children. The relationship may be due to common aetiological factors, the impact of attentional and regulatory difficulties on relationships with peers and the importance of how the parent and child relationship must be salient to this. The early experience of life-threatening illness in the child coupled with potentially traumatic reaction in the parents may impact on parent-infant interaction and the developing relationship in a variety of ways. This will be discussed more fully in the following sections.

These findings indicate that preterm infants are at risk of a range of neurodevelopmental, social-communication and social-emotional difficuties across early and middle childhood and into adolescence. The relative contribution of the neurological complications of prematurity and environmental factors remains uncertain. Some authors have pointed to the variance of outcomes for children with known cerebral insults and the potential for the postnatal environment to ameliorate or exacerbate neurodevelopmental outcome (Milgrom et al., 2010; Tronick et al., 2008;)Also the potential for neural plasticity in brain reorganisation is an area of much research and optimism (Ansermet & Magistretti, 200).

The literature on attachment and preterm birth suggests that, while there are differences in the quality of mother-infant interactions, preterm infants across gestational ages can and do form secure attachments. Studies however indicate that for infants whose neonatal course is complicated by significant illness there is an increased risk of insecure attachment. Some studies have found specific patterns of association such as the insecure resistant (ambivalent) pattern predominantly (Plunkett et al 1996), whereas other studies have not distinguished between the insecure patterns, usually due to small sample sizes. Studies have also highlighted the potential impact of neurological impairment as a particular risk factor in predicting attachment security (Brisch et al. 2003 & 2005). There may be a particular association between neurological impairment, the developing infant-parent relationship and the emergence of disorganized attachment which needs further exploration in larger studies. Several authors have described the transaction between infant and mother, whereby the infant's neurological and associated neurobehaviour and communication attempts are perhaps challenging for the mother to attune to and interpret. The mother may have indeed experienced the birth as a trauma and so her capacity to contain and respond to the infant may be impaired. The transactions then are disturbed and the relationship suffers perhaps leading to the insecure and disorganized patterns observed in these studies.

However the literature also suggests that preterm infants form secure attachments, with several studies finding equivocal results or comparative patterns of attachment between preterm and full term samples. These conflicting findings may be due to the methodological differences across the studies on mother-infant interaction and infant attachment. In some studies preterm infants may be relatively healthy, of higher birth weight and gestational age, while other studies have chosen to focus on those infants of higher medical risk. Definition of medical risk also varies between studies. It is of note that more recent studies which include higher risk, lower birth weight and infants born extremely preterm tend to show more attachment insecurity. In addition factors such as socioeconomic status appear to mediate and influence mother-infant interaction, maternal representations of attachment and infant attachment security. The method of assessment of attachment may be significant. Field (1980) has commented also that there are limitations to the Strange Situation procedure, even though this is the gold standard in attachment assessment. In a review of the relationship between early interaction, attachment in the SSP and later social-emotional behaviour in normative and clinical samples including preterm infants she has highlighted that a more complex paradigm which takes into account ecological factors in stressful and non-stressful situations would provide insight into the functional significance of attachment. In addition timing of the assessments may be significant as has been pointed out in studies such as Manglesdorf et al.

(1996) who found that infants attachment security was unstable from the first to the second year, possibly related to a delay in attachment consolidation in preterm samples or possibly due to increasing stress in the second year for some families as their infant's difficulties become more obvious and as support services may diminish. As Muller Nix also noted infant maladaptive interactional behaviour may develop over time and only emerge fully as development ensues (Muller Nix et al. 2004). These interactional difficulties may compound felt maternal stress or trauma and have repercussions for the ongoing mother-infant relationship. Provision of long term support and longitudinal follow-up to establish the trajectory of these findings are recommended.

V. Relationship Focused Interventions for Preterm Infants

Why Intervene in the Relationship between a Preterm Infant and their Parents?

In the preceding sections of the chapter we have seen how the stage upon which the 'dance' between infant and parent takes place may be affected by preterm birth. The mother's emotional state and her experiences of the birth and the NICU, have been shown to affect her mood, cognitions, perceptions and behaviours. This may impact on her developing role as the mother of her baby, in her sensitive attunement and responsiveness to her infant and her sense of competence and efficacy in this role. For the baby, physiological and physical immaturity and ill-preparedness for the extra-uterine environment, particularly when born extremely preterm, are critical. This neurobehavioural immaturity and dependence on intensive care and technology for survival make early social interaction between infant and parent challenging. Yet we know that infants, even those born very prematurely make gestures of communication, and that their relationship to their parents is vital for their development (Trevarthen, 2010; Milgrom, 2010). With this in mind several approaches to early prevention and intervention for preterm infants and their parents have been developed.

This section of the chapter will focus on those early interventions which are relationship focused. These interventions have developed from a variety of theoretical perspectives however many include elements which address the evolving parent-infant relationship. For some the relationship is the core focus of intervention. Interventions may be provided immediately following birth (Melnyk et al., ,) and during the NICU admission (Rauh et al., 1990;), the rationale being that supporting the early parent-infant relationship will prevent maladaptive patterns of interaction forming and thus improve outcomes in the future. Other interventions have been conducted in the community through home visiting programmes which provide education, relationship guidance, child care and other social supports. These have been of varying lengths and intensities (IHDP, Avon). Interventions that provide visual, tactile and kinaesthetic stimulation, during the NICU admission and afterwards, to enhance the developmental potential of the preterm infant (Scarr-Salaptek & Williams, 1973; Resnik et al., 1987) have also been developed. While these interventions have found modest effects on cognitive development they are not relationship focused and will not be discussed further in this chapter.

The theoretical background to relationship-focused interventions will first be discussed followed by a critique of the relevant research studies. The findings of three meta-analyses of early interventions which included samples of preterm infants and their parents will be considered. This will lead to a discussion of the provision of mental health consultation to Neonatal Intensive Care, drawing on the work of several infant mental health and child and adolescent psychotherapists who have written about their work with infants, parents and staff in these units (Zeanah et al., 1984; Cohen, 2003; Negri, 1994, Mendelsohn, 2005; McFaddyen,). The chapter will close with a summary of the findings and directions for future research.

Theoretical Background and Examples of Intervention Programmes

The understanding of the physiological and neurobehavioural immaturity of the preterm infant and the recognition of the impact of the environment of the NICU upon him has increased significantly in the past 3 decades. Als has described the potentially "deleterious effects vigorous stimulation has on the integrative functioning of the fragile systems of the preterm infant" (Als et al., 1986). The infant's inability to habituate to repetitive stimuli such as light, noise and tactile experiences, results in sleep cycle disturbance and energy expenditure. The psychological impact of excessive, painful and stressful procedures experienced by the preterm infant has been a concern of many clinicians working with these most vulnerable infants (Lucey, 1977). The impact on the stress response system has been documented with elevations of cortisol demonstrated following endotracheal intubation and screening for retinopathy of prematurity. These findings have led to the development of approaches which address the environmental adaptation and developmental care needs of the premature baby (Slevin et al., 2000; Als et al., 1994,). The concern being that early and excessive noxious stimulation alters the rapidly developing brain. Findings from animal studies and now being replicated in humans have found that the very presence of the mother following the birth is protective, with corresponding regulation of the stress response system (Milgrom, 2010). The potential for family focused care to promote a functioning dyadic relationship between mother and infant is exquisitely important for these most vulnerable infants.

One such programme which attends to the individual developmental needs, the environment of the preterm infant and also takes a family based approach is the Newborn Individualized Developmental Care and Assessment Programme (NIDCAP, Als, 1986; 1994). The approach involves naturalistic observations of the preterm infant before, during and after care-giving procedures. The focus of the observation is the baby's capacities to organise and modulate the five interactive sub-systems described by Als as critical to the infant's overall organisation and development. How the infant responds to and copes with stimuli from the environment in each of these subsystems, autonomic, physiological, motor, state organisational, attention-interactive and self-regulatory systems is observed and noted. The programme involves training staff and parents to recognise and respond appropriately to the infant's behavioural and developmental cues, such as changes in skin colour and breathing, alert periods when the infant is available for interaction and signals indicating disorganization and the 'shutting out' of excessive stimuli. The approach helps to reduce unexpected sensory stimulation and pain which can overwhelm the immature neonate. The programme aims at promoting mother-infant interactions through more accurate interpretations and responses to the baby's communications and including the parents in the daily cares. The process involves positioning and handling of the infant so as to maintain his homeostasis and promote regulation.

The Newborn Individualized Developmental Care and Assessment Programme (NIDCAP, Als 1983) provides a framework for a family centred, developmentally supportive approach to the preterm infant. Als reported positive effects of the NIDCAP intervention on medical outcome and length of stay (Als et al.,1986, 1994). Kleberg et al. (2000) found positive effects on behavioural indices at 3 years of age. In a further study, Kleberg et al., (Kleberg et al., 2002) found improved cognitive development at one year, corrected age, on the Bayley Scales of Infant Development (BSID) in their sample of VLBW infants, randomized to the NIDCAP intervention. They also found that the probability of being alive with an MDI >80 (mental developmental index on the BSID) was 7 times greater in the intervention group. A major limitation of the study however was the small sample size of only 20 infants in total. The hypothesis for supporting the environmental adaptation and developmental care approach is to support the developing brain during a period of rapid cellular proliferation and neuronal organisation. There are interesting findings in terms of neurophysiological studies, which have shown improvements in preterm infant brain evoked potentials in high risk and low risk infants (Als et al., 1994; Beuhler et al., 1995). Ariagno (Ariagno, 1997) reported no statistically significant beneficial effects of the programme on the BSID at 12 months or at 2 years, while there was a trend toward improved mental indices in this sample. In a more recent study van der Pal et al., (van der Pal et al., 2008) have found that in a randomised trial of NIDCAP compared with basic developmental care, which included nesting and covering the incubator for rest periods, provided to 128 babies, children who received prolonged intervention, more than 1.5 months were found to have improved social-relatedness at 12 months. There was no difference between the groups on infant temperament or infant problem behaviour. Parental qualitative reports about the NIDCAP intervention were positive but there was no statistically significant difference in parental stress between the groups. Several authors have concluded that it is yet too early to draw conclusive evidence of the beneficial effects of NIDCAP over standard developmental care given the cost implications for implementation (Westrup et al., 2002). However it is important that the subtle relational and interactional effects of developmental care are further studied, in longitudinal designs and randomized trials which follow children into childhood and beyond. It is also important that a range of outcomes of infant social-emotional development and parent-infant wellbeing are evaluated to truly appreciate the potential effectiveness and cost effectiveness of the intervention.

The unique insights that the newborn infant's behavioural responses to stimuli from the environment can give clinicians into the infant's capacities for self regulation have been pivotal in shaping several interventions for preterm infants and their parents. These interventions are based on the developmental principles of the Boston Children's Hospital Medical Centre and the work of Brazelton (Rauh et al 1990). The NBAS consists of …..

The Neonatal Behavioural Assessment Scale has become a developmental intervention in itself, in addition to influencing the development of programmes such as NIDCAP. The importance of sharing this developmental understanding of the infant with parents for the parent infant relationship has been shown. The scale has been used as a means for cliniciansto develop a therapeutic relationship with the parents through the child, by illustrating the child's capacities and limitations and by together beginning to understand the child (Nugent & Brazelton, 1989). The beneficial use of this scale has also been shown to be particularly helpful to parents of high risk infants including preterm infants (Britt& Myers, 1994;Beeghley et al., 1995; Rauh et al. 1990). Warren et al. developed a multidisciplinary early intervention programme for low birth weight infants, based on the NBAS self regulation scores and interviews with the parents (Warren et al., 1989). The results of the programme were positive and highlight the importance of using the assessment to ground further interventions for these infants and that supporting effective parent-infant interaction is a way to overcome the early problems following preterm birth. Das Eiden has conducted a meta-analysis of the intervention studies using the NBAS finding small to medium effect sizes for this intervention on subsequent parenting quality. This meta-analysis included three publishes studies including preterm infants and their mothers with effect sizes of 0.03, 0.12 and 0.28. The authors conclude that while there are areas for further investigation, such as potential moderators of the effectiveness of the programmes, such as socioeconomic status, these positive findings for the NBAS as intervention are encouraging.

The Mother Infant Transaction Program (Rauh et al., 1990) was designed to foster the mother's appreciation of her infant's unique characteristics, his temperament and potential for development and to sensitize her to signals of exhaustion, or when the infant became overwhelmed and disorganised as well as to signs that the infant was available for social interaction. A specially trained nurse used the NBAS to help the mother identify the infants reflex systems, state organisation and motor control. The baby's capacity for social interaction was highlighted and there was a focus on how the mother could integrate her knowledge of her baby's capacities into her daily care for him. This programme aimed to help the mother to respond appropriately to her infant's cues, when to pause, console, to alert and to attune to her infant having identified his individual temperament, capacities and sensitivity to environmental stimuli. The mother learned how to create opportunities for mutually satisfying interaction and play. A key focus was to encourage the mother's enjoyment of her baby and to emphasize the baby as a unique person. The intervention was conducted over seven daily sessions in the week prior to the infant's discharge as well as four home based sessions spread over 3 months following discharge. In the original study (Rauh et al., 1988) the low birth weight preterm infants were randomised to the intervention or control groups. In the intervention study, there were significant effects at 6 months on maternal measures of self confidence and role satisfaction and the mother's perceptions of her infant's temperament. There were significant differences at 36 and 48 months on the McCarthy scales. These effects were maintained at 9 years (Achenbach et al..) A number of studies have replicated these findings. Newnham et al., (2008) found that in their early intervention based on the MITP, intervention dyads showed enhanced mother-infant interactions, temperamentally infants in the intervention group were more approaching and easier and had fewer regulatory problems. These infants also had more advanced communication skills. Mothers were less stressed by their infants at 3 months. Kaarensen et al., studied the effects of an intervention programme based on the MITP at 2 years for preterm infants who were randomised to the programme (Kaaresen, et al., 2008). They found no difference in cognitive or motor development at 2 but there were significantly less behaviour problems and parenting stress for the infants and parents who received the programme. Nordhov et al.(2011) found that parents of the preterm born children who received the intervention described fewer behavioural problems at age 5.

Skin to skin contact, also termed Kangaroo care, where the infant is placed naked against the mother's chest, has been shown to promote bonding, and there is some evidence that it also may enhance maternal sensitivity (Tessier et al. 1998;). The protective presence of the mother and father has been more recently the focus of observations and interventions to reduce pain and distress in preterm neonates. The use of kangaroo care during and after blood tests and non-nutritive sucking may help reduce the associated physiological changes and emotional distress caused by these necessary yet very distressing procedures.

Attachment Oriented Interventions

Attachment theory as described in the introduction to the chapter holds that the sensitivity and responsiveness of the mother, or main care givers, in the first months of life provides the infant with the basis for the establishment of a secure attachment relationship. The mother provides a secure base from which the infant can explore the environment, play and learn and to whom he can return for comfort and protection. The emotional regulation provided within the setting of the secure attachment confers a resiliency to stress and a capacity to embrace challenging situations and novelty. Bowlby (1969, 1980) hypothesized that as the child develops, internal representations, or mental models of these early relationship experiences are created, which guide subsequent interpersonal experiences. Subsequent research has shown that adults' representations of attachment experience influence the attachment patterns of their infants. More recent research has also highlighted that parent's representations of their relationship with their infants, both prenatally and in infancy predicts the attachment of the child (Zeanah et al., 1994). Insecure and disorganised attachments are predictive of problems with stress management, emotional regulation and behaviour (Juffer et al. 2005). As outlined previously, preterm birth may affect the quality of mother-infant interaction, in particular maternal sensitivity and mother- infant synchrony. Sensitivity appears to be a crucial factor in determining later attachment security.

Attachment theory has led to the development of interventions based on the concepts of 1. sensitivity and responsiveness, qualities of parenting behaviour, 2. maternal representations of attachment and also on the 3. social support systems of vulnerable parents which in turn represent attachments. Bakermans-Kranenberg et al., conducted a meta-analysis of 70 published studies of attachment interventions, with 88 intervention effects on sensitivity and attachment. The total sample included over 7000 participants, involving samples with non-clinical and clinical populations, including parents at risk for insensitive parenting, children at risk of developmental problems and attachment difficulties and multi-risk families. Sensitivity and attachment security were measured as outcomes using standardised objective measures such as the Ainsworth sensitivity rating scales (Ainsworth, Bell & Stayton, 1974) and the Strange Situation procedure among others. The studies involved interventions where the focus was on changing the behaviour of parents towards more sensitive parenting (eg Teti et al., 1977), changing the representations of parents with regard to attachment (eg Robert-Tissot et al. 1996), providing social support (Barnett et al., 1987) or a combination of the three approaches described (Barnett et al., 1987; Egeland and Erisckson., 1993)

The meta-analysis included 12 studies of preterm infants and their parents which will be discussed below. The meta-analyses highlighted several important findings. Sensitivity focused intervention is as effective as the combined types of intervention, while all interventions which focused on sensitivity, representation or a combined approach showed substantial effect sizes (d = 0.46). In addition interventions with video feedback were more effective. Interventions with fewer sessions were also more effective, with interventions with fewer than 5 sessions being as effective as sessions with 5 – 16 sessions.

The start of the treatment was also important as it showed that starting intervention after 6 months was more effective. With regard to interventions for preterm infants however almost all of these commenced at or shortly after birth or discharge from hospital thus differing from other studies which commenced later in infancy. A number of authors have highlighted the need for such early intervention in the case of preterm birth, the rationale being that researchers have questioned whether home based interventions, even those which are intensive and extending into the preschool period may not be able to ameliorate patterns of interaction and distress which have already been established early in the post-natal period (Johnson et al., 2004).

The authors conclude that a 'less is more' approach may be most beneficial when designing attachment based interventions and that intervention which focuses predominantly on enhancing sensitivity of parents to their children's cues may confer most advantage in terms of later attachment security.

Several studies have shown positive effects on sensitivity, parent-infant interaction or infant attachment in preterm infants (eg. Barerra et al. 1986; Beckwith, 1988; Bustan & Sagi, 1984; Field et al., 1980; Kang et al., 1995; Meyer et al., 1994; Sajaniemi et al., 2001; Spiker et al., 1993; Tessier et al., 1998; Teti et al., 2009; Wijnroks 1994; Zahr et al. 1992; Zahr, 2000). Examples of these studies are described below.

In the study by Bustan & Sagi (1984), 8 preterm infants and their mothers received an individualised standardised intervention during their hospital stay, which included three discussions with NICU staff regarding the mother's feelings, provision of information about prematurity and a manual giving further information about prematurity. The intervention group was compared to a control group who did not receive the intervention. The intervention positively affected infant mother interactions, infants were perceived by their mothers to cry less and vocalise more.

Kang et al. (1995) The authors tested a hospital based intervention programme which taught mothers to read the behavioural cues of their infants and how to optimise the infants states of consciousness during feeding and a home based programme over 5 months following the infant's discharge. The effects were greater for the hospital based programme for mothers with higher educational attainment and for the combined programme for mothers with lower educational attainment.

Two studies which provided home based long term intervention were the Infant Health and Development Project (Spiker et al., 1993) and the Avon Premature Infant Project (Johnson et al., 1998; Johnson et al., 2005). The IHDP study was a multi-centre randomised trial of an early intervention programme, consisting of home visits, developmental education, support, full-day childcare after age 2 and referrals to relevant paediatric specialists for preterm infants across gestational ages and birth weights. The children in the intervention group had significantly better cognitive development scores than the control group at 2 and 3 years, in particular for the heavier birth weight infants. There were also small differences in behavioural outcomes, although these and the cognitive advantages attenuated over time. Heavier infants showed continuing modest gains in cognition over time. This study combines an educational component with relationship focused support programme. In terms of attachment the IHDP study found positive gains in parent infant synchrony, maternal support and child cooperation.

The Avon Premature Infant Project (1998) was a randomised trial of a 2 year developmental educational programme (Portage) or a social support intervention, non-directive counselling, provided at home to 284 preterm infant born at < 33 weeks gestation. At 2 years this study found there to be small positive effects of the developmental educational intervention and after planned secondary analysis significant effects were found for those children without severe disability and after correction for social confounding variables. A further follow-up of 187 (66%) of the original cohort at 5 years revealed no statistical significant effects for the intervention on cognitive or other outcome measures.

Other home based interventions focused on the parent-infant or parent-therapist relationship include those of Field, (1980), Wijnroks (1994), Beckwith (1988) and Barerra, (1986). These studies have all demonstrated positive effects and small to moderate effect sizes.

Studies which have assessed infant attachment as an outcome measure include those by Brisch et al. (2003), Sajaniemi et al (2001) and Cassiba et al.,(2009). An interesting study by Brisch et al., investigated a comprehensive NICU based intervention, including attachment oriented individual and supportive group intervention, parental sensitivity training with video feedback and a home visit following discharge to consolidate the intervention. The authors found that the rates of secure and insecure attachment in their very low birth weight sample were similar to those found in term infants and there was no statistical difference in the attachment quality of the intervention versus the control group. However there was a significant effect of the intervention for those infants who were neurologically impaired who were more secure. Sajaniemi et al. found their home based Occupational Therapy intervention improved disorganised attachment in their sample at age 4 years. The study by Cassiba et al found their video informed sensitivity intervention, which included a discussion of maternal attachment representations to enhance the sensitivity of insecure mothers of preterm infants, while it did not improve those mothers who were secure, as assessed prior to the intervention on the adult attachment interview. The authors caution that the intervention with secure mothers may have negative effects in stirring up doubts about their parenting. A previous study found that mothers of secure infants rated their infants as more insecure (). This is an important question in the provision of interventions generally to populations at risk. Careful design application of intervention programmes is warranted.

The transactional model of development has been critical in influencing the approaches to interventions with preterm infants and parents (Brisch et al. 2003. Other approaches used have utilised other theoretical models such as coping (Melnyk et al., 2001), trauma-prevention (Jotzo & Poets, 2005) and the work of Bandura (Bandura, 1986) on self efficacy of parents (Beckwith, 1988; Teti et al., 2009).

While most intervention studies have focused on mothers, the importance of the role of fathers is being increasingly recognised. The recognition of the impact of the preterm birth and subsequent medical complications of the infant for fathers and their important role in the infant's social-emotional development, in addition to supporting the mother must translate into evaluations of psychosocial interventions for fathers also.

Psychotherapeutic understanding has been applied more broadly also to the provision of NICU by several authors. Zeanah et al. have described clinical approaches to parents of preterm infants in the setting of the NICU. They highlight that parents may require a flexible approach which may consist of crisis intervention, supportive psychotherapy and insight oriented psychotherapy, depending on their emotional responses to the challenge of adaptation following the potential trauma of preterm birth. Crisis intervention has a role in helping parents restore psychological functioning and to cope when this is a temporary disturbance. Supportive psychotherapy promotes the parent's adaptation to their and their baby's predicament. Insight-oriented psychotherapy aims at bringing unconscious and past conflicts to consciousness, these unconscious processes potentially interfering with the developing relationship between parent and infant. In addition to working psychotherapeutically with parents, child psychotherapists and mental health professionals have used their skills in psychoanalytic infant observation to understand the infant's experience. Based on the work of Bick (1952) this work has not only informed the care of individual infants and their families but also formed the basis of successful interventions (Negri, 1994). Cohen (1993) has described the impact of her work in terms of understanding the most profound of human qualities, personal integrity and respect in the context of the 'extraordinary' setting of the NICU.

Conclusion and Future Directions

. Increasing awareness of the traumatic nature of preterm birth, of the emotional sequelae and grief associated with the experience and the potentially long term mental health implications for infants indicate that supports are needed to contain and understand parental experiences and to offer individualised intervention where appropriate. The importance of maternal and indeed paternal attachment representations of the current relationship with their baby is also gaining increased recognition in the literature. The salience of the parent-infant relationship to the infant's capacity for emotion regulation, security of attachment and infant mental health has also been highlighted.

Researchers such as De Wolff and Van IJzendoorn (1997) have called within attachment research for a "move to the contextual level.... to interpret the complex transactions between context and sensitivity in less stable and more stressful settings". The potential for several factors acting at differing levels of impact to influence the variability of outcomes in these clinical populations such as preterm infants and their parents must be considered. At a neurobiological level several studies have shown that early adversity does not fully determine outcome. Resilience and the neural plasticity of the brain are particularly important when considering adaptation in preterm infants (Ansermet & Magistretti, 2007). The impact of stress and the variability of the individual to respond to, adapt and cope with stress need to be further explored. Further study of the link between neurological vulnerability and the protective effects of the parent-infant relationship, as suggested by the research of Milgrom et al. (2010) is essential.

At a dyadic interactional and systemic level Tronick has noted that the "dyad faced with uncertainty and confusion at the beginning may make several changes in direction before stability emerges" (Tronick, 2008). At a transactional level (Sameroff, 1973) the impact of multiple influences and ecology on the system must be taken into account. Just as preterm infant-parent relationship and attachment research may clarify issues of pathological significance it also may also clarify questions about resilience and the potential for recovery.

Tronick has highlighted the development of trust in the experience of reparation following disruption in the mother-infant interaction (Tronick et al., 2007). Stern (2002) has described how the earliest mother-infant interactions are the real lived experiences upon which the representational world of the infant develops and how this representational world may be subjectively experienced for the baby. The the potential for mis-regulations and mis-steps to occur which lead to the various forms of mother-infant relationship problems is increasingly being recognised. These early interactional difficulties may be areas of preventive therapeutic intervention for infant and mother. In addition the association of socioeconomic status and developmental outcome for preterm infants and parents indicates that much still needs to be done to support the most disadvantaged infants and parents.

Early NICU based intervention has shown to have positive effects which can be found both early and also some years following the intervention. The attenuation of the positive effects of other programmes by middle childhood makes the case that individualized interventions, flexible in duration, and specialized services for preterm infants and parents may make therapeutic and economic sense. These issues require further research.

FUNDING

Supported by a grant from the National Children's Research Centre, Our Lady's Children's Hospital, Crumlin, Dublin 12, Ireland.

REFERENCES

Achenbach T.M, Phares, V., Howell, C.T., Rauh, V.A., Nurcombe, B (1990) 7 year Outcome of the Vermont Intervention Program for Low-Birthweight Infants. Child Develeopment. Vol 61 (6) 1672-1681

Achenbach, T.M et al. 9 year Outcome of the Vermont Intervention Programme for Low-Birthweight Infants.

Ainsworth, M.D.S., Bell, S.M., Stayton, D. (1971) Individual Differences in Strange Situation behaviour of one-year-olds. In H.R. Schaeffer (Ed,), *The origins of human social relations*. Pp 17-57. London: Academic Press.

Ainsworth, M. D. S., Bell, S. M., & Stayton, D. (1974). Infant-mother attachment and social development. In M. P. Richards (Ed.), *The introduction of the child into a social world* (pp.99-135). London: Cambridge University Press.

Als, H. (1986). A synactive model of neonatal behavioural organization: Framework for the assessment of neurobehavioural development in the premature infant and for support of infants and parents in the neonatal intensive care environment. In J.K. Sweeney (Ed.), *The high-risk neonate: Developmental therapy perspectives* (pp. 3-55). New York: Haworth Press.

Als, H.A., Lawton, G., Duffy, F., McAnulty, G., Gibes-Grossman, R., Blickman., F (1994) Individualised Developmental Care for the Very Low Birth Weight Preterm Infant – Medical and Neurofunctional effects. Journal of the American Medical Association. 272 (11) 853-858

Als, H. A., Lester, B. M., Tronick, E. Z., & Brazelton, T. B. (1982). Manual for the assessment of preterm infants' behaviour (APIB). In H.E. Fitzgerald, B. M. Lester, & M. W. Yogman (Eds.), *Theory and research in behavioural pediatrics* (pp. 65-132). New York: Plenum Press.

Als. H., Duffy, F.H., McAnulty, G.B., Rivkin, M. J., Vajapeyam, S., Mulkern, R.V., et al. (2004). Early experience and brain function and structured. *Pediatrics,* 113 (4), 846-857.

American Psychiatric Association.(2000). *Diagnostic and statistical manual of mental disorders DSM-IV-TR* (4th ed., text rev.). Washington, DC: Author.

Ansermet & Magistretti (2007) Biology of Freedom Neural Plasticity, Experience and the Unconscious. Karnac.

Ariagno R.L., Thoman, E.B., Boeddiker, M.A., Kugener, B., Constantinou, J.C., Mirmiran, M., Baldwin, R (1997). Developmental Care Does Not Alter Sleep and Development of Premature Infants. *Paediatrics,* 100 (6)

Bakeman R, Brown JV. (1980) Early interaction, consequences for social and mental development atthree years. *Child Development.;* 51: 437-447.

Bakermans-Kranenburg, M.J., van IJzendoorn, M.H., Juffer, F. (2003) Less is more: Meta-analyses of sensitivity and attachment interventions in early childhood. Psychological Bulletin Vol 129 (2) 195-215. Bandura A., (1986) Social Foundations of Thought and Action: A social cognitive theory. Engelwood Cliffs, NJ: Prentice Hall

Barrera M.E., Doucet, D.A., Kitching., K.J. (1990) Early Home Intervention and Socio-Emotional Development of Preterm Infants. *Infant Mental Health Journal,* Vol 11, No. 2

Beckwith, L. (1988) Intervention with Disadvantaged Parents of Sick Preterm Infants. Psychiatry Vol. 51. PP 242-247.

Beeghly, m., Brazelton, T.B., Flannery, K., Nugent, J.K., Barret, D.E., Tronick, E.Z. (1995)' Specificity of paediatric intervention effects in early infancy.' *Journal of Developmental and Behavioural Paediatrics.*

Behrman R.E., & Stith Butler, A.(2006). *Preterm birth: Causes, consequences, and prevention.* Washington, DC: The National Academic Press.

Buehler, DM Als, H. Duffy, FH et al. Effectiveness of individualized developmental care for low risk preterm infants: behavioral and electrophysiological evidence. *Pediatrics*, 96 (1995), pp. 923–932.

Bick, E., Notes on Infant Observation in Psychoanalytic Training (1964) In Surviving Space, Papers on Infant Observation Ed. Briggs, A. The Tavistock Clinic Series.

Binder, W.S; Zeltzer, L.K; Simmons, C.F., Mirocha, J., Pandya, A. (2011) The Father in the Hallway: Posttraumatic Stress Reactions in Fathers of NICU Babies. *Psychiatric Annals.* Vol 41 (8).

Borghini, A., Pierrehumbert, B., Miljkovitch, R., Muller Nix, C., Forcada Guex, M., & Asermet, F. (2006). Mother's attachment representations of their premature infant at 6 and 18 months after the birth. *Infant Mental Health Journal,* 27(5), 494-508.

Botting, N., Powls, A., Cooke, R.W., & Marlow, N. (1997) Attention deficit hyperactivity disorder and other psychiatric outcomes in very low birthweight children at twelve years. *Journal of Child Psychology and Psychiatry,* 38(8), 931-941.

Botting, N., et al., Attention deficit hyperactivity disorders and other psychiatric outcomes in very low birthweight children at 12 years. *Journal of Child Psychology and Psychiatry and Allied Disciplines,* 1997. 38(8): p. 931-941.

Botting, N., et al., Cognitive and educational outcome of very-low-birthweight children in early adolescence. *Developmental Medicine & Child Neurology,* 1998. 40(10): p. 652-60.

Bowlby, J. (1969. 1980) *Attachment and Loss.* Vol (1). Brazelton, T., & Nugent, J. (1995). *Neonatal behavioural assessment scale.* London:Mac Keith Press.

Bretherton I. (1992). The Origins of Attachment Theory. *Developmental Psychology* (1992), 28, 759-775.

Brisch K.H., Bechinger, D., Betzler, S., Heinemann, H. (2003) Early preventive attachment-oriented psychotherapeutic intervention program with parents of a very low birthweight premature infant: esults of attachment and neurological development. *Attachment & Human Development* Vol 5 No 2 pp 120-135.

Brisch KH, Bechinger D, Betzler S, Heinemann H, Kachele H, Pohlandt F et al. Attachment quality in very low birth weight premature infants in relation to maternal attachment representations and neurological development. *Parenting: Science and Practice*. 2005; 5(4):311-331.

Britt, G.C. & Myers, B.J (1994a) The effects of Brazelton Intervention: a review. Infant Mental Health Journal, 15, 293-304.

Bruschweiler-Stern, N. (2009). The Neonatal Moment of Meeting—Building the Dialogue, Strengthening the Bond. *Child and Adolescent Psychiatric Clinics of North America*, Volume 18, Issue 3, Pages 533-544

Butcher PR, Kalverboer, AF, Minderaa RB, van Doormal EF, ten Wolde Y. (1993) Rigidity, sensitivity and quality of attachment: the role of maternal rigidity in the early socio-eotional development of premature infants. *Acta psychiatrica scandinavica.;* 375 (88):1-30.

Bustan,D&Sagi,A.(1984). Effects of early hospital-based intervention on mothers and their preterm infants. *Journal of Applied Developmental Psychology*, 5, 305–17

Clafin,C., Bozynski, M., Meisels, S,. Dichtellmilller, M., & Burns, C. (1992) Relationship of extremely low birth weight infant morbidity patterns to maternal reports of family impact during the first two years of life. *Paper presented at the International Conference on Infant Studies.* Miami, FL.

Cohen, M. (2003) *Sent Before My Time.*A Child Psychotherapists view of life on a Neonatal Intensive Care Unit. Karnac.

Coppola, G., Cassiba, R. (2007). What can make the difference?: Premature birth and maternal sensitivity at 3 months of age: The role of attachment organization, traumatic reaction and baby's medical risk. *Infant behaviour and Development.* Vol 30 (4) pp 679-684.

Cox, S.M., Hopkins, J., Hans, S.L. (2000) Attachment in preterm infants and mothers: neonatal risk status and maternal representations. *Infant Mental Health Journal,* Vol. 21(6), 464-480.

Crittenden, P. M. (1979-2004) *CARE-index coding manual*. Unpublished manuscript Miami, FL., available from the author.

Crnic KA, Ragozin, AS, Greenberg, MT, Robinson, NM, Basham, RB, (1983). Social interaction and developmental competence of preterm and full term infants during the first year of life. *Child Development,* Vol 54, 1199-1210.

Das Eiden & Reifman, A. (1996). Effects of Brazelton demonstrations on later parenting: A meta-analysis. *Journal of Pediatric Psychology,* 21, 857–868.

De Wolff, M.S., van Ijzendoorn, M.H. (1997) A meta-analysis on parental antecedents of Infant Attachment. *Child Development.* Vol 68 (4) pp 571-591.

DeMier, R., Hynan, M., Hatfield, R., Varner, M., Harris, H., & Maniello, R. (2000). A measurement model of perinatal stressors: Identifying risk for postnatal emotional distress in mothers of high-risk infants. *Journal of Clinical Psychology, 56*(1), 89-100.

DiVitto, B& Goldberg, S, (1979) 'The effect of newborn medical status on early parent infant interaction' in T Field, Sostek, Goldberg and Shuman (Eds) *Infants born at risk.*

Doyle, L.W. and D. Casalaz, *Outcome at 14 years of extremely low birthweight infants: a regional study.* Archives of Disease in Childhood, 2001. 85(3): p. F159-F164.

Easterbrooks MA, (1989), Quality of attachment to mother and to father: effects of perinatal risk status. *Child Development*, 60, 825-830.

Goldberg, Perotta, Minde, & Corter (1986) Maternal behaviour and attachment in low birth weight twins and singletons, *Child Development.*

Holditch-Davis, D., Bartlett, T.R., Blickman, Al. & Miles, M.S.(2003). Post-traumatic stress symptoms in mothers of premature infants. *Journal of Obstetric, Gynaecologic, and Neonatal Nursing,* 32 (2), 161-171

Hoy& Sykes, The Social Competence of Very-Low-Birth-Weight Children - Teacher, Peer, and Self-Perceptions. *Journal of Abnormal Child Psychology,* 1992. **20**(2): p. 123-150.

Hughes, M. A. & McColluM, j. (1994). Neonatal Intensive Care: mothers and fathers perceptions of what s stressful. *Journal of Early Intervention.*

Indredavik, M.S., et al., Psychiatric symptoms in low birth weight adolescents, assessed by screening questionnaires. *European Child & Adolescent Psychiatry,* 2005. **14**(4): p. 226-236.

Johnson et al (2010) Psychiatric Disorders in Extremely Preterm Children: Longitudinal Finding at Age 11 Years in the EPICure Study. *Journal American Academy of Child and Adolescent Psychiatry.*

Jotzo, M & Poets, C.F. (2005) Helping Parents Cope with the Trauma of Premature Birth: An evaluation of a trauma preventive psychological intervention. *Pediatrics.* Vol 115.

Joyce A. *The Psychodynamics of Human Development.*

Juffer, F., van IJzendoorn, M.H., Bakermans-Kranenburg, M.J., *Attachment based interventions in early childhood*(2005) In: Promoting Positive Parenting. Ed.

Kaaresen, P.I., Ronning, J.A., Tunby, J., Nordhov, S.M., Ulvund, S.E., Dahl., L.B. (2008) A randomized controlled trial of an early intervention program in low birth weight children: Outcome at 2 years. *Early Human Development.* Vol. 84, 201-209.

Kang, R; Barnard, K; Hammond, M; Oshio, S; Spencer, C, Thibodeaux, B; Williams, J. Preterm Infant Follow-up Study: A Multi-Site Field Experiment of Hospital and Home Intervention Programs for Mothers and Preterm Infants. *Public Health Nursing,* Vol 12 (3), 171-180. 1995.

Kleberg, A., Westrup, B., Stjernqvist, K., Lagercrantz, H., Indications of improved cognitive development at one year of age among infants born very prematurely who received care based on the Newborn Individualized Developmental Care and Assessment Programme (NIDCAP).(2002) *Early Human Development* 68 PP 83-91.

Kuban, K.C., et al., Positive Screening on the Modified Checklist for Autism in Toddlers (M-CHAT) in Extremely Low Gestational Age Newborns. *The Journal of Pediatrics,* 2009. 154(4): p. 535-540.

Larsson, H.J., et al., Risk factors for autism: perinatal factors, parental psychiatric history, and socioeconomic status. *American Journal of Epidemiology,* 2005. 161(10): p. 916-925.

Levy-Schiff, R., et al., *Emotional and Behavioral-Adjustment in Children Born Prematurely. Journal of Clinical Child Psychology,* 1994. 23(3): p. 323-333.

Limperopoulos, C., et al., Positive Screening for Autism in Ex-preterm Infants: Prevalence and Risk Factors. *Pediatrics,* 2008. 121: p. 758-765.

Lucey, J.F. Is Intensive Care becoming too intensive? (1977) Paediatrics; 59 Suppl: 1064-5.

Main, M., Goldwyn, R., (1984). Predicting rejection of her infant from mother's representation of her own experience: implications for the abused-abusing intergenerational cycle. *Child Abuse and Neglect.* Volume 8, Issue 2, pp 203-217.

Main, M., Kaplan, N., Cassidy, J. (1985). Security in infancy, childhood and adulthood: A move to the level of representation. In I Bretherton & E. Waters (Eds.), Growing points in attachment theory and research. *Monographs of the Society for Reseach in Child Development,* 50 (1-2), Serial No. 209), 66-104.

McCormick, M. C., Brooks-Gunn, J., Workman-Daniels, K., Turner, J., Peckham, G.J. (1992). The health and Developmental Status of Very Low-Birth-Weight Children at School Age. *Journal Of The American Medical Association* 267(16):2204-2208.

Melnyk. B.M., Alpert-Gillis, L., Fischbeck Feinstein, N., Fairbanks, E., Schultz-Czarniak, J., Hust, D., Sherman, L., LeMoin, C., Moldenhauer, Z., Small, L., Bender, N., Sinkin, R.A. (2001) Research in Nursing and Health, 2001 Vol 24 pp 373-389.

Mendelsohn, A. (2005) Recovering Reverie: Using infant observation in interventions with traumatized mothers and their premature babies. *Infant Observation: International Journal of Infant Observation and its applications.* Vol 8 (3).

Miles M.S, Holditch-Davis, D., Schwarz, T; Scher, M., (2007) Depressive Symptoms in Mothers of Prematurely Born Infants. *Journal of Developmental and Behavioural Pediatrics* Vol 28 (1).

Milgrom, J., Newnham, C., Anderson, P., Doyle, L., Gemmill, A., Lee, K., Hunt, R., Bear, M., Inder, T. (2010) Early Sensitivity Training for Parents of Preterm Infants: Impact on the Developing Brain. *Pediatric Research.* Vol 67 (3) pp 330-335.

Minde, K., Perrotta, M., Marton, P. (1985) Maternal Caretaking and Play with Full-Term and Premature Infants. *Journal of Child Psychology and Psychiatry.* Volume 26, Issue 2, pp 231-244.

Muller-Nix & Forcada-Guex (2009). Perinatal Assessment of Infant, Parents and Parent-Infant Relationship: Prematurity as an Example. *Child Adoles Clin North America*, Volume 18(3) 545-557.

Muller-Nix, C & Ansermet, F., 2009 Prematurity, Risk Factors and Protective Factors, pp 180-196, in Zeanah, C. (Ed.) *Handbook of Infant Mental Health,* 2009 The Guilford Press.

Negri, R. (1994) *The Newborn in the Intensive Care.* Clunie Press.

Newnham, C., Milgrom, J., Skouteris, H. (2009). Effectiveness of a Modified Mother-Infant Transaction Program on Outcomes for Preterm Infants from 3 to 24 months of age. *Infant Behaviour and Development* Vol 32, (1) pp 17-26.

Padden, T., & Glenn, S., (1997) Maternal experience of preterm birth and neonatal intensive care. *Journal of Reproductive and Infant Psychology,* Vol 15, (2), 1997.

Pianta, R.C., Marving, R.S., & Morong, M.C (1999). Resolving the past and present: Relations with attachment organization. In J. Solomon & C. George (Eds), *Attachment Disorganization* (pp. 379 – 398). New York, London: Guilford Press.

Pierrehumbert, B., Nicole, A., Muller-Nix, C., Forcada-Guex, M., Ansermet, F. (2003) Parental post-traumatic reactions after premature birth: implications for sleeping and eating problems in the infant. *Archives of Disease in Childhood: Fetal & Neonatal* Vol 88 (5) pp400-404.

Pietrini J.R., Dias T., McCormick M., Massolo M., Green N., Escobar G. Increased Risk of Adverse Neurological Development for Late Preterm Infants. *Journal of Pediatrics* 2009; 154, (2) pp169-176.

Rauh, V.A., Nurcombe, B., Achenbach, T., Howell, C (1990) The Mother-Infant Transaction Program. The content and implications of an intervention for the mothers of low birth weight infants. *Clinics in Perinatology* 17(1): 31-45.

Resnik M.B., Eyler F.D., Nelson, R.M., Eitzman, D.V., Bucciarelli, R.L. Developmental Intervention for Low Birth Weight Infants: Improved Early Developmental Outcome. (1987) Paediatrics 80. 68.

Rode, Chang, Niau, Fisch & Sroufe, 1981; Attachment patterns in infants separated at birth. *Developmental Psychology* 17, 188-191.

Saigal, S., et al., Transition of extremely low-birth-weight infants from adolescence to young adulthood - Comparison with normal birth-weight controls. *Jama-Journal of the American Medical Association,* 2006. 295(6): p. 667-675.

Sajaniemi, N., Makela, J., Salokorpi, T., von Wendt, L., Hamalainen, T., Hakamies-Blomqvist, L. (2001) Cognitive performance and attachment patterns at 4 years of age in extremely low birth weight infants after early intervention. *European Child and Adolescent Psychiatry* 10:122-129.

Scarr-Salaptek, S & Williams, M.L (1973) The effects of early stimulation on Low Birth Weight Infants. Child Development. Vol 44, 94-101.

Shah, P.E., Clements, M., Poehlmann, J. (2011) *Pediatrics* 127(2) pp284-292.

Singer, L., Salvator, M.S., Shenyang, G., Collin, M., Lawrence, L., Bayley, J. (1999) Maternal Psychological Distress and Parenting Stress After the Birth of a Very Low-Birth-Weight Infant. *Journal of the American Medical Association* 281 (9): 799-805.

Slevin, M, Farrington, N., Duffy, G, Daly, L, Murphy, J.F.A. Altering the NICU and measuring infants' responses. (2000) Acta Paediatica; 89: 577-81.

Spiker, D., Ferguson, J., Brooks-Gunn, J(1993) Enhancing Maternal Interactive Behavior and Child Social Competence in Low Birth Weight, Premature Infants. Child Development 64 :754-68.

Spittle A.J., Treyvaud, K., Doyle. L.W, Roberts, G., Lee, K., Inder, Cheong, J., Hunt, R., Newnham, C., Anderson, P. (2009) *Journal of the American Academy of Child and Adolescent Psychiatry.* Vol 48, (9) pp 909-918.

Sroufe, A. (2005) *The Development of the Person.* Guilford Press.

Stern, D. (2002) *The First Relationship.* Harvard Press. *Stern, D. The interpersonal world of the infant.*

Tessier, R., Cristo, M., Velez, S., Giron, M., Figueroa de Calume, Z., Ruiz-Palaez, J.G., ET AL.(1998).1998 Kangaroo mother care and the bonding hypothesis. *Pediatrics.* 102 e17*.

Teti, D.M., Black., M.M., Viscardi, R., Glass, P., O'Connell., M., Baker., L., Cusson., R., Reiner Hess., Christine. Intervention With African American Premature Infants: Four Month Results of An Early Intervention Programme. (2009) Journal Of Early Intervention Vol 31: 146

Trevarthen, C. (1979) Communication and cooperation in early infancy: a description of primary intersubjectivity. In M. Bullowa (Ed.) *Before speech: the beginning of interpersonal communication.* Cambridge University Press.

Trevarthen, C. (2010) What is it like to be a person who knows nothing? Defining the active intersubjective mind of a newborn human being. *Infant and Child Development.* Vol 20 (1) pp 119-135.

Treyvaud, K., Anderson, V.A., Howard, K., Bear, M., Hunt., R.W., Doyle. L.W, Inder. T., Woodward, L., Anderson, P. (2009)Parenting Behaviour is Associated With the Early Neurobehavioural Development of Very Preterm Children. *Pediatics Vol.* 123 (2)ppp555-561.

Tronick, E. (2007) *The neurobehavioural and social-emotional development of infants and children* Ed. Norton & Company.

van der Pal S., Maguire, C.M., Le Cessie, S, Veen, S., Wit, J.W., Walther, F.J., Bruil, J. (2008) Parental Stress and Child Behaviour and Temperament in the First Year After the Newborn Individualized Developmental Care and Assessment Program. Journal of Early Intervention 2008 30: 102.

Warren 1989

Westrup, B., Stjernqvist, K., Kleberg, A., Hellstrom-Westas, L., Lagercrantz H. Neonatal IndividualiZED Care in practice: A Swedish experience. Seminars in Neonatology 2002; 7 (6): 447-547

Whitfield MF. (2005) Family Centered Developmentally Supportive Care of the High Risk Infant and Family: Comments on Als, Westrup, Mallik and Spiker. In: Tremblay RE, Barr RG, Peters RDeV, Eds. Encyclopaedia on Early Childhood Development (online). Montral, Quebec: Centre of Excellence for Early Childhood Development: 1-4.

Wijnroks, L. (1999). Maternal recollected anxiety and mother–infant interaction in preterm infants. *Infant Mental health Journal.* Vol 20 (4). Pp 393-409.

Wille, D.E. (1991) Relation of Preterm Birth with Quality of Infant-Mother Attachment at One Year. *Infant Behaviour and Deveopment.* 14, pp 227-240.

Winnicott, D.W., (1949a) 'Birth Memories, Birth Trauma and Anxiety'. In: *Through Paediatrics to Psychoanalysis* – Collected Papers. Karnac. pp 174-193.

Winnicott, D.W., (1949b) 'Mind and its relation to the psyche-soma'. In: *Through Paediatrics to Psychoanalysis* – Collected Papers. Karnac. pp 243-254.

Winnicott, D.W., (1956) 'Primary Maternal Preoccupation'. In: Through Paediatrics To Psychoanalysis – Collected Papers. Karnac. pp 300-305.

Zahr, L. (2000) Infant Mental Health Journal. Home Based Intervention After Discharge For Latino Families of Low Birth Weight Infants. Infant Mental Health Journal, Vol. 21(6), 448-463

Zeanah, C., Benoit, D., Barton, M.(1986) *Working Model of the Child Interview.* Unpublished manuscript.

Zeanah, C., Doyle-Zeanah, P. (2009). The scope of infant mental health. *Handbook of Infant Mental Health.* Third Edition. Ed. Zeanah, C. The Guilford Press.

Zeanah, C.. (2007). Constructing a relationship formulation for mother and child. In *Attachment theory in clinical work with children. Bridging the gap between research and practice.* Eds. Oppenheim, D. & Goldsmith, D. F. The Guilford Press.

Zeanah, C.H., Canger, C. I., Jones, J. D., (1984). Clinical approaches to traumatised parents: *Psychotherapy in the intensive care nursery. Child Psychiatry and Human Development,* 14(), 159-169.

In: Preterm Infants
Editors: Diogo Contreiras and Johann Sampaio ISBN 978-1-62081-819-0

Chapter 2

LATER PRETERM BIRTH AND THE DEVELOPING BRAINSTEM

Ze Dong Jiang*
Department of Paediatrics, University of Oxford,
John Radcliffe Hospital, Oxford, UK

ABSTRACT

Carefully monitoring the neurologic status and development in early life is important for preterm infants. A decrease in gestational age is often associated with an increased incidence of neurodevelopmental abnormalities or deficits such as cerebral palsy, even for those infants born at late pregnancy or late preterm. Of all preterm births, late preterm birth comprises about 70%. Therefore, late preterm infants are an important population in preterm infants. Numerous previous studies have shown that infants who are born at very or extremely preterm are predisposed to brain damage and neurological impairment. By comparison, there is relatively limited information available for brain function and neurodevelopment in late preterm infants. Over the last decade, there is an increased interest in studying neurodevelopment in these infants.

Recently, there are investigators who studied brainstem auditory evoked response (BAER) in late preterm infants using the maximum length sequence technique (MLS). In those who had no major perinatal conditions or problems, MLS BAER was basically normal, except for a moderate abnormality at high-rate click stimulation. This finding implies that low-risk late preterm infants have a mild delay in neural conduction in the brainstem and that late preterm birth has limited or no major effect on the immature brain. In late preterm infants who had major perinatal conditions or problems, there were some major abnormalities in those MLS BAER components that mainly reflect functional status of the more central or rostral brainstem. The abnormalities indicate that the functional integrity of the auditory brainstem, mainly in the central regions, is impaired in late preterm infants with perinatal problems. Since late preterm birth *per se* does not exert any significant effect on the immature auditory brainstem, the major MLS BAER abnormalities and, in turn, this functional impairment must be predominately caused by the perinatal problems that are associated with the late preterm birth. This is consistent

* Correspondence address: Department of Paediatrics, John Radcliffe Hospital, Headington, Oxford OX3 9DU, UK. E-mail address: zedong.jiang@paediatrics.ox.ac.uk.

with some clinical observation that perinatal problems associated with late preterm birth contribute to the overall risk of brain injury in late preterm infants. These findings shed some lights on functional integrity of the brain, specifically the auditory brainstem, in high-risk late preterm infants. Further research into brain development and injury in these infants will help develop focused plans to optimize their management and prevent adverse neurological outcomes.

INTRODUCTION

Of all preterm births, late preterm birth comprises about 70% (Barros et al., 2005; Buitendijk et al., 2003; Davidoff et al., 2006; Moser et al., 2007). Therefore, late preterm infants are an important population in preterm infants. During late gestation, there are dramatic and nonlinear developmental changes in the brain, including the brainstem. This may predispose the immature brain to various perinatal risk factors, resulting in brain injury. The brainstem development in infants born at late gestation has been found to be less mature than in infants born at full term (Darnall et al., 2006). Neurodevelopmental abnormalities or deficits such as cerebral palsy can occur in infants who are born at late pregnancy or late preterm (Petrini et al., 2009). As documented by neuroimaging and autopsy studies, some neuropathology, e.g. periventricular leukomalacia, occurs not only in very preterm infant, but also in late preterm infants (Kinney, 2006). In both very preterm and late preterm infants gray matter injury is associated with periventricular leukomalacia (Billiards et al., 2006; Kinney, 2006). Recently, there is an increased interest in studying neurodevelopment and outcome in late preterm infants (Baron et al., 2009; Inder, 2010; Petrini et al., 2009; Picone and Paolillo, 2010; Romeo et al., 20010,2011; Saluja et al., 2010; Talge et al., 2010; Wuttikul et al., 2008).

There are numerous previous reports that infants who are born at very or extremely preterm are predisposed to brain damage and neurological, including auditory, impairment (Marlow et al., 2005; Romeo et al., 2010; Xoinis et al., 2007). On the other hand, limited information is available for brain function and neurodevelopment in early life in infants who are born at late preterm (Adams-Chapman, 2006; Billiards et al., 2006; Cohen-Wolkowiez et al., 2009; Darnall et al., 2006; Hunt, 2006; Kinney 2006; Sarici et al., 2004). In recent years, there is an increased interest in studying neurodevelopment in late preterm infants (Petrini et al., 2009; Romeo et al., 20010; Talge et al., 2010). For instance, Talge et al (2010) reported that children born at late preterm birth is associated with behavioral problems and lower IQ, independent of maternal IQ, residential setting, and sociodemographics. Research into brainstem development and injury in these infants will not only enhance our understanding of brainstem maturation during later preterm period, but also help develop focused plans to optimize management and prevent adverse neurological outcomes.

The functional status and development of the auditory brainstem in low-risk children born preterm has been studied using the brainstem auditory evoked response (BAER) that reflects the electrophysiological activity of auditory neurons in the brainstem following acoustic stimuli (Wilkinson and Jiang, 2006). The BAER is widely used to study functional integrity and development of the, specifically auditory, brainstem and detect neuropathology that involves in the brainstem auditory pathway, particularly in pediatric neurology (Eggermont and Salamy, 1988; Wilkinson and Jiang, 2006). The BAER has been studied in preterm infants by many authors (e.g. Henderson-Samrt etal., 1991; Krumholz et al., 1985; Ken-Dror et al., 1987; Pasman et al., 1992,1996; Jiang and Wilkinson, 2008). Some reported an increase in BAER wave latencies and intervals at time of testing (Krumholz et al., 1985), whereas the others reported a decreased I-V interval (Henderson-Samrt etal., 1991). A more recent study of conventional BAER in late preterm infants found no appreciable abnormality (Jiang and Wilkinson, 2008). Thus, the reported BAER findings in preterm infants are somewhat controversial, and further studies are needed to clarify brainstem development in late preterm infants and the effect of late preterm birth on the brainstem.

In order to improve the detectability of neuropathology by the BAER that uses conventional averaging techniques (i.e. conventional BAER), the maximum length sequence technique (MLS) has been introduced to study the BAER in infants (Jiang, 2008,2010,2012; Jiang et al., 1999,2000,2003,2005,2006,2007,2008,2009a-c,2010,2012; Li et al., 2011; Wilkinson and Jiang, 2006 ; Wilkinson et al., 2007; Yin et al., 2008). The MLS is a relatively new technique to study auditory evoked potentials (Bell et al., 2001,2002,2006; Jirsa, 2001; Lasky, 1997; Lasky et al., 1998; Lina-Granada et al., 1994; Musiek and Lee, 1997; Nagle and Musiek, 2009; Picton et al., 1992). Compared to conventional averaging techniques, the higher repetition rates of click stimuli provided by the MLS technique present a much stronger temporal/physiological challenge to auditory neurons in the brainstem, potentially increasing the detection of pathology in the auditory brainstem (Jiang, 2008,2012). In recent years, MLS BAER has been studied in infants with various perinatal problems or conditions. These studies demonstrated that the higher repetition rates provided by the MLS technique improves the detection of brain damage or neuropathology in some perinatal problems, typically hypoxia-ischemia (Jiang, 2008,2010; Jiang et al., 2000, 2003,2005,2007,2008,2009a-c,2010; Wilkinson and Jiang, 2006). The use of MLS BAER is particularly valuable for detection of some (early or subtle degrees of) neuropathology that cannot be shown by conventional BAER and other examinations (Jiang, 2012; Jiang et al., 2006,2007).

In recent years, we have studied the MLS BAER, mainly at term equivalent date, in late preterm infants to detect any functional abnormalities in the auditory brainstem. Changes in MLS BAER variables with the increase in repetition rate of stimuli (i.e. stimulus rate-dependent changes) were examined for the efficacy of synaptic transmission along the auditory brainstem (Jiang, 2012). We further compared MLS BAER results between high-risk late preterm infants (i.e. those who had associated perinatal problems or unfavorable conditions) and low-risk late preterm infants (i.e. those who did not have associated perinatal problems or unfavorable conditions) to help clarify whether any MLS BAER abnormalities in high-risk late preterm infants are caused by late preterm birth or by associated perinatal conditions. The findings should shed light on functional development of the brainstem in late preterm infants and any effect of late preterm birth and associated perinatal conditions on the immature brain.

Part I. Low-Risk Late Preterm Infants and the Auditory Brainstem

During the early life, development of BAER overlaps or parallels the critical period of brainstem myelination, axonal sprouting, formation of central synaptic connections, improvement of synaptic efficiency, development of central dendritic properties (Henderson-Smart et al., 1991; Krumholz et al., 1985; Ponton et al., 1996; Moore et al., 1997). A recent study of MLS BAER revealed some abnormalities in low-risk very preterm infants who were born at 30-32 week gestation (Jiang et al., 2006). Wave V latency and I-V interpeak interval tended to increase at all click rates, and differed significantly from the controls at the highest click repetition rate 910/s. III-V interpeak interval was increased significantly at all click rates 91-910/s, particularly at very high rates 455/s and 910/s. The slope for III-V interval-rate function was also increased significantly. On the other hand, I-III interpeak interval tended to decrease. These findings suggest that there is a delayed development in both neural conduction and synaptic transmission in the more central part of the auditory brainstem, which could not be shown by conventional BAER (Jiang et al., 2006). In order to address whether there are similar changes or abnormalities in the MLS BAER in late preterm infants, we recorded and analyzed MLS BAER, mainly at term equivalent date, in infants born at 33-36 week gestation without any major perinatal conditions or problems, i.e. low-risk late preterm infants (Li et al., 2011).

Mild Delay in Neural Conduction in the Rostral Part of the Auditory Brainstem

At term equivalent date, there was an increase in the III-V interval at 227-910/s clicks, though not at the lowest rate 91/s, in low-risk late preterm infants. The III-V interval, the more central component of the I-V interval, reflects functional status of the rostral or more central part of the auditory brainstem. This abnormality, which occurred only at high-rate stimulation that cannot be achieved with conventional averaging techniques, suggests that low-risk late preterm infants have a mild delay in neural conduction in the rostral or more central part of the auditory brainstem. Compared with that in infants born at 30-32 weeks gestation (Jiang et al., 2006), the delay in late preterm infants is relative less significant.

Late Preterm Birth Has No Marked Effect on Early Brainstem Auditory Development

Compared with those in normal term infants, there were no appreciable abnormalities in the latencies of wave I, III and V in low-risk late preterm infants. The I-V interpeak interval in these infants was increased slightly at all click rates 91-910/s, but did not differ significantly from that in the normal term controls. The I-III interval in later preterm infants was similar to that in the controls. No significant difference was found in the III-V intervals between the two groups at the lowest rate 91/s, although the interval in late preterm infants was increased significantly at all higher rates 227-910/s, particularly at 455 and 910/s. The amplitudes of wave I, III and V in the infants were all similar to those in the controls, without any significant differences.

All wave latencies and interpeak intervals in the late preterm infants were correlated significantly and positively with the repetition rate of clicks, while all wave amplitudes were correlated significantly and negatively with click rate. As the rate was increased from 91/s to 910/s, wave I, III and V latencies and the I-III, III-V and I-V interpeak intervals were all increased, while all wave amplitudes decreased. These findings in late preterm infants were generally similar to those in the controls. All wave latencies and amplitudes and interpeak intervals in preterm infants had a linear regression with click rate, which is similar to that in the normal term controls. The slopes of all latency, interval and amplitude-rate functions in late preterm infants were similar to those in the controls. No statistical significant differences were found between the two groups of infants in any slopes of these functions.

As a more peripheral component of the I-V interval, the I-III interval reflects functional status of the more caudal or peripheral part of the auditory brainstem. The interval in preterm infants born at 30-32 weeks was decreased significantly at 227 and 455/s gestation (Jiang et al., 2006). Very preterm birth exposes such infants to sound environment *extra utero* earlier than term infants. The earlier exposure can accelerate the development of the more peripheral part of the auditory brainstem (Jiang et al., 2002). Therefore, the decrease in the I-III interval in preterm infants born at 30-32 weeks reflects a slight acceleration in the maturation of the more peripheral part of the auditory brainstem due to the preterm birth that exposes such infants to sound environment *extra utero* slightly earlier than term infants. The acceleration leads to an increase in neural conduction and, in turn, a decrease in the I-III interval. In infants born at 33-36 weeks gestation, the I-III interval was basically normal, with only a slight decrease at 227 and 455/s, suggesting that neural conduction in the more peripheral part of the auditory brainstem in late preterm infants is essentially normal, even following a physiological challenge (i.e. high-rate stimulation). Apparently, late preterm birth is unlikely to significantly affect or accelerate the development of the more peripheral part of the auditory brainstem.

The stimulus rate-dependent change is an important BAER parameter that primarily reflects neural processes concerning the efficacy of synaptic transmission and metabolic status of auditory neurons following a physiological challenge (Jiang, 2012; Ken-Dror et al., 1987). This change in the BAER is reflected by the slope of each BAER variable-rate function. In preterm infants born at 30-32 weeks, the slopes of latency-rate functions for waves I, III and V were reported to be similar to term infants at term age (Jiang et al., 2006). This was also the case of the slopes of interval-rate function for the I-V and I-III intervals. However, the slope for III-V interval-rate function was increased significantly, reflecting an increased rate-dependent change in the III-V interval. This finding suggests a decrease in the efficacy of synaptic transmission along the more central part of the auditory brainstem in very preterm infants (Jiang et al., 2006). By comparison, the slopes of the latency-, amplitude- and interval-rate functions in late preterm infants were all similar to those in the term controls. Apparently, the rate-dependent changes, and, in turn, the efficacy of synaptic transmission along the auditory brainstem are essentially normal in low-risk late preterm infants.

Some authors reported that development of the brainstem in late preterm infants is less mature than that in infant born at full term (Darnall et al., 2006). The MLS BAER study in low-risk late preterm infants found no major abnormalities, suggesting that neural conduction and the efficacy of synaptic transmission in the auditory brainstem are essential similar to those in normal term infants. Nevertheless, there was an increase in the III-V interval at high-rate stimulation, although the rate-dependent change is basically normal. These results suggest that there is a mild delay in neural conduction in the more central part of the auditory brainstem in low-risk late preterm infants. Compared with those reported in very preterm infants (Jiang et al., 2002,2006), the delay in later preterm infants is less significant. The mild delay in low-risk later preterm infants may be a developmental phenomenon in early life in such infants. It is possible that this pattern of early development may 'catch up' toward normal during postnatal development, which has been shown in our current follow-up study of these late preterm infants.

PART II. HIGH-RISK LATE PRETERM INFANTS AND THE AUDITORY BRAINSTEM

As described in Part I, MLS BAER in low-risk late preterm infants (i.e late preterm infants who have any major perinatal problems or conditions) was basically normal, except for an increase in III-V interval at high-rate stimulation (Li et al., 2011). Such finding implies that low-risk late preterm infants only have a mild delay in neural conduction in the auditory brainstem. However, whether high-risk late preterm infants (i.e. later preterm infants who have major perinatal problems or conditions) have any abnormalities in the auditory brainstem is still open to speculation. Thus, we further studied the MLS BAER in high-risk late preterm infants to detect any abnormalities in the auditory brainstem (Jiang et al., 2012). These infants had various perinatal problems or conditions, including hypoglycaemia, metabolic acidosis, patent ductus arteriosus, apnea, preterm rupture of membranes, respiratory distress syndrome, sepsis, pneumonia, periventricular leukomalacia, hyperbilirubinemia at a serum level requiring exchange transfusion, pneumonia, and bacterial meningitis. Some of these infants had more than one problem or complication. Perinatal asphyxia or hypoxia-ischemia affects the MLS BAER, indicating that perinatal asphyxia damage functional integrity of the auditory brainstem (Jiang et al., 2009b,c). To exclude the known effect and better understand the effect of perinatal problems other than asphyxia on the auditory brainstem, any infants who had perinatal asphyxia were excluded from the study.

Brainstem Impairment in High-Risk Late Preterm Infants

As shown in the sample MLS BAER recordings in Fig. 1, with the increase in click rate all wave latencies and interpeak intervals were increased and all wave amplitudes were reduced in high-risk late preterm infants. This was generally similar to that in low-risk late preterm infants and normal term infants, although there were some differences. When compared with normal term controls, high-risk late preterm infants showed an increase in wave V latency at 227, particularly, 455 and 910/s, although no significant abnormalitiy was found in wave I and III latencyies (Table 1).

The I-V interpeak interval in high-risk late preterm infants was increased at all 91-910/s clicks, and the difference from the controls was increased with the increase in click rate (Table 1). Fig. 2 shows sample distribution of the data points of the I-V interval, obtained with 455/s clicks, in individual infants for each of the high-risk and low-risk late preterm infants, and normal term infants. The interval in the high-risk late preterm infants is distributed much higher than those in the normal term controls, and also higher than those in the low-risk late preterm infants. Such differences are more significant at younger age than at older age, reflected by the differences in data points at different PCA in Fig. 2. Similar differences are seen in the distribution of data points of wave V latency, III-V interval and III-V/I-III interval ratio at click rates 455 and 910/s. The III-V interval in high-risk late preterm infants was also increased at all rates used, which was more significant at higher than at lower rates (Table 1). The differences from the controls in the two intervals were both increased with the increase in click rate. By comparison, the I-III interval in high-risk late preterm infants was only slightly increased, without significant difference from the controls at any click rates. The III-V/I-III interval ratio in the high-risk infants was slightly increased at the lowest click rate 91/s, but significantly increased at all higher rates 227-910/s.

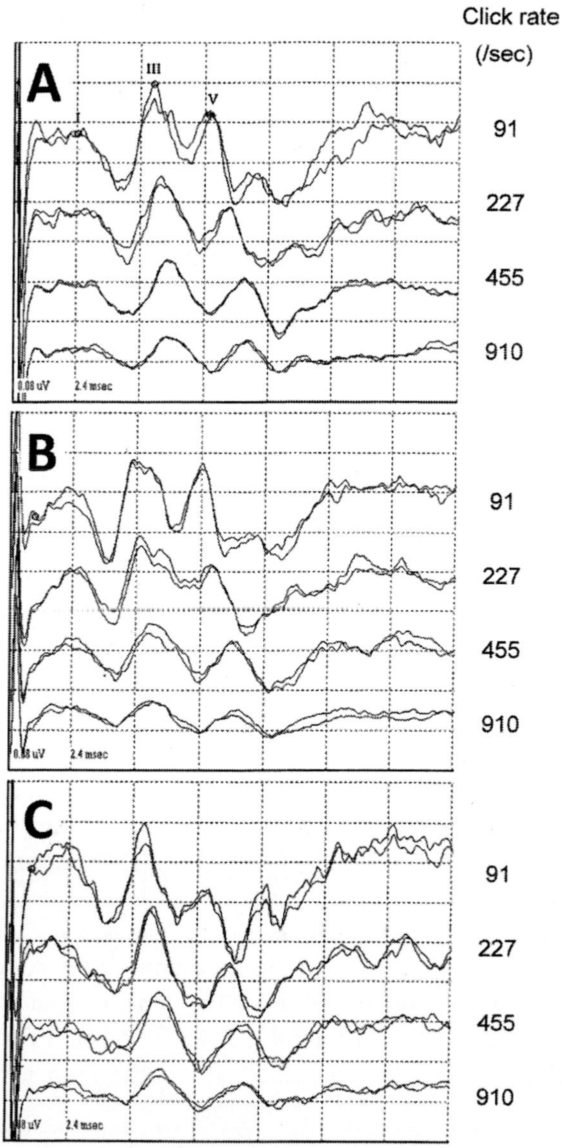

Figure 1. Sample MLS BAER recordings in infants from each of the normal term group (A), low-risk late preterm group (B) and high-risk late preterm group (C). There are no apparent differences in MLS BAER waveforms between normal term infants (A, female, 39 week gestation) and low-risk late preterm infant (B, female, 33 week gestation). However, the high-risk late preterm infant (C, male, 34 week gestation, with sepsis) shows an increase in wave V latency and I-V interval, particularly at higher click rates.

Table 1. Means and standard deviations (SD) of MLS BAER wave latencies and interpeak intervals (≥ 40 dB above BAER threshold of each subject) and comparisons of high-risk late preterm (LP) with low-risk LP and normal term infants

BAER Variables	Subjects	91/s mean ± SD	227/s mean ± SD	455/s mean ± SD	910/s mean ± SD
I (ms)	Normal	2.40 ± 0.17	2.58 ± 0.16	2.71 ± 0.16	2.75 ± 0.16
	Low-risk LP	2.40 ± 0.23	2.56 ± 0.24	2.71 ± 0.23	2.76 ± 0.22
	High-risk LP	2.32 ± 0.26	2.51 ± 0.26	2.62 ± 0.26	2.66 ± 0.26
III (ms)	Normal	5.23 ± 0.24	5.60 ± 0.24	5.86 ± 0.23	5.92 ± 0.21
	Low-risk LP	5.27 ± 0.24	5.57 ± 0.26	5.90 ± 0.29	5.94 ± 0.27
	High-risk LP	5.20 ± 0.35	5.57 ± 0.34	5.85 ± 0.34	5.92 ± 0.21
V (ms)	Normal	7.53 ± 0.27	8.16 ± 0.27	8.72 ± 0.24	8.78 ± 0.24
	Low-risk LP	7.62 ± 0.32	8.21 ± 0.36	8.88 ± 0.38	8.90± 0.36
	High-risk LP	7.58 ± 0.37	8.31 ± 0.42*	8.99 ± 0.44**+	9.05 ± 0.41***+
I-III (ms)	Normal	2.83 ± 0.16	3.03 ± 0.18	3.16 ± 0.18	3.18 ± 0.17
	Low-risk LP	2.87 ± 0.17	3.01 ± 0.21	3.20 ± 0.21	3.19 ± 0.21
	High-risk LP	2.86 ± 0.21	3.06 ± 0.23	3.23 ± 0.24	3.24 ± 0.19
III-V (ms)	Normal	2.31 ± 0.16	2.57 ± 0.16	2.85 ± 0.17	2.86 ± 0.16
	Low-risk LP	2.36 ± 0.15	2.64 ± 0.17	2.97 ± 0.18*	2.97 ± 0.18*
	High-risk LP	2.39 ± 0.16*	2.74 ± 0.22***+	3.13 ± 0.26***++	3.13 ± 0.28***++
I-V (ms)	Normal	5.14 ± 0.21	5.60 ± 0.21	6.01 ± 0.20	6.03 ± 0.20
	Low-risk LP	5.23 ± 0.26	5.65 ± 0.32	6.16 ± 0.28*	6.18 ± 0.27*
	High-risk LP	5.25 ± 0.29*	5.80 ± 0.35**+	6.37 ± 0.38***++	6.37 ± 0.33***+
III-V/I-III	Normal	0.82 ± 0.07	0.85 ± 0.08	0.90 ± 0.08	0.90 ± 0.07
	Low-risk LP	0.82 ± 0.07	0.88 ± 0.06	0.91 ± 0.08	0.92 ± 0.08
	High-risk LP	0.84 ± 0.08	0.90 ± 0.09*	0.97 ± 0.10***+	0.96 ± 0.10***+

* P <0.05, ** P <0.01, *** P <0.001, in ANCOVA for comparison between LP and normal term infants; + P <0.05, ++ P <0.01 for comparison between high-risk and low-risk LP infants.

In regression analysis, the slopes of wave I and III latency-, and I-III interval-rate functions in the high-risk late preterm infants were similar to those in term controls. However, the slopes of wave V latency-, and I-V and III-V interval-rate functions were significantly greater than those in the controls. The slope of the III-V/I-III interval ratio-function was also greater than in the controls.

There were only slight differences between high-risk late preterm infants and normal term controls in the amplitudes of MLS BAER wave components. All amplitudes of waves I, III and V in high-risk late preterm infants were slightly smaller than in the controls at almost all 91-910/s clicks (Table 2). None of the amplitudes differed significantly from the controls at any click rates. Neither the V/I nor the V/III amplitude ratio in high-risk late preterm infants differed significantly from those in the controls.

In summary, high-risk late preterm infants demonstrated a significant increase in wave V latency at 227-910/s clicks, and III-V and I-V intervals at all 91-910/s. There was also a significant increase in the III-V/I-III interval ratio at 277-910/s clicks. All these increases were more significant at higher than at lower click rates. On the other hand, there was no appreciable abnormality in the I-III interval, although the interval was slightly increased. All wave amplitudes were slightly reduced at higher click rates. The slopes of wave V latency-, I-V and III-V interval- and III-V/I-III interval ratio-rate functions were significantly increased.

These results indicate that brainstem auditory function is abnormal in high-risk later preterm infants, and the abnormalities is more evident following more stressful high-rate stimulation. For these infants, there may be a need of some neuroprotective measures targeting to the central regions of the brainstem.

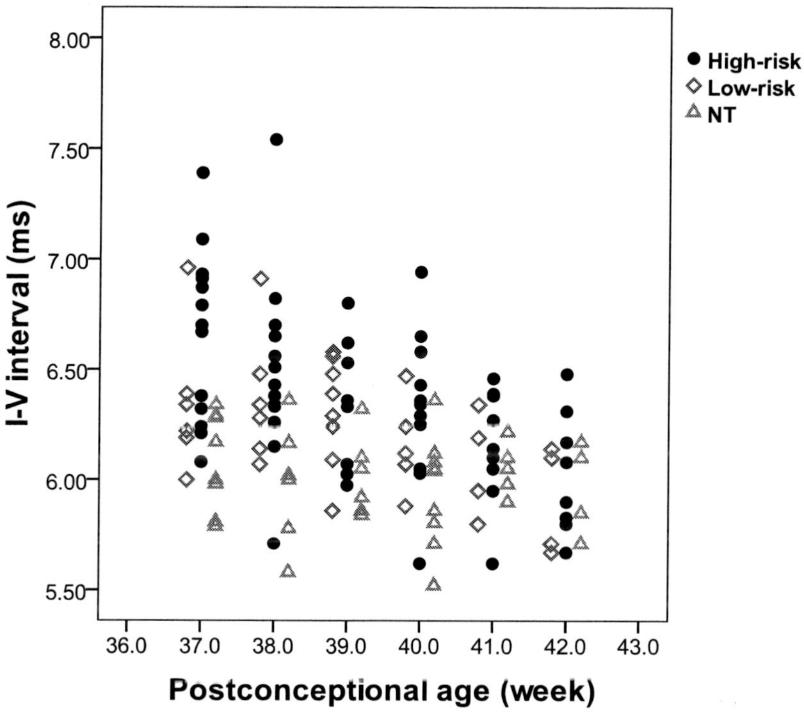

Figure 2. Scatterplot of data points of I-V interval in individual infants in each of high-risk and low-risk late preterm infants, and normal term infants (NT) in MLS BAER recorded with 455/s clicks. The data points in high-risk group are distributed much higher than those in normal term group, and also higher than those in low-risk group. This is particularly obvious in younger infants.

The I-V interval, the major MLS BAER variable that reflects brainstem auditory function, is comprised of the earlier I-III interval and the later III-V intervals. In high-risk late preterm infants, the III-V and I-V intervals were significantly increased at all click rates used, while the I-III interval did not show any appreciable abnormality. This indicates that the significant increase in the I-V interval (and wave V latency) is predominantly produced by the significant increase in the III-V interval, which is further supported by the increase in the III-V/I-III interval ratio in high-risk late preterm infants. In the BAER, the I-V interval is an important index of reflecting functional status of the auditory brainstem. The I-III interval reflects functional status of the more caudal or peripheral of the auditory brainstem, whereas the III-V interval reflects functional status of the more rostral or central regions (Jiang, 2012). As a major, fundamental abnormality in the MLS BAER in high-risk late preterm infants, the significant increase in the III-V interval indicates that the functional abnormality occurs predominately in the more central regions of the auditory brainstem.

Table 2. Means and standard deviations (SD) of BAER wave amplitudes and amplitude ratios at term (≥ 40 dB above BAER threshold of each subject) and comparisons of high-risk late preterm (LP) with low-risk LP and normal term infants

BAER Variables	Subjects	91/s mean ± SD	227/s mean ± SD	455/s mean ± SD	910/s mean ± SD
I (μV)	Normal	0.127 ± 0.041	0.084 ± 0.029	0.051 ± 0.018	0.036 ± 0.015
	Low-risk LP	0.120 ± 0.038	0.098 ± 0.030	0.061 ± 0.017	0.040 ± 0.023
	High-risk LP	0.122 ± 0.053	0.083 ± 0.033	0.050 ± 0.024+	0.034 ± 0.021
III (μV)	Normal	0.188 ± 0.055	0.140 ± 0.041	0.088 ± 0.028	0.059 ± 0.026
	Low-risk LP	0.181 ± 0.056	0.129 ± 0.044	0.086 ± 0.030	0.057 ± 0.025
	High-risk LP	0.191 ± 0.064	0.131 ± 0.044	0.086 ± 0.031	0.055 ± 0.022
V (μV)	Normal	0.160 ± 0.059	0.109 ± 0.047	0.082 ± 0.033	0.053 ± 0.025
	Low-risk LP	0.172 ± 0.058	0.141 ± 0.046*	0.087 ± 0.043	0.051 ± 0.027
	High-risk LP	0.174 ± 0.054	0.110 ± 0.041+	0.076 ± 0.031	0.044 ± 0.020
V/I	Normal	1.425 ± 0.563	1.458 ± 0.810	1.731 ± 0.836	1.691 ± 1.212
	Low-risk LP	1.710 ± 1.022	1.535 ± 0.552	1.597 ± 0.854	1.413 ± 0.554
	High-risk LP	1.652 ± 0.767	1.488 ± 0.552	1.772 ± 0.881	1.653 ± 0.981
V/III	Normal	0.929 ± 0.406	0.803 ± 0.286	0.911 ± 0.316	0.906 ± 0.299
	Low-risk LP	1.042 ± 0.299	1.137 ± 0.340*	1.068 ± 0.375	0.972 ± 0.425
	High-risk LP	0.975 ± 0.360	0.951 ± 0.458	0.947 ± 0.392	0.891 ± 0.367

* P <0.05 in ANCOVA for comparison between LP and normal term infants; + P <0.05 for comparison between high-risk and low-risk LP infants.

The significant increase in the slopes of wave V latency-, I-V and III-V interval- and III-V/I-III interval ratio-rate functions in high-risk late preterm infants implies that the click rate-dependent changes in these MLS BAER variables are increased in these infants. In the BAER, the rate-dependent change reflects the efficacy of synaptic transmission along the auditory brainstem (Jiang, 2008,2012; Lasky, 1997). The increase in the rate-dependent changes in high late preterm infants suggests a decrease in the efficacy of synaptic transmission in the auditory brainstem, mainly the more central regions or a decreased ability of central neurons to recover in time to transmit the next stimulus-evoked response. The efficacy of synaptic transmission is related to the mechanisms for synthesis, release and uptake of neurotransmitters that are known to play a crucial role in the regulation of neural development as distinct from their differentiated function as neural signal modulators (Jiang, 2008; Lasky, 1997). It is presumable that some perinatal conditions in high-risk late preterm infants may disturb the metabolism of neurons and depresses the electrophysiological function of synapses which, in the developing brain, transmit developmental as well as regulatory signals between neurons.

Brainstem Impairment in Late Preterm Infants is Mainly Produced by Perinatal Problems

As described in Part I, in infants born at 33-36 week gestation and without any major perinatal conditions, i.e. low-risk late preterm infants, no apparent abnormalities were found in wave latencies and amplitudes, and I-V and I-III intervals at all click rates 91-910/s. There was also no abnormality in any of the slopes of MLS BAER variables-rate functions. The only abnormal finding in low-risk late preterm infants was an increase in the III-V interval at higher rates. Similar findings are also observed in the present study of low-risk late preterm infants, as presented in Table 1. These mild abnormalities in the brainstem in low-risk late preterm infants are indicative of a slight delay in neural conduction in the more central regions of the auditory. Thus, late preterm birth *per se* only has a mild or very limited effect on functional development of the developing auditory brainstem. In contrast, high-risk late preterm infants demonstrated some major abnormalities in MLS BAER, suggesting that the functional integrity of the more central regions of the auditory brainstem is impaired in these infants.

We compared MLS BAER results between high-risk and low-risk late preterm infants. Wave I and III latencies and I-III interval in high-risk infants were all similar to those in low-risk infants. On the other hand, wave V latency in high-risk infants was increased at the higher rates 227-910/s, and differed significantly from low-risk infants at 455/s and 910/s (Table 1). The III-V and I-V intervals in high-risk infants were increased, and differed significantly from those in low-risk infants at 227-910/s, particularly 455/s (Table 1). The III-V/I-III interval ratio in high-risk infants was increased significantly at 455/s and 910/s (Table 1). The amplitudes of waves I and V in high-risk infants both tended to be smaller than those in low-risk infants at higher rates, and differed significantly at 455/s for wave I amplitude and at 227/s for wave V amplitude (Table 2). None of wave III amplitude, V/I and V/III amplitude ratios had any significant difference between the two groups of preterm infants.

The high-risk infants showed significant greater slopes for wave V latency-, and I-V and III-V interval-rate functions than in low-risk infants (Table 3). This was generally similar to the result of comparison with normal term controls. The slopes of other MLS BAER variable-rate functions high-risk infants were all similar to or slightly greater than those in low-risk infants, without any significant differences. No significant differences were found between the two groups of infants in any of the slopes for waves I, III and V latency-rate functions.

Apparently, compared with those in low-risk late preterm infants, MLSBAER variables that mainly reflect central auditory function were abnormal in high-risk late preterm infants. Since late preterm birth *per se* does not exert any significant effect on the immature auditory brainstem, the major MLS BAER abnormalities and, in turn, the functional impairment of the auditory brainstem in high-risk late preterm infants must be predominately caused by the perinatal problems that occurred in these infants. This is consistent with some clinical observation that perinatal problems associated with late preterm birth contribute to the overall risk of brain injury in late preterm infants (Adams-Chapman, 2006).

It would be very interesting to identify what perinatal factor(s) in high-risk late preterm infants play(s) a major role in the damage to the late preterm brainstem. Some previous investigators studied auditory impairment in infants or children, and tried to identify the causes for the impairment. They found that there were often several potential causative factors for the impairment and no one simgle cause could be identified (Meyer et al., 1999; Newton, 2001). We assume that there might be collective adverse effects, produced by more than one perinatal condition or risk factor, that contribute to the MLS BAER abnormalities found in high-risk late preterm infants. Further studies are needed in large populations to reliably and accurately identify major perinatal risk factors.

Table 3. Linear regression between MLS BAER variables and rate (91-455/s) in high-risk late preterm (LP) and normal term infants

MLS BAER Variable	Subjects	Intercept Mean	SE	Slope (/decade)		T	*P*
I (ms)	Normal	2.344	0.030	0.008	0.001	8.102	<0.001
	Low-risk LP	2.349	0.042	0.008	0.002	4.64	<0.001
	High-risk LP	2.266	0.040	0.009	0.001	6.261	<0.001
III (ms)	Normal	5.124	0.044	0.017	0.002	11.105	<0.001
	Low-risk LP	5.142	0.060	0.017	0.002	8.074	<0.001
	High-risk LP	5.069	0.059	0.019	0.002	8.991	<0.001
V (ms)	Normal	7.307	0.049	0.032	0.002	14.747	<0.001
	Low-risk LP	7.361	0.080	0.034	0.003	12.576	<0.001
	High-risk LP	7.295	0.072	0.039	0.003	15.165	<0.001
I-III (ms)	Normal	2.781	0.033	0.009	0.001	7.653	<0.001
	Low-risk LP	2.799	0.039	0.008	0.001	6.245	<0.001
	High-risk LP	2.802	0.039	0.010	0.001	7.168	<0.001
III-V (ms)	Normal	2.189	0.031	0.015	0.001	14.540	<0.001
	Low-risk LP	2.223	0.040	0.015	0.001	12.989	<0.001
	High-risk LP	2.227	0.036	0.020	0.001	15.442	<0.001
I-V (ms)	Normal	4.966	0.040	0.024	0.001	17.632	<0.001
	Low-risk LP	5.014	0.065	0.026	0.002	11.802	<0.001
	High-risk LP	5.028	0.059	0.030	0.002	14.181	<0.001
I amp (μV)	Normal	0.139	0.006	-0.002	0.000	-10.293	<0.001
	Low-risk LP	0.134	0.007	-0.002	0.000	-6.841	<0.001
	High-risk LP	0.130	0.006	-0.002	0.000	-9.625	<0.001
III amp (μV)	Normal	0.183	0.008	-0.003	0.000	-10.039	<0.001
	Low-risk LP	0.199	0.011	-0.003	0.000	-7.204	<0.001
	High-risk LP	0.193	0.008	-0.003	0.000	-8.672	<0.001
V amp (μV)	Normal	0.169	0.009	-0.002	0.000	-6.790	<0.001
	Low-risk LP	0.109	0.011	-0.002	0.000	-6.330	<0.001
	High-risk LP	0.181	0.009	-0.002	0.000	-8.099	<0.001

Perinatal hypoxia-ischemia has a major effect on MLS BAER in term infants (Jiang, 2008; Jiang et al., 2000,2003,2008). More recent studies show that perinatal hypoxia-ischemia also significantly affect MLS BAER in preterm, including late preterm, infants (Jiang, 2008; Jiang et al., 2009b,c). By comparison, the MLS BAER abnormalities found in high-risk late preterm infants with perinatal problems other than hypoxia-ischemia are relatively less significant. It appears that brainstem auditory impairment due to perinatal problems other than hypoxia-ischemia is less severe than that due to severe hypoxia-ischemia.

Our on-going follow-up study of late preterm infants have shown that the abnormalities initially detected in high-risk late preterm infants gradually recovered with the improvement of clinical conditions and the increase in age. At 1 and 3 months of corrected postnatal age, there were still some, though less significant, differences between high-risk late preterm infants and low-risk late preterm and term infants. Obviously, brainstem auditory abnormalities in high-risk late preterm infants have largely, but not completely, recover during the first 3 months of postnatal life.

CONCLUSION

So far, there are limited clinical, physiologic, neuroanatomic, and neurochemical studies in late preterm infants. The studies of MLS BAER in high-risk late preterm infants revealed an increase in wave V latency and I-V and III-V intervals and III-V/I-III interval ratio. The increase was more significant at higher than at lower click rates. The slopes of wave V latency-, I-V and III-V interval- and III-V/I-III interval ratio-rate functions were significantly increased. These results indicate that the functional integrity of the auditory brainstem, mainly in the central regions, is impaired in late preterm infants with perinatal problems. The findings shed some lights on functional integrity of the auditory brainstem in high-risk late preterm infants and provide valuable information for perinatal management of these infants. Further research into brain development and injury in these infants will help develop focused plans to optimize their management and prevent adverse neurological outcomes.

REFERENCES

Adams-Chapman I. Neurodevelopmental outcome of the late preterm infant. *Clin Perinatol* 2006;33:947-64.

Baron IS, Erickson K, Ahronovich MD, Coulehan K, Baker R, Litman FR. Visuospatial and verbal fluency relative deficits in 'complicated' late-preterm preschool children. *Early Hum Dev* 2009;85:751-4.

Barros FC, Victora CG, Barros AJ, Santos IS, Albernaz E, Matijasevich A, Domingues MR, Sclowitz IK, Hallal PC, Silveira MF, Vaughan JP. The challenge of reducing neonatal mortality in middle-income countries: findings from three Brazilian birth cohorts in 1982, 1993, and 2004. *Lancet* 2005;365:847-54.

Bell SL, Allen R, Lutman ME. The feasibility of maximum length sequences to reduce acquisition time of the middle latency response. *J Acoust Soc Am* 2001;109:1073-81.

Bell SL, Allen R, Lutman ME. Optimizing the acquisition time of the middle latency response using maximum length sequences and chirps. *J Acoust Soc* Am 2002;112:2065-73.

Bell SL, Smith DC, Allen R, Lutman ME. The auditory middle latency response, evoked using maximum length sequences and chirps, as an indicator of adequacy of anesthesia. *Anesth Analg* 2006;102:495-8.

Billiards SS, Pierson CR, Haynes RL, Folkerth RD, Kinney HC. Is the late preterm infant more vulnerable to gray matter injury than the term infant? *Clin Perinatol* 2006;33:915-33.

Buitendijk S, Zeitlin J, Cuttini M, Langhoff-Roos J, Bottu J. Indicators of fetal and infant health outcomes. *Eur J Obstet Gynecol Reprod Biol* 2003;111(suppl 1):S66-S77.

Cohen-Wolkowiez M, Moran C, Benjamin DK; Cotten CM; Clark RH, Benjamin DK Jr, Smith PB. Early and Late Onset Sepsis in Late Preterm Infants. *Pediatr Infect Dis J* 2009;28:1052-6.

Darnall RA, Ariagno RL, Kinney HC. The Late Preterm Infant and the Control of Breathing, Sleep, and Brainstem Development: A Review. *Clin Perinatol* 2006;33:883-914.

Davidoff MJ, Dias T, Damus K, Russell R, Bettegowda VR, Dolan S, Schwarz RH, Green NS, Petrini J. Changes in the gestational age distribution among U.S. singleton births: impact on rates of late preterm birth, 1992 to 2002. *Semin Perinatol* 2006;30:8-15.

Eggermont JJ, Salamy A. Maturational time course for the ABR in preterm and full term infants. *Hear Res* 1988;33:35-48.

Henderson-Smart DJ, Pettigrew AG, Edwards DA, Jiang ZD. Brain stem auditory evoked responses: physiological and clinical issues; in Hanson MA (ed): *The Fetal and Neonatal Brain Stem: developmental and clinical issues.* Cambridge, Cambridge University Press, 1991, p. 211-29.

Hunt CE. Ontogeny of autonomic regulation in late preterm infants born at 34-37 weeks postmenstrual age. *Semin Perinatol* 2006;30:73-6.

Inder T. Imaging insights of alterations and adaptations in the preterm and late preterm brain. *J Pediatr* 2010;156:867-8.

Jiang ZD. Brainstem electrophysiological changes after perinatal hypoxia ischemia. In: Hämäläinen E, editor. *New Trends in Brain Hypoxia Ischemia Research*. New York: Nova Science Publishers; 2008. p. 203-220.

Jiang ZD. Damage of chronic sublethal hypoxia to the immature auditory brainstem. In: Fiedler D, Krause R, editors, *Deafness, Hearing Loss, and the Auditory System.* New York: Nova Science Publishers; 2010, p. 159-80.

Jiang ZD. Maximum length sequence technique improves detection of neuropathology involving infant brainstem. *Pediatric Neurology*. New York: Nova Science Publishers; 2012 (in press).

Jiang ZD, Brosi DM, Wilkinson AR. Brainstem auditory evoked response recorded using maximum length sequences in term neonates. *Biol Neonate* 1999;76:193-9.

Jiang ZD, Brosi DM, Shao XM, Wilkinson AR: Maximum length sequence brainstem auditory evoked response in infants after perinatal hypoxia-ischaemia. *Pediatr Res* 2000;48:639-45.

Jiang ZD, Brosi DM, Wilkinson AR. Auditory neural responses to click stimuli of different rates in the brainstem of very preterm babies at term. *Pediatr Res* 2002;51:454-9.

Jiang ZD, Brosi DM, Wang J, Xu X, Chen GQ, Shao XM, Wilkinson AR: Time course of brainstem pathophysiology during first month in term infants after perinatal asphyxia, revealed by MLS BAER latencies and intervals. *Pediatr Res* 2003;54:680-7.

Jiang ZD, Brosi DM, Li ZH, Chen C, Wilkinson AR. Brainstem auditory function at term in preterm babies with and without perinatal complications. *Pediatr Res* 2005;58:1164-9.

Jiang ZD, Brosi DM, Wilkinson AR. Maximum length sequence BAER at term in low-risk babies born at 30-32 week gestation. *Brain Dev* 2006;28:1-7.

Jiang ZD, Xu X, Brosi DM, Shao XM, Wilkinson AR. Suboptimal function of the auditory brainstem in term neonates with transient low Apgar scores. *Clin Neurophysiol* 2007;118:1088-96.

Jiang ZD, Wilkinson AR. Normal brainstem responses in moderately preterm infants. *Acta Paediatr* 2008;97:1366-9.

Jiang ZD, Brosi DM, Shao XM, Wilkinson AR. Sustained depression of brainstem auditory electrophysiology during the first month in term infants after perinatal asphyxia. *Clin Neurophysiol* 2008;119:1496-505.

Jiang ZD, Brosi DM, Chen C, Wilkinson AR. Brainstem auditory response amplitudes in neonatal chronic lung disease and differences from perinatal asphyxia. *Clin Neurophysiol* 2009a;120:967-73.

Jiang ZD, Brosi DM, Wilkinson AR. Depressed brainstem auditory electrophysiology in preterm infants after perinatal hypoxia-ischemia. *J Neurolog Sci* 2009b;281:28-33.

Jiang ZD, Brosi DM, Wilkinson AR. Impairment of perinatal hypoxia-ischaemia to the preterm brainstem. *J Neurolog Sci* 2009c;287:172-7.

Jiang ZD, Brosi DM, Wilkinson AR. Differences in impaired brainstem conduction between neonatal chronic lung disease and perinatal asphyxia. *Clin Neurophysiol* 2010;121:725-33.

Jiang ZD, Pin LL, Wilkinson AR. Functional abnormality of the auditory brainstem in high-risk late preterm infants. *Clin Neurophysiol* 2012; 123:993-1001.

Jirsa RE. Maximum length sequences-auditory brainstem responses from children with auditory processing disorders. *J Am Acad Audiol* 2001;12:155-64.

Ken-Dror A, Pratt H, Zeltzer M, Sujov P, Katzir J, Benderley A. Auditory brainstem evoked potentials to clicks at different presentation rates: estimating maturation of pre-term and full-term neonates. *Electroencephalog Clin Neurophysiol* 1987;68:209-18.

Kinney HC. The near-term (late preterm) human brain and risk for periventricular leukomalacia: a review. *Semin Perinatol.* 2006;30:81-8.

Krumholz A, Felix JK, Goldstein PJ, McKenzie E. Maturation of the brain stem auditory evoked potential in premature infants. *Electroenceph Clin Neurophysiol* 1985;62:124-34.

Lasky RE. Rate and adaptation effects on the auditory evoked brainstem response in human newborns and adults. *Hear Res* 1997;111:165-76.

Lasky RE, Barry D, Veen V, Maier MM. Nonlinear functional modelling of scalp recorded auditory evoked responses to maximum length sequences. *Hear Res* 1998;120:133-42.

Li ZH, Chen C, Jiang ZD. Maximum length sequence brainstem auditory evoked response in low-risk late preterm babies. *J Metern-Fet Neonat Med* 2010; 24:536-40.

Lina-Granada G, Collet L, and Morgon A. Auditory-evoked brainstem responses elicited by maximum-length sequences in normal and sensorineural ears. *Audiology* 1994;33:218–36.

Marlow N, Wolke DM, Bracewell MA, Samara M. Neurologic and developmental disability at six years of age after extremely preterm birth. *N Engl J Med* 2005; 352: 9-19.

Meyer C, Witte J, Hildmann A, Hennecke KH, Schunck KU, Maul K, Franke U, Fahnenstich H, Rabe H, Rossi R, Hartmann S, Gortner L. Neonatal screening for hearing disorders in infants at risk: incidence, risk factors and follow-up. *Pediatrics* 1999;104;900-4

Moore JK, Guan, YL, Shi SR. Axogenesis in the human fetal auditory system, demonstrated by neurofilament immunohistochemistry. *Anat Embryol Berl* 1997;195:15-30.

Moser K, Macfarlane A, Chow YH, Hilder L, Dattani N. Introducing new data on gestation-specific infant mortality among babies born in 2005 in England and Wales. *Health Stat Q.* 2007;35:13-27.

Musiek FE, Lee WW. Conventional and maximum length sequences middle latency response in patients with central nervous system lesions. *J Am Acad Audiol* 1997;8:173–80.

Nagle S, Musiek FE. Morphological changes in the middle latency response using maximum length sequence stimuli. J Am Acad Audiol. 2009;20:492-502.

Newton V. Adverse perinatal conditions and the inner ear. *Semin Neonatol* 2001;6:543-51.

Pasman JW, Rotteveel JJ, de Graaf R, Stegeman DF, Visco YM. The effect of preterm birth on brainstem, middle latency and cortical auditory evoked responses (BMC AERs). *Early Hum Dev* 1992;31:113-29.

Pasman JW, Rotteveel JJ, de Graaf R, Maassen B, Visco YM. The effects of early and late preterm birth on brainstem and middle-latency auditory evoked responses in children with normal neurodevelopment. *J Clin Neurophysiol.* 1996 May;13(3):234-41.

Petrini JR, Dias T, McCormick MC, Massolo ML, Green NS, Escobar GJ. Increased risk of adverse neurological development for late preterm infants. *J Pediatrics* 2009;154:169-76.

Picton TW, Champagne SC, Kellett AJC. Human auditory potentials recorded using maximum length sequences. *Electroencephalogr Clin Neurophysiol* 1992;84:90–100.

Ponton CW, Moore JK, Eggermont JJ. Auditory brain stem response generation by parallel pathways: differential maturation of axonal conduction time and synaptic transmission. *Ear Hear* 1996;17;402-10.

Romeo DM, Stefano AD, Conversano M, Ricci D, Mazzone D, Romeo MG, Mercuri E. Neurodevelopmental outcome at 12 and 18 months in late preterm infants. *Eur J Paediatr Neurol* 2010;14:503-7.

Saluja S, Agarwal A, Kler N, Amin S. Auditory neuropathy spectrum disorder in late preterm and term infants with severe jaundice. *Int J Pediatr Otorhinolaryngol* 2010;74:1292-7.

Sarici SU, Serdar MA, Korkmaz A, Erdem G, Oran O, Tekinalp G, Yurdakok M, Yigit S. Incidence, course, and prediction of hyperbilirubinemia in near-term and term newborns. *Pediatrics* 2004;113:775-80.

Talge NM, Holzman C, Wang J, Lucia V, Gardiner J, Breslau N. Late-Preterm Birth and Its Association With Cognitive and Socioemotional Outcomes at 6 Years of Age. *Pediatrics* 2010;126:1124-31.

Wilkinson AR, Jiang ZD. Brainstem auditory evoked response in neonatal neurology. *Semin Fet Neonatol Med* 2006;11:444-51.

Wilkinson AR, Brosi DM, Jiang ZD. Functional impairment of the brainstem in infants with bronchopulmonary dysplasia. *Pediatrics* 2007;120:362-71.

Wuttikul C, Taoka T, Akashi T, Nakagawa H, Miyasaka T, Sakamoto M, Takayama K, Wada T, Kitano S, Takahama J, Marugami N, Kichikawa K. Prominent signal intensity of T1/T2 prolongation in subcortical white matter of the anterior temporal region on conventional screening MRI of late preterm infants with normal development. *Magn Reson Imaging* 2008;26:1374-80.

Xoinis K, Weirather Y, Mavoori H, Shaha SH, Iwamoto LM. Extremely low birth weight infants are at high risk for auditory neuropathy. *J Perinatol* 2007;27:718-23.

Yin R, Wilkinson AR, Chen C, Brosi DM, Jiang ZD. No close correlation between brainstem auditory function and peripheral auditory threshold in preterm infants at term age. *Clin Neurophysiol* 2008;119:791-5.

In: Preterm Infants
Editors: Diogo Contreiras and Johann Sampaio

ISBN 978-1-62081-819-0

Chapter 3

READINESS OF PRETERM INFANTS TO START BREASTFEEDING

Thaíla C. Castral*[*,1], *Cristina I. Fujinaga*[2], *Fay Warnock*[3], *Andreara A. Silva*[4], *Laiane M. Ribeiro*[4], and *Carmen G. S Scochi*[4]

[1]University of Goias, School of Nursing, Goiânia, GO, Brazil
[2]Speech, Language and Hearing Science Department of Universidade Estadual do Centro, Oeste, Irati-PR, Brazil
[3]British Columbia University, School of Nursing, Vancouver, BC, Canada
[4]University of Sao Paulo at Ribeirao Preto College of Nursing, WHO Collaborating Centre for Nursing Research Development, Ribeirao Preto, SP, Brazil

An estimated 3.1 million neonatal deaths occur annually worldwide, accounting for more than 40% of all deaths in children younger than five years of age [1]. Complications of preterm birth (before 37 weeks of gestation) are the leading direct cause and major risk factor for neonatal deaths, accounting for 27% or approximately 1 million neonatal deaths annually. However, there is a marked regional difference in these rates, with 99% of the neonatal deaths occurring in low and middle-income countries [2].

There are approximately 13 million preterm infants born each year worldwide. Data from a systematic review conducted between 1997 to 2007 [3] revealed a world preterm birth rate of 9.6%, with more developed countries having a rate of 7.5% compared to 8.8% in less-developed countries and 12.5% in least-developed countries.

Neonatal morbidity and mortality rates are greater in preterm infants than term infants, with preterm infants having higher risk of temperature stability, respiratory distress, infections, apnea, hypoglycemia, seizures, jaundice, kernictures, feeding difficults, necrotizing enterocolitis, periventricular leukomalacia, peri-intraventricular hemorrhage and rehospitalizations [4]. Furthermore, preterm infants also have a nutritional risk related to low levels of body nutrients, quick growth and physiological immaturity of gastrointestinal tract, potentially leading to neurodevelopmental problems, memory and learning deficits [5].

[*] Corresponding author. Address: Av. Bandeirantes 3900 Ribeirao Preto – SP CEP: 14040-902 Brazil Phone: 55 – 16 – 36023411 (office) Fax number: 55 – 16 – 36333271. E-mail: thaccastral@gmail.com.

Neonatal mortality rates increase proportionally with decreasing gestational age (and hence decreasing birth weight) and are greatest among infants born at less than 32 weeks of gestation [2].

In the past three decades, infant mortality rates have reduced substantially [6] as a result of modern neonatal units with high technological equipments, skilled human resources and early pre-natal care and follow-up.

However, neonatal deaths are still high. One goal of The United Nations Millennium Development Goals is to reduce two-thirds of under five deaths between 1990 and 2015 [7] (More information available at http://www.undp.org/content/undp/en/home/ mdgoverview. html). Given this priority and considering the high impact that neonatal deaths have on child mortality, evidence-based interventions to prevent preterm delivery and to improve survival of preterm newborns are urgently needed.

One key intervention to help reduce child mortality and morbidity related to common childhood illnesses is breastfeeding, particularly in low and middle-income countries, in view of its acknowledged benefits in decreasing neonatal deaths [6,8] and promoting optimal later child neurobiological and psychosocial development [9]. Since 1980s there have been a number of international initiatives to increase the number of women starting and continuing to breastfeed. In 1981, the World Health Assembly adopted the International Code of Marketing of Breast Milk Substitutes to contribute to the provision of safe and adequate nutrition for infants by the protection and promotion of breastfeeding, and by ensuring the proper use of artificial food, where these are necessary. In the next decade, the World Health Organization (WHO) and The United Nations Children's Fund (UNICEF) launched The Baby Friendly Hospital Initiative, that provide clinical guidelines to protect, promote and support breastfeeding. They recommended infants be exclusive breastfeed until six months (meaning only breast milk and no other liquids or solids, not even water) and to continue until two years of age or more [10,11,12].

Specific to high-risk infants, including infants born preterm, a policy statement by the American Academy of Pediatrics (AAP) advocates that "hospitals and physicians should recommend human milk for premature and other high risk infants either by direct breastfeeding or using mother´s own expressed breast milk". The statement also recommended maternal support and education, mother infant skin-to-skin contact, and direct breastfeeding as early as possible as keys to success [13].

Breastfeeding has several benefits for the preterm infant. Babies who are breastfed are generally healthier and achieve optimal growth and development compared to those who are fed with formula [14]. Preterm infants exclusively fed with formula have more chance to develop necrotizing enterocolitis than infants fed with breast milk [15]. In addition, preterm infants have a higher energetic expenditure when fed with formula compared to those fed with breast milk which can easily destabilize the infant [16].

Breast milk of mothers who have a preterm infant has a composition, uniquely adapted to the needs of the preterm infant [17]. Compared to mothers' milk of term born infants in the first four weeks of lactation, mothers' milk of preterm infants contains higher concentrations of nitrogen, immune active proteins, lipids, sodium, chlorides, magnesium, iron, copper, zinc and vitamins A, D and E [18]. Besides its nutritional quality, breastfeeding has an important role in the maturation of the gastrointestinal system, facilitation of digestion and nutrients absorption, establishment of attachment and mother-child bond, increase in neurobehavioral performance, protection against necrotizing enterocolitis, and lower incidence of infection and re-hospitalization due to its anti-infection properties [18]. It may also reduce acute pain in infants with mature breastfeeding abilities [19,20,21].

Long term benefits of breastfeeding or breast milk ingestion include a lower incidence of retinopathy of prematurity [22], better fine motor, adaptability, and communication skills at age 1 and 3 years [23] and higher Bayley Mental Developmental Index scores, higher Bayley behavior score percentiles for emotional regulation, and fewer rehospitalizations between discharge and 30 months [24]. If the vast majority of babies were exclusively fed with breast milk in their first six months of life, it is estimated this would reduce the annual child mortality by at least 1.2 million worldwide and that continued breastfeding up to two years and beyond would greatly improve the long term health and development of millions of children [25].

Although the many benefits of breastfeeding are well documented and clinical guidelines have been available for clinicians, the prevalence of breastfeeding in preterm infants is low and early weaning commonly occurs during hospitalization in neonatal units [26] or before six months of age [27].

According to UNICEF, less than half (43%) of newborns in the developing world are united with their mothers for breastfeeding within one hour of birth. Regional averages range from a high of 54% in Eastern and Southern Africa to a low of 39% in South Asia and West and Central Africa. Social-economical status, among other factors, contribute to these differences (http://www.childinfo.org/breastfeeding_status.html). Infants born in hospitals that have adopted the UNICEF breastfeeding guidelines show higher proportion of exclusive breastfeeding and longer duration of breastfeeding than infants born elsewhere [28]. These rates however are lower for the preterm population in view of the immature feeding behaviors of these infants among other related factors.

In Europe, a population-based cohort study conducted in 2003 that involved very preterm infants at discharge from neonatal units reported overall breastfeeding rates to range from 19% to 70% [29]. In that study, exclusive breastfeeding ranged from 6% to 29% and mixed rates (breastfeeding combined with formula) ranged from 5% to 52%. At a university hospital in Brazil, 76.7% of preterm infants at hospital discharge were reported to be breastfeed, supplemented with formula (48,3%) or not (28,4%) [30]. A better scenario was found in Denmark, where 60% of very preterm infant (gestational age 24 weeks +1 to 32 weeks and birth weight 520g – 2255g) were exclusively breastfeed at hospital discharge (mean postmenstrual age of 37 weeks + 2 and mean weight was 2634g), 35% were bottle-fed and 5% were both bottle- and breast-feed [31].

These statistics show breastfeeding is a common practice in neonatal units worldwide, but rates are far from desirable. Given the multiple benefits that early breastfeeding affords the preterm infant, it is critical that health professionals have basic knowledge and skills to give appropriate advice and counsel to mothers to help solve feeding difficulties, and to know when and where to refer a mother who experiences more complex feeding problems [32]. Health professionals need to provide accurate information regarding the benefits and methods of breastfeeding, so that the mother can make an informed choice. A standardized care plan could guide practitioners in making decisions to assist establishment of breastfeeding in the preterm infant [33].

In order to help clinicians to better decide when and how to successfully initiate and maintain breastfeeding in preterm infants, in this chapter, we provide information on factors that create challenges in breastfeeding a preterm infant and discuss some strategies to help the infant transition from tube feeding to oral feeding. We also show evidence on how to systematically assess readiness of the preterm infant to start breastfeeding.

Challenges in Breastfeeding a Preterm Infant

Preterm infants have less glycogen [34] and nutrients reserve (e.g.: calcium, iron) [35] than term newborns at birth since deposit of these elements only occur in the third semester of gestation. Adverse medical conditions and frequent exposure to pain and stress requires a great amount of energy for the preterm infant to self stabilize, demanding frequent weight and daily adjustment of liquid tolerance [36,37]. Also, physiological immaturity of the gastrointestinal tract and the limited gastric capacity of the preterm infant [38] result in lower motility and decrease enzymatic activity what can complicate digestion and absorption [39].

Besides gastrointestinal immaturity, very preterm infants commonly have immature suckling, swallowing and vomit reflex due to lack of integration in muscle activities of the lips, cheeks, jaw, tongue, palate, pharynx and larynx; they are very small and have no energy to suck [40] ; have problems in coordinating suck-swallow-breathing; stay little time in a alert state to be fed; have greater risk of aspiration and do not show sign of hungry and satiety [41,42].

Maturation of feeding skills are essential to initiate oral feeding. Sucking is a very primitive reflex appearing as early as 15 to 16 weeks' gestation. The fetus swallows amniotic fluid and the newborn can coordinate suck and swallow while breastfeeding as early as 28 weeks' gestation. An increasing level of organization of nutritive sucking occurs with increasing gestational age, maturity, and experience. By 32 to 34 weeks postconceptual age, there is a change in sucking burst, although respiration may still not be well coordinated. Consistent coordination is generally achieved by 35 to 37 weeks' postconceptual age [43]. Lack of infant's coordination in suck-swallow-breathing may cause the infant stress (e.g. color change, tachypnea, nasal flaring and gagging) and lead to more energy expenditure [44,45].

Breastfeeding is the most physiologic method to help the infant to develop coordination in suck-swallow-breathing. Preterm infants who are breastfeed show higher oxygen saturation and body temperature when compared to those who were bottle-feed, causing less stress [42,46]. Postnatal complications (chronic lung disease, intraventricular hemorrhage, seizures, and so on) are associated with delays in the onset of the first feeding, as well as with delays in achieving full enteral intake [47].

The condition of the infant's mother is another important issue to consider when breastfeeding preterm infants. There is some speculation on when mothers of preterm infants are prepared to breastfeed. Lactogenesis II may be truncated with the birth of preterm infants, specially the very low birth weight preterm infant, as it affects the hormone balance stimulated by labor. In addition, increased milk volume is related to increased frequency of expression [48]. It is unclear how much breast tissue is necessary to support full lactation, however, many other maternal factors other than breast size affect milk production, such as stress and fatigue, both of which are increased when a preterm infant is born [43].

The stress that mothers experience following a premature birth may include not only their concerns over premature birth and its possible consequences to the infant's health, but also their own health and/or lifestyle [49]. This may lead to maternal psychological distress that can be displayed as anxiety, depression and/or psychological stress. Stress, whether psychological or physical, may affect lactation through physiological or hormonal responses that prevent the development of milk, milk release and/or maternal behavior [50]. Maternal wellbeing is thus an important attribute to the success of lactation.

One crucial factor for exclusive breastfeeding preterm infant is milk production [51], which depends on early initiation and frequent pumping [52,53]. However, pumping and maintaining milk supply can also prove to be difficult for the mother when she does not have frequent stimulation from her new infant to help increase her lactation. Consequently, it is recommended to introduce oral breast milk (preferable of the infant's own mother) as early as possible when the preterm infant is stable [54]. Formula should be used with caution because it may interfere in mothers' feeling of capacity when caring for her infant. Giving the mother the opportunity to breastfeed her preterm infant or offer breast milk via tube feeding is a efficient method to provide contact between mother-infant and to involve the mother [55].

Facilitating Breastfeeding in Preterm Infants

It is important that health professionals choose a safe and adequate method to help the preterm infant to transition from tube to breast-feeding, facilitating quick and non stressful learning [41,56].

Breastfeeding was originally thought to result in more energy expenditure, weight loss, and alterations in cardio respiratory and thermal systems than bottle feeding for the preterm and low birth weight infant [57]. However, Silva et al. [42] show that preterm infant are able to better coordinate breathing during breastfeeding than bottle feeding and have less physiological instability.

Bottle feeding may cause nipple confusion, interfering in preterm infant's ability to breastfeed, and should be avoided [58]. Milk flow in bottle feeding is high, so the infant only needs to apply slight pressure to the nipple to extract the milk. Moreover, bottle-fed infants show higher decrease in oxygen saturation than breast-fed infants as a possible result of the anatomical position of the tongue during bottle-feed and a more frequent swallowing, thus, interrupting breath more frequently [59].

An alternative method to bottle-feeding is cup feeding, where a cup filled with milk (preferable from the infant's mother) to at least three fourths of its capacity is placed in an angle at the lower lip so that milk touches the infant's lips, stimulating tongue protrusion and "lapping" of the milk by the infant. Maintaining the cup in a position that makes milk available to the infant while not accidentally placing milk in the infant's mouth necessitated close observation and coordination [60]. Cup feeding is found to cause lower incidence of oxygen desaturation and heart rate increase when compared to bottle feeding [61]. Although cup feeding is considered simple, inexpensive and practical to feed preterm infants [62,63], there should be caution on the indiscriminate use of this technique because it can delays hospital discharge and does not increase breastfeeding rates [64,65]. Additionally, there is no evidence to support safety of cup feeding overtime and its possible negative developmental effects on breastfeeding in preterm infants [60].

A more valuable method to be considered is translactation, which consist in an adaptation of the relactation technique. Through this procedure, maternal milk is expressed and offered using a tube connected to a syringe fixed at the level of mother's breasts, with the other end of the tube positioned alongside the areola during breastfeeding [66]. The infant ingest milk that comes from the breast and from the syringe only through suction, making it more physiological and allowing mothers participation [62,67].

In order to promote early breastfeeding in preterm infants, mother-based interventions, such as maternal kangaroo care (MKC), also called skin-to-skin care, should be provided in neonatal units. This intervention consist in positioning the unclothed newborn infant vertically between the mother's breasts and under her clothing, as long as necessary or pleasant for both. At least 6 hours/day of MKC improved exclusive breastfeeding rates in preterm infants at end of three months follow-up study compared to incubator care (88% vs. 72%, respectively) [68]. Short periods of MKC also resulted in longer duration of any breastfeeding for 1 month after discharge [risk ratio (RR) 4.76, 95% confidence interval (CI) 1.19 to 19.10] and for more than 6 weeks (RR 1.95, 95% CI 1.03 to 3.70) among clinically stable infants in industrialized settings [69]. An increased volume of milk in mothers of ventilated low birth weight infants compared to a retrospective control group of mothers not exposed to MKC may be pointed as an additional benefit [70].

Nonnutritive sucking with a gloved finger or pacifier has also been shown to be beneficial for several important indicators during preterm infant's hospitalization (length of stay, transition from gavage to oral feeding and improvements in digestion). It facilitates the development of sucking behavior, as reflected in the neurobehavioral organization and maturation of preterm infants [71,72].

A more natural choice to promote nonnutritive suckling in preterm infants who are not ready to breastfeed is the nonnutritive breastfeeding (also referred as recreational breastfeeding) [59]. The mother pumps her both breasts until there is no more milk flow before putting the infant to breast. Even though the breast is never complete empty because of posterior milk production, the preterm infant is not able to effectively suck to withdraw milk from the breast [73]. This intervention provides sucking experience for preterm infants without interfering with their nutritional intake and consequent weight gain, and encourages subsequent breast feeding [74].

An individual assessment of preterm infant's condition (e.g. physiological stability, oro-motor development, presence of anomalies etc.) is necessary to select adequate strategies for transition from tube to breast-feeding. Translactation should be the preferable method to initiate breastfeeding in preterm infants because it can provide additional stimuli for milk production through suction, eliciting same mechanisms involved in breastfeeding. Moreover, it offers additional contact between mother-infant and allows mother active participation while caring for her infant, enhancing her feeling of capacity. To help promote breastfeeding among preterm infants, MKC and non-nutritive suckling are safe interventions that can be implemented in neonatal units.

When to Initiate Breastfeeding a Preterm Infant

The health care team has great difficulties to establish the ideal time to transition preterm infants′ feeding from gastric to oral, which involves a comprehensive evaluation, especially of the sucking behavior of the infant.

Initiation of oral feeding has been predominantly established by infant's clinical stability defined by infant's weight (> 1500g) or maturity (gestational age > 34 weeks) [51,75]. Therefore, transition from gastric to oral feeding is an important issue when caring of preterm infants in view that health professionals base their decision on isolated factors to start breastfeeding, without a comprehensive assessment of infant general condition, oral-motor and psychomotor ability [76].

Measures of nonnutritive sucking organization and suck consistency constitute useful candidate predictors of feeding performance by premature infants [77]. There are in the literature five protocols available to assess preterm infant suckling behavior [78-82] but these are accessible only in Portuguese, were developed using bottle feeding as a method for transition from tube to oral feeding, which involves different suckling mechanisms when compared to breastfeeding, and none were validated or have a user guide. These limitations highlight a need of a systematic approach to assess when is the adequate time to initiate breastfeeding in preterm infants.

Fujinaga et al. [83] developed a tool, the Preterm Oral Feeding Readiness Assessment Scale (POFRAS) (Figure 1), and a user guide for clinicians to assess the readiness of the preterm infant to initiate transition from gastric to oral feeding. The instrument comprises 18 items structured in five categories (corrected neonatal age, neurobehavioral state, oral posture, oral reflex and non-nutritive suckling), scoring from 0 to 2, with a maximum score of 36. It has proven content and face validity [83], with inter-rater agreement of 0.85 or higher [84]. The instrument global accuracy was 74.38%, and the highest sensitivity and specificity were obtained for three cut-offs: 28, 29 and 30 [85].

Differently from existing protocols that evaluate infant suckling behavior, POFRAS was validated with the method of translactation (described previously in this chapter). As a result, the total volume of 5ml ingested by the infant direct from mother's breast with suckling movements and no signs of stress at first contact was considered the gold standard [85]. This technique demonstrated to be adequate to measure total volume of milk ingested by the infant without causing stress. Research currently underway aims to test the concurrent validity of POFRAS using the same criterion described.

In using the POFRAS in the clinical setting, the accompanying clinical guideline (Figure 2) recommends to initially position the preterm infant in flexed lateral decubitus, outside the incubator, while providing gentle stimuli (e.g.: talk, eye gaze and touch). Next, the infant is observed for two minutes to determine neurobehavioral state and oral posture. There is no need to manipulate the infant to rate these items, except for tongue posture that it is necessary to lower the jaw to visualize the tongue. The following steps include rating oral reflexes for one minute and infant behavior during one minute of non-nutritive suckling using the little finger with a glove embebed in maternal milk. Then, each individual item scored by the infant is summed to obtain the final score. A score of more than 30 indicates that the infant is able to start transition to breastfeeding.

To ensure an instrument is feasible for use in clinical practice it has to involve a quick and objective assessment [86]. Thus, a brief version of the POFRAS was developed containing seven items (neurobehavioral state, lip posture, suckling reflex, tongue movement, suckling strength and maintenance of neurobehavioral state). Psychometric testing of the brief version is now under way.

Taking in consideration preterm infants are at risk for several diseases that cause millions of deaths annually, global efforts should be made by clinicians and policy makers aimed at increasing breastfeeding rates and duration in this particular population. Research being currently conducted will help to establish guidelines to a safe and early transition from tube to oral feeding in preterm infant, and will contribute to a more systematic and objective assessment. Moreover, this unique instrument could be easily used by health professionals in clinical practice and help early identification of those infants at risk for delayed oral feeding who would benefit from interventions aimed at feeding skill and also promote early oral feeding and breastfeeding successful establishment.

PRETERM INFANT ORAL FEEDING READINESS ASSESSMENT SCALE (POFRAS)

Date o f assessment: __/__/__ Time: _____
Infant´s name: ____________________________
Hospital file number:________
Birth Date: __/__/__
Gestational age: ___ Postnatal age: ___Corrected gestational age: ___
Tube feeding: ( ) Yes ( ) No ( ) Nasogastric( ) Orogastric Volume: ____ml

CORRECTED GESTATIONAL AGE(2) 34 WEEKS OR MORE
(1) between 32 and 34 weeks
(0) 32 weeks or less

Behavioral Organization

Behavioral state	(2) alert	(1) drowsy	(0) sleep
Global posture	(2) flexed	(1) partly flexed	(0) extended
Global tonus	(2) normotonia	(0) hypertonia	(0) hypotonia

Oral Posture

Lips posture	(2) closed	(1) half-open	(0) open	
Tongue posture	(2) flat	(0) elevated	(0) retracted	(0) protruded

Oral Reflexes

Rooting reflex	(2) present	(1) weak	(0) absent
Sucking reflex	(2) present	(1) weak	(0) absent
Biting reflex	(2) present	(1) exacerbated presence	(0) absent
Gag reflex	(2) present	(1) present in anterior region	0) absent

Nonnutritive Sucking

Tongue movement	(2) adequate	(1) altered	(0) absent
Tongue cupping	(2) present	(0) absent	
Jaw movement	(2) adequate	(1) altered	(0) absent
Sucking strain	(2) strain	(1) weak	(0) absent
Sucking and pause	(2) 5 to 8	(1) >8	(0) <5
Maintenance of rhythm	(2) rhythmic	(1) arrhythmic	(0) absent
Maintenance of alert state	(2) yes	(1) partial	(0) no
Stress signs	(2) absent	(1) up to 3	(0) more than 3

Saliva accumulation	( ) absent	( ) present
Nose wings trembling	( ) absent	( ) present
Skin color changes	( ) absent	( ) present
Apnea	( ) absent	( ) present
Tonus variation	( ) absent	( ) present
Posture variation	( ) absent	( ) present
Tongue or jaw tremors	( ) absent	( ) present
Hiccupping	( ) absent	( ) present
Crying	( ) absent	( ) present

Score: ____ Maximum score: 36

PRETERM INFANT ORAL FEEDING READINESS ASSESSMENT SCALE (POFRAS) - INSTRUCTION GUIDE

Assessment of infant oral feeding readiness should occur close to feeding hours. First, position the preterm infant in a flexed lateral decubitus, outside the incubator, while providing gentle stimuli (e.g.: talk, eye gaze and touch). The optimal state for feeding is an awake, alert, or active state, although some infants can feed adequately in a drowsy state.

Corrected Gestational Age

It is calculated by subtracting the number of weeks born before 40 weeks of gestation from the chronological age. Gestational age can be obtained through the medical chart. It is calculated by the ultrasound, considered the most reliable method when performed before 20 weeks of gestation. Other methods can also be used to calculate the gestational age such as first day of the mother's last menstrual period or assessment of newborn's neuromuscular and physical characteristics (e.g. Dubowitz, Capurro, Ballard and New Ballard).

- ✓ 32 weeks or less.
- ✓ Between 32 and 34 weeks.
- ✓ 34 weeks or more.

Behavioral Organization

Observe the infant during 1 minute to rate the items below. Do not manipulate the infant during this period.

Behavioral State

- ✓ Alert: eyes open and shining, responsive to stimulation, some spontaneous activity.
- ✓ Drowsy: eyes open and close, confused and dull look, takes time to respond to stimulation, varied spontaneous activity.
- ✓ Sleep: eyes closed, non-responsive to stimulation; no motor activity.

Global Posture

- ✓ Flexed: flexed upper, lower limbs and neck position median line in relation to trunk.
- ✓ Partly flexed: flexed lower limbs and neck position in median line in relation to trunk.
- ✓ Extended: upper and lower limbs and neck extended in relation to trunk.

Global Tonus

Consider what is expected for preterm infant's maturity.

- ✓ Normotonic: light resistance to passive flexion and extension movements, slightly stronger in the latter.
- ✓ Hypertonic: increased resistance to passive flexion and extension movements.
- ✓ Hypotonic: decreased resistance to passive flexion and extension movements.

Oral Posture

Observe the infant during 1 minute to rate the items below. Do not manipulate the infant to assess lips posture. Lower the infant's jaw to view the tongue to rate tongue posture.

Lips Posture

- ✓ Closed: upper and lower lip side by side.
- ✓ Half-open: upper and lower lip partially separated.
- ✓ Open: upper and lower lip totally separated.

Tongue Posture

- ✓ Flat: tongue in flat position inside oral cavity, with a rounded tip.
- ✓ Elevated: tip of the tongue in elevated position, pressing the palate.
- ✓ Retracted: tongue in retracted position in the oral cavity.
- ✓ Protruded: tongue in protruded position in the oral cavity, beyond labial border.

Oral Reflexes

Use a gloved little finger to evoke oral reflexes and observe infant response up to 1 minute.

Rooting reflex: Gentle touch or stroke infant's perioral region at the four main cardinal points.

- ✓ Present: infant *immediately* seeks stimulated region, directing the head towards the stimulus and/or opening the mouth.
- ✓ Weak: infant *slowly* seeks the stimulated region, directing the head towards the stimulus and/or opening the mouth.
- ✓ Absent: absence of response.

Sucking reflex: Gentle introduce a gloved little finger into infant's month.

- ✓ Present: readily sucks own hand or examiner's gloved finger.
- ✓ Weak: takes some time to start sucking own hand or examiner's finger.
- ✓ Absent: absence of response.

Biting reflex: Exert gentle pressure into infant's gingival line of oral cavity with a gloved little finger.

- ✓ Present: jaw clenching, followed by relaxing.
- ✓ Exacerbated presence: maintaining jaw clenching.
- ✓ Absent: absence of response.

***Gag reflex*:** Gentle introduce a gloved little finger into infant's month and touch tongue.

- ✓ Present: responds to stimulus with nauseas or vomiting when the middle-posterior portion of the tongue is touched.
- ✓ Present in anterior region: responds to stimulus with nauseas or vomiting when the anterior portion of the tongue is touched.
- ✓ Absent: absence of response.

Nonnutritive Sucking

Use a gloved little finger embebed in maternal milk to perform nonnutritive suckling and observe infant response during 1 minute.

Tongue Movement

- ✓ Normal: intraoral stimulus generates anterior-posterior and coordinated tongue movement.
- ✓ Altered: intraoral stimulus generates posterior-anterior or uncoordinated movement.
- ✓ Absent: absence of movement.

Tongue Cupping

- ✓ Present: elevated tongue sides and presence of groove in central tongue region.
- ✓ Absent: absence of response.

Jaw Movement

- ✓ Normal: reduced jaw excursion, rhythmic and spontaneous jaw movement.
- ✓ Altered: wide jaw excursion and/or arrhythmic jaw movement and/or jaw clenching.
- ✓ Absent: absence of movement.

Sucking Strain

- ✓ Strain: strain compression against palate and negative intraoral pressure with resistance to withdrawal of examiner's finger from oral cavity.
- ✓ Weak: weak compression against palate and negative intraoral pressure without resistance to withdrawal of examiner's finger from oral cavity.
- ✓ Absent: absence of response.

Sucking and Pause

Use the average obtained in three groups of suck/pause.

- ✓ Between 5 and 8 sucks per respiratory pause.
- ✓ More than 8 sucks per respiratory pause.
- ✓ Less than 5 sucks per respiratory pause.

Maintenance of Rhythm of Sucking and Pause

Use the number of sucks/pause obtained in three groups of suck/pause and verify if this number varied between set intervals.

- ✓ Rhythmic: maintains the number of sucks per pause expected in one and the same interval (less than 5, between 5 and 8 or more than 8 sucks per pause).
- ✓ Arrhythmic: changes the number of sucks per pause between intervals (less than 5, between 5 and 8 or more than 8 sucks per pause).
- ✓ Absent: absence of sucking.

Maintenance of Alert State

- ✓ Yes: continues alert throughout the nonnutritive sucking test.
- ✓ Partial: continues alert only at beginning or end of nonnutritive sucking test.
- ✓ No: does not continue alert during the nonnutritive sucking test

Stress Signs

- ✓ Absent: absence of stress signs.
- ✓ Up to 3 stress signs.
- ✓ More than 3 stress signs.

  The following stress signs must be observed during assessment:

  - Saliva accumulation
  - Nose wings trembling
  - Color changes
  - Apnea
  - Tonus variation
  - Posture variation
  - Tongue or jaw tremors
  - Hiccupping
  - Crying

References

[1] Lawn JE, Cousens S, Zupan J. 4 million neonatal deaths: when? Where? Why?. *Lancet.* 2005; 365(9462):891-900.

[2] Simmons LE, Rubens CE, Darmstadt GL, et al. Preventing preterm birth and neonatal mortality: exploring the epidemiology, causes, and interventions. *Semin Perinatol.* 2010; 34(6):408-15.

[3] Beck S, Wojdyla D, Say L, et al. The worldwide incidence of preterm birth: a systematic review of maternal mortality and morbidity. *Bull World Health Organ.* 2010; 88(1):31-8.

[4] Saygal S, Doyle LW. An overview of mortality and sequelae of preterm birth from infancy to adulthood. *Lancet.* 2008; 371(9608):261-9.

[5] Oliveira AG, Siqueira PP, Abreu L. C. [Nutritional care of very low birth weight preterm infants]. *Rev Bras Crescimento Desenvolv Hum.* 2008; 18(2): 148-154.

[6] Victora CG, Aquino EM, do Carmo Leal M, et al. Maternal and child health in Brazil: progress and challenges. *Lancet.* 2011; 377(9780): 1863-76.

[7] United Nations Millennium Declaration of 2000, *Pub. L.* No.55/2, 1-9. (Sep. 08, 2000).

[8] Kramer MS, Chalmers B, Hodnett ED, et al. Promotion of Breastfeeding Intervention Trial (PROBIT): a randomized trial in the Republic of Belarus. *JAMA.* 2001; 285(4): 413-20.

[9] World Health Organization. *Child and adolescent health and development: nutrition, infant and young child, exclusive breastfeeding. 1989.* Available at: http:www.who.int/child-adolescent-health/nutrition/infat_exclusive.htm. Accessed February 10, 2012.

[10] World Health Organization. *The optimal duration of exclusive breastfeeding.* 2001. Available at: http://www.who.int/inf-pr-2001/en/note2001-07.html. Accessed February 10, 2012.

[11] World Health Organization. *Global strategy for infant child feeding. Geneva,* Switzerland: World Health Organization; 2003.

[12] American College of Obstetricians and Gynecologists, Committee on Health Care for Underserved Women. ACOG committee opinion No. 361: breastfeeding—maternal and infant aspects. *Obstet Gynecol.* 2007; 109(2):479–480.

[13] American Academy Of Pediatrics. Breastfeeding and the use of human milk. *Pediatrics.* 2005; 115(2): 496-506.

[14] McGuire W, Anthony MY. Formula milk versus preterm human milk for feeding preterm or low birth weight infants. *Cochrane Database Syst Rev.* 2001; (3): CD002972.

[15] McGuire W, Anthony MY. Donor human milk versus formula for preventing necrotising enterocolitis in preterm infants: systematic review. *Arch Dis Child Fetal Neonatal Ed* 2003;88:F11e4.

[16] Lubetzky R, Vaisman N, Mimouni FB, Dollberg S. Energy expenditure in human milk-versus formula-fed preterm infants. *J Pediatr.* 2003; 143(6): 750-3.

[17] Feferbaum R, Quintal VS, Araujo MCK. Nutrição enteral do recém-nascido de baixo peso. In: Feferbaum R, Falcão MC. *Nutrição do recém nascido.* São Paulo: Atheneu; 2005.

[18] Nascimento MBR, Issler H. Breastfeeding: making the difference in the development, help and nutrition of term and preterm newborns. *Rev. Hosp. Clin. Fac. Med. S. Paulo.*2003; 58(1): 49-60, 2003.

[19] Campbell-Yeo M, Fernandes A, Johnston C. Procedural pain management for neonates using nonpharmacological strategies: part 2: mother-driven interventions. *Advances in Neonatal Care.* 2011; 11(5): 312-8.

[20] Leite AM, Linhares MB, Lander J, et al. Effects of breastfeeding on pain relief in full-term newborns. Clin J Pain. 2009; 25(9): 827-32.

[21] Shah PS, Aliwalas L, Shah V. Breastfeeding or breastmilk to alleviate procedural pain in neonates: a systematic review. *Breastfeed Med.* 2007; 2(2): 74–82.

[22] Hylander MA, Strobino DM, Pezzullo JC, Dhanireddy R. Association of human milk feedings with a reduction in retinopathy of prematurity among very low birthweight infants. *Perinatol.* 2001; 21(6):356-62.

[23] Oddy WH, Robinson M, Kendall GE, Li J, Zubrick SR, Stanley FJ. Breastfeeding and early child development: a prospective cohort study. *Acta Paediatr.* 2011; 100(7): 992-9. doi: 10.1111/j.1651-2227.2011.02199.x.

[24] Vohr BR, Poindexter BB, Dusick AM, et al. Persistent beneficial effects of breast milk ingested in the neonatal intensive care unit on outcomes of extremely low birth weight infants at 30 months of age. *Pediatrics.* 2007;120:e953-e959.

[25] United Nations Children's Fund. *Facts of life.* New York; UNICEF, WHO, UNESCO, UNFPA, UNDP, UNAIDS, WFP, World Bank; 2010.

[26] Taylor LK, Lim K, Neville SE. Newborn feeding practices at the time of discharge from hospital in NSW in 2007: a descriptive study. *N S W Public Health Bull.* 2009;20(11-12):177-81.

[27] Jones JR, Kogan MD, Singh GK, Dee DL, Grummer-Strawn LM. Factors Associated With Exclusive Breastfeeding in the United States. *Pediatrics.* 2011; 128(6): 1117-1125.

[28] Merten S, Dratva J, Ackermann-Liebrich U. Do baby-friendly hospitals influence breastfeeding duration on a national level? *Pediatrics.* 2005; 116(5): e702-8.

[29] Bonet M, Blondel B, Agostino R, et al. Variations in breastfeeding rates for very preterm infants between regions and neonatal units in Europe: results from the MOSAIC cohort. *Arch Dis Child Fetal Neonatal* Ed. 2011; 96(6): F450-2.

[30] Scochi CGS, Ferreira FR, Goés FSN, et al. Alimentação láctea e prevalência do aleitamento materno em prematuros durante internação em um hospital amigo da criança de RibeirãoPreto-SP. Ciência, *Cuidado e Saúde.* 2008; 7(2): 145-54, 2008.

[31] Zachariassen G, Faerk J, Grytter C, Esberg B, Juvonen P, Halken S. Factors associated with successful establishment of breastfeeding in very preterm infants. *Acta Paediatr.* 2010; 99(7):1000-4.

[32] World Health Organization. *Infant and young child feeding: model chapter for textbooks for medical students and allied health professionals.* Geneva, Switzerland: World Health Organization; 2009.

[33] Borrero-Pachón Mdel P, Olombrada-Valverde AE, Martínez de Alegría MI. [Role of nursing in the development of breastfeeding in the premature newborn]. *Enferm Clin.* 2010 ;20(2):119-25.

[34] Hay WW. Early postnatal nutritional requirements of the very preterm infant based on a presentation at the NICHD-AAP workshop on research in neonatology. *J Perinatol.* 2006; 26 Suppl 2:S13-8.

[35] Elizabeth KE, Krishnan V, Zachariah P. Auxologic, biochemical and clinical (ABC) profile of low birth weight babies- a 2-year prospective study. *J Trop Pediatr.* 2007; 53(6):374-82.

[36] Oliveira AG, Siqueira PP, Abreu L. C. [Nutritional care of very low birth weight preterm infants]. R*ev Bras Crescimento Desenvolv Hum.* 2008; 18(2): 148-154.

[37] Ziegler EE, Thureen PJ, Carlson SJ. Aggressive nutrition of the very low birthweight infant. *Clin Perinatol.* 2002; 29:225-244.

[38] Auler F, Delpino FS. Terapia nutricional em recém-nascidos prematuros. *Revista Saúde e Pesquisa.* 2008; 1(2): 209-216.

[39] Sousa AB, Sakai MC, Takagi CA, Friedrich M. Physicochemical analysis of pasteurized human milk and commercial premature formulas fortified with phosphorus solution or commercial fortifier. *Rev Ciênc Farm Básica Apl.*2009;30(1):31-34.

[40] Gewolb IH, Vice FL, Schweitzer-Kenney EL, Taciak VL, Bosma JF.Developmental patterns of rhythmic suck and swallow in preterm infants. *Dev Med Child Neurol.* 2001; 43: 22-7.

[41] Aquino RR, Osório MM. [The feeding of preterm newborns: alternative methods for the transition from tube-feeding to breastfeeding]. *Revista Brasileira Saúde Materno Infantil.* 2008a; 8(1):11-6.

[42] Silva MHA, Fujinaga CS, Leite AM, et al. [Bottle and breast sucking effects in premature infants]. *Revista RENE.* 2011; 12(1): 81-87.

[43] Gardner SL, Snell BJ, Lawrence RA. Breastfeeding the neonate with special needs. In: Merenstein GB, Gardner SL. *Handbook of Neonatal Intensive Care.* 6th ed. Mosby Elsevier: Missouri; 2006. p.467-519.

[44] Mizuno K, Ueda A. The maturation and coordination of sucking, swallowing, and respiration in preterm infants. *J Pediatr.* 2003;142(1):36-40.

[45] Gewolb IH, Bosma JF, Reynolds EW, Vice FL. Integration of suck and swallow rhythms during feeding in preterm infants with and without bronchopulmonary dysplasia. *Dev Med Child Neurol.* 2003;45(5):344-8.

[46] Meier PP, Brown LP, Hurst NM. et al. Nipple shields for preterm infants: effect on milk transfer and duration of breastfeeding. *J Hum Lact.* 2000; 16(2): 106-14.

[47] 47. Lemons PK. From gavage to oral feedings: just a matter of time. *Neonatal Netw.* 2001; 20(3): 7-14.

[48] Henderson JJ, Hartmann PE, Newnham JP, Simmer K. Effect of preterm birth and antenatal corticosteroid treatment on lactogenesis II in women. *Pediatrics.* 2008; 121(1):e92-100.

[49] Lindberg B, Ohrling K. Experiences of having a prematurely born infant from the perspective of mothers in northern Sweden. *Int J Circumpolar Health.* 2008; 67(5):461-71.

[50] Zanardo V, Gambina I, Begley C, Litta P, Cosmi E, Giustardi A, Trevisanuto D. Psychological distress and early lactation performance in mothers of late preterm infants. *Early Hum Dev.* 2011; 87(4):321-3.

[51] Buckley KM, Charles GE. Benefits and challenges of transitioning preterm infants to at-breastfeedings. *International Breastfeeding Journal.*2006; 1(13): 1-7.

[52] Flacking R, Ewald U, Nyqvist KH, Starrin B. Trustful bonds: a key to "becoming a mother" and to reciprocal breastfeeding. Stories of mothers of very preterm infants at a neonatal unit. *Soc Sci Med.*2006; 62(1): 70-80.

[53] Jones E, Spencer AS. Optimising the provision of human milk for preterm infants. *Arch. Dis. Child. Fetal Neonatal.*2007;92:F236-8.

[54] Schanler RJ, Shulman RJ, Lau C, Smith EO, Heitkemper MM. Feeding strategies for premature infants: randomized trial of gastrointestinal priming and tube-feeding method. *Pediatrics.* 1999;103(2):434-9.

[55] Serra OA, Scochi CSG. [Mother's difficulties in breastfeeding premature babies in the neonatal ICU]. *Rev. Latino-Am.* 2004; 12(4): 597-805.

[56] Gupta A, Khanna K, Chattree S. Cup feeding: an alternative to bottle feeding in a neonatal intensive care unit. *J Trop Pediatr.*1999; 45(2): 108-10.

[57] Pickler RH, Reyna B.A. A descriptive study of bottle-feeding opportunities in preterm infants. *Advances in neonatal care.* 2003; 3(3): 139-46.

[58] Black A. Breastfeeding the premature infant and nursing implications. *Adv Neonatal Care.* 2012; 12(1): 10-1.

[59] Sridhar S, Arguello S, Lee HC. Transition to Oral Feeding in Preterm Infants. *Neoreviews.* 2011; 12:e141-e147.

[60] Dowling DA, Meier PP, DiFiore JM, Blatz M, Martin RJ. Cup-feeding for preterm infants: mechanics and safety. *J Hum Lact.* 2002;18(1):13-20.

[61] Rocha NM, Martinez FE, Jorge SM. Cup or bottle for preterm infants: effects on oxygen saturation, weight gain, and breastfeeding. *J Hum Lact.* 2002; 18(2): 132-8.

[62] Aquino RR, Osório MM. [The feeding of preterm newborns: alternative methods for the transition from tube-feeding to breastfeeding]. *Rev. Bras. Saúde Matern. Infant.*2008; (1): 11-16.

[63] Marinelli KA, Burke GS, Dodd VL. A comparison of the safety of cupfeedings and bottlefeedings in premature infants whose mothers intend to breastfeed. *J Perinatol.* 2001; 21(6):350-5.

[64] Collins CT, Makrides M, Gillis J, McPhee AJ. Avoidance of bottles during the establishment of breast feeds in preterm infants. *Cochrane Database Syst Rev.* 2008; (4): CD005252.

[65] Flint A, New K, Davies MW. Cup feeding versus other forms of supplemental enteral feeding for newborn infants unable to fully breastfeed. *Cochrane Database Syst Rev.* 2007; (2): CD005092. Review.

[66] World Health Organization. Department of child and adolescent health and development. *Relactation: a review of experience and recommendations for practice.* Geneva, Switzerland: World Health Organization; 1998.

[67] Aquino RR, Osório MM. Relactation, translactation, and breast-orogastric tube as transition methods in feeding preterm babies. *J. Hum Lact.*2009; 25(4): 420-426.

[68] Gathwala G, Singh B, Singh J. Effect of Kangaroo Mother Care on physical growth, breastfeeding and its acceptability. *Trop Doct.* 2010; 40(4):199-202.

[69] Renfrew MJ, Dyson L, McCormick F, et al. Breastfeeding promotion for infants in neonatal units: a systematic review. *Child Care Health Dev.* 2010; 36(2): 165-78.

[70] Hurst NM, Valentine CJ, Renfro L, Burns P, Ferlic L. Skin-to-skin holding in the neonatal intensive care unit influences maternal milk volume. *J Perinatol.* 1997; 17:213–217

[71] Pinelli J, Symington A. Non-nutritive sucking for promoting physiologic stability and nutrition in preterm infants. *Cochrane Database Syst Rev.* 2005;(4):CD001071.

[72] Fucile S, Gisel EG, Lau C. Effect of an oral stimulation program on sucking skill maturation of preterm infants. *Dev Med Child Neurol.* 2005; 47(3):158-62.

[73] Venson Crisiane, Fujinaga Cristina Ide, Czluniak Gilsane Raquel. [Non-nutritive sucking stimulation on the "emptied breast" in preterm infants: case report]. *Rev. Soc. Bras. Fonoaudiol.* 2010; 15(3): 452-457. Available at: http://www.scielo.br/ scielo. php?script=sci_arttext&pid=S1516803420100003000022&lng=pt. http://dx.doi.org/10.1590/S1516-80342010000300022. Accessed March 02, 2012.

[74] Narayanan I, Mehta R, Choudhury DK, Jain BK. Sucking on the 'emptied' breast: non-nutritive sucking with a difference. Arch Dis Child. 1991;66(2):241-4.

[75] Meier P. Bottle and breastfeeding: effects on transctaneous oxigen pressure and temperature in preterm infants. *Nurs. Research.* 1998; 37(1): 36-41.

[76] Thoyre SM. Developmental transition from gavage to oral feeding in the preterm infant. *Annual review of nursing research.* 2003; 21:61-92.

[77] Bingham PM, Ashikaga T, Abbasi S. Prospective study of non-nutritive sucking and feeding skills in premature infants. *Arch Dis Child Fetal Neonatal Ed.* 2010; 95(3):F194-200.

[78] Bernardis KC, Marchi SON. Sucção não-nutritiva em recém-nascidos a termo e pré-termo: um estudo descritivo comparativo. *Pró-Fono Revista de Atualização Científica.* 1998; 10(2): 8-15.

[79] Hernandez AM. Atuação fonoaudiológica com recém-nascidos e lactentes disfágicos.. In: Hernandez AM, Marchesan I. *Atuação fonoaudiológica em ambiente hospitalar.* São Paulo: Revinter; 2001. p.1-37.

[80] Neiva FCB. Proposta de um formulário de avaliação da sucção de recém-nascidos. *Pró-fono.* 2000; 12(2): 113-19.

[81] Quintella T, Silva AA, Botelho MIMR. Distúrbios da deglutição (e aspiração) na infância. In: Furkin AM, Santini CS. *Disfagias orofaríngeas.* Carapicuíba: Pró-fono; 1999. p.61-96.

[82] Xavier C. *Avaliação de alimentação de recém nascidos em fase de hospitalização* (Escala de avaliação motora oral da Irmandade Santa Casa de Misericórdia de São Paulo). Pró-Fono Revista de Atualização Científica. 1995; 7(2): 69-74.

[83] Fujinaga CI, Scochi CGS, Santos CB, Zamberlan NE, Leite AM. [Content validation as a tool for evaluating oral feeding readiness in preterm babies]. *Rev. Bras. Saude Mater. Infant.*2008; 8(4): 391-9.

[84] Fujinaga CI, Zamberlan NE, Rodarte MDO, Scochi CGS. *Reliability of an instrument to assess the readiness of preterm infants for oral feeding. Pró-Fono.* 2007; 19(2): 143-50. Available at: http://www.scielo. br/scielo.php?script=sci_arttext&pid= S010456872007000200002&lng=en. http://dx.doi.org/10.1590/S0104-568720070002 00002.

[85] Fujinaga CI. [Preterm readiness for oral feeding: reliability and clinical validation of an evaluation instrument]. *Thesis.* Ribeirão Preto: College of Nursing, University of São Paulo, Ribeirão Preto; 2005. Available at: http://www.teses.usp.br

[86] Nyqvist KH. Early attainment of breastfeeding competence in very preterm infants. *Acta Paediatrica.* 2008; 97(6): 776-81.

In: Preterm Infants
Editors: Diogo Contreiras and Johann Sampaio
ISBN 978-1-62081-819-0

Chapter 4

HORMONAL DYSREGULATION OF THE HYPOTHALAMIC-PITUITARY-ADRENAL AND HYPOTHALAMIC-PITUITARY-THYROID AXES IN PRETERM INFANTS

Sze May Ng
Department of Paediatrics
Southport and Ormskirk NHS Trust
Honorary Lecturer, Department of Women's and Children's Health
Institute of Translational Medicine
University of Liverpool, UK

Survival for infants born prematurely now exceeds 80% [1]. These infants are at high risk of abnormal neurodevelopment with disabilities affecting 1 in 8 survivors [2]. Hormonal dysregulation is common in prematurity. In adaptation, maternal factors and the placenta control many aspects of the fetal endocrine milieu. After preterm birth, the infant suddenly has to cope and adapt to the external environment. Abnormal values of endocrine tests such as the thyroid and cortisol axes are commonly encountered in preterm infants and infants with more extreme endocrine disturbances are at increased risk of abnormal development.

The optimal way to manage endocrine problems in preterm infants is not clear. In part, this is because infants born at extreme prematurity have different physiology from term infants and older children. What constitutes a "normal" physiological hormone level of a preterm infant at different gestations remains unclear. Examples of delayed adaptation have been evident in the hypothalamic-pituitary-thyroid axis (HPT) and the hypothalamic-pituitary-adrenal (HPA) axes in preterm infants.

The developmental origins theory proposes that events and stress in fetal life provokes adaptive changes in endocrine and metabolic function which can be permanently programmed resulting in an adverse impact in late adult health [3-5]. Reduced birth weight has been associated with risk for type 2 diabetes mellitus, hyperlipidaemia, hypertension and syndrome X in adulthood [6-8]. Maternal exposure to exogenous glucocorticoids leads to increased fetal brain exposure to excess glucocorticoids which may result in permanent modification of hypothalamo-pituitary-adrenal (HPA) axis and can have life-long effects on later neuro-endocrine function [9]. Maternal hypothyroxinaemia has been reported to be a serious risk factor for neurodevelopmental difficulties that can be identified in neonates as young as 3 weeks of age [10].

Hypothalamic-Pituitary-Thyroid Axis in Preterm Infants

The question as to whether the hypothalamic–pituitary–thyroid (HPT) axis in premature infants is already established remains debated. Congenital hypothyroidism in the newborn causes neurodevelopmental disability if not optimally treated [11]. In very premature infants between 23–31 weeks' gestation, there was no increase in TSH at 24 hours, 72 hours and at the first week of life [12]. Conversely, healthy premature infants born at 30 – 37 weeks' gestation appeared to produce a substantial TSH surge at 30 – 90 minutes which was comparable to term infants and the TSH surge did not correlate with gestational age [13]. Infants as premature as 29 weeks' gestation are able to produce a marked TSH increase (>51 IU/mL) in response to a transient hypothyroidism [14]. There was therefore evidence that HPT axis in premature babies was sufficiently established to be able to produce TSH and such an infant with hypothyroidism should be revealed on a TSH profile. Observational studies have found that low thyroid hormone levels in the first few weeks of life in preterm infants have been linked with poor neurodevelopmental outcome (see Table 1).

Table 1. Low thyroid hormone levels are linked with poor neurodevelopmental outcome

Study	Participants	Outcome
Reuss et al [15]	463 infants born below 33 weeks' gestation	4-fold increased risk of disabling cerebral palsy at 2 years of age associated with hypothyroxinaemia group
Den Ouden et al [16]	563 infants born below 32 weeks' gestation	Higher incidence of neurological dysfunction at 5 years and 9 years of age associated with hypothyroxinaemia group after adjustments for other perinatal factors
Leviton et al [17]	1414 infants weighing 500 to 1500 g	Double the risk of cerebral white matter changes associated with hypothyroxinaemia group.
Paul et al [18]	343 infants weighing less than 1500 grams	Increased mortality and increased incidence of intraventricular haemorrhage associated with hypothyroxinaemia group.
Lucas et al [19]	279 infants born below 36 weeks' gestation	Reduction in IQ at 8 years of age associated with low T3 after adjustment for potential confounding factors
Meijer et al[20]	563 infants born below 32 weeks' gestation and/or birthweight less than 1500 g	Negative score on the three milestones of development at 2 years of age associated with hypothyroxinaemia group.

Animal studies have shown that a deficiency of thyroxine results in impaired neurological pathways during early neurogenesis which results in abnormalities of the cytoarchitecture of specific brain structures such as the cerebellum, hippocampus, temporal and sensorimotor cortex [21-25]. Lavado Autric et al have shown that hypothyroxinaemia causes migration defects of the cerebral cortex which are associated with neurological deficits. [25] Eayrs and colleagues have shown in early studies [26, 27] that perinatal hypothyroidism in rats alter the density and size of neurones and fibre density in specific brain regions and the orientation of cortical layers. Berbel et al [28, 29] also described effects on spine density of pyramidal neurones in the cerebral cortex, organisation of callosal connection and maturation of dendrite connections as a result of hypothyroidism. Thyroid hormones are also demonstrated to increase proliferation of cerebellar granule cells as well as affect apoptosis which is important in suppression of proliferation and downgrading of these cells [30, 31]. Thyroid hormones are essential for normal axonal myelination and for normal interhemispheric commisure development [32, 33]. Thyroid hormones are important in the control of gene expression and regulating transcription of specific genes expressed in the developing brain [34, 35]. This suggests an important role for thyroid hormone in the complex developing brain throughout gestation.

In preterm infants, hypothyroxinaemia of prematurity as characterised by low blood thyroxine (T4) and triiodothyronine (T3) concentrations with normal plasma thyroid stimulating hormone (TSH) concentrations has been commonly reported [36-38]. The severity of the hypothyroxinaemia in these infants is observed to be inversely related to gestational age and birth weight [36, 39].

Increments in T3 was observed at 1 hour relative to cord levels in all infants and were unrelated to the peak TSH levels, which differed markedly between gestational ages. This may be explained by increased thyroidal T3 secretion, peripheral T4 to T3 conversion and reduction in T3 clearance and degradation by decrease in D3 expression. Cord reverse T3 (rT3) levels were also the highest in infants 24-27 weeks' gestation compared to the more mature infants, and there was a marked decrease in rT3 levels after the first hour in all preterm infants which was most evident in the most extreme preterm group, probably reflecting the deficit in available T4 during the same period. These features critically define the 24-27 weeks' gestational age group as distinct, suggesting failed response to the HTP axis at this age group. Klein et al observed significant increases in cord plasma T4, FT4, thyroid binding globulin (TBG) levels between 26 and 33-36 weeks gestational age, with no significant changes seem thereafter to term [40].

In earlier analyses between gestational ages 11 and 40 weeks, T4 and FT4 appeared to increase continuously to term but TSH were unchanged between 22 weeks to term[199]. Parallel changes observed in T4 and TBG levels suggests that between 26 weeks to term, the changes observed in T4 were largely reflecting changes seen in TBG levels. However, increasing FT4 levels imply that circulating T4 pool increased more rapidly than the TBG pool resulting in a saturation of TBG-T4 binding sites [40]. However, the increases in T4 and FT4 levels without the detected changes in TSH levels between 26-33 weeks gestation suggest that the pituitary negative feedback control of TSH release remains insensitive. Plasma TSH fails to suppress as FT4 levels increases indicates that the set point for negative feedback control of TSH secretion is also increasing at the pituitary level during this period of maturity.

These observations suggest that the HPT axis and its maturation throughout gestation is a complex process and is not yet complete until 1-2 months of postnatal life. In addition, the increase in FT4 and FT3 in the last trimester of pregnancy suggest that there may be a change in pituitary thyrotroph conversion capacity of T4 to active T3, or a possible increase in the pituitary thyrotroph nuclear T3 receptor numbers or affinity or responsiveness. TRH stimulation tests have been used to assess the maturity of the pituitary-thyroid axis involving postnatal administration of TRH and subsequent measurement of TSH, T3 and T4. Roti et al[41] reported that human term fetal pituitary TSH response to exogenous TRH stimulation was exaggerated and prolonged which was a response characteristic of hypothalamic hypothyroidism.

The rising FT4, TSH, FT3/TSH ratios in the developing fetus can reflect a progressive increase in level of TRH stimulation in the fetal pituitary gland. However, a fall in plasma TSH in the neonatal period occurs whether or not the newborn is full term or premature and this suggest that extra uterine environmental influences also contribute to the maturation of the HPT axis. This environmental effect is likely to be mediated via an increased T4 and T3 conversion capacity in peripheral non-thyroidal non-pituitary tissues after delivery, but other maturational events may also contribute to this. The fact that FT4 levels increases in the face of stable plasma TSH levels suggests that thyroid gland sensitivity to TSH stimulation increases with gestational age as observed in the hypothyroxinaemia phenomena of prematurity. This is consistent with the ontogenic pattern of increasing thyroid gland sensitivity to TSH with increasing fetal age observed in fetal sheep during the last trimester of pregnancy [25]. Obtundation of neonatal TSH surge particularly in prematurity may also reflect a reduced capacity for hypothalamic responsiveness to cooling which is an environmental trigger of being "born" into extra uterine environment. There is considerable evidence that neonatal TSH surge is stimulated by the cooling effect, mediated via the hypothalamic control [40, 42].

Other factors which may contribute to abnormal thyroid function in very preterm infants include: immaturity of the thyroid gland, immaturity of the hypothalamic-pituitary-thyroid axis, disruption of maternal transfer of T4 through the placenta, relative immaturity of type 1 deiodothyronine monodeiodinase enzyme systems and reduction in thyroid binding globulin (TBG) due to hepatic immaturity [37, 43, 44]. Non thyroidal illness syndrome or “sick euthyroid syndrome” which is often described as a condition that alters thyroid function by lowering T4 and/or T3 concentrations but not necessarily FT4 concentrations may also be associated in prematurity [37, 45]. Medical complications of prematurity such as respiratory distress syndrome, infection, necrotising enterocolitis are associated with non-thyroidal illness syndrome [46]. Premature infants have elevated cytokines as a result of cardiopulmonary and infectious disorders. The increased cytokines are thought to inhibit thyroid hormone production contributing to the hypothyroxinaemia phenomenon seen in these infants [47-49].

Medication like dopamine which is frequently given as first line agent in the clinical management of hypotension in preterm infants, had been reported in clinical studies to cause anterior pituitary hormone suppression [50]. Animal experiments have shown that the basal secretion of TSH from pituitary thyrotropes was inhibited by dopamine in a dose-dependent manner in adult humans although no work on the effects of dopamine on the HPT axis has been done in embryonic animals [51]. In a randomised controlled trial of dopamine versus dobutamine, dopamine was observed to reduce serum levels of growth hormone, TSH, T4 and prolactin levels from 12 hours of administration in very low birth weight infants [50]. Dopamine was also a potent inhibitor of GH and prolactin which were reversible on withdrawal of the dopamine [52]. The mechanisms by which this occurs in humans are not understood and the consequences of the iatrogenic disruption of the endocrine functions have not been studied. Dopamine receptors are expressed in thyroid, pituitary and hypothalamus. Basal secretion of TSH and PRL from thyrotrophs and lactotrophs were rapidly and significantly inhibited by dopamine in a dose-dependent manner in rat anterior pituitary cells [53]

Infection also disrupts the HPT axis in clinical situations [54]. This has been demonstrated in adult rats, when the administration of bacterial lipopolysaccharide (LPS) resulted in rapid suppression of thyroxine releasing hormone (TRH) and thyroid stimulating hormone (TSH) mRNA levels [55]. However, the long term effects of thyroidal disruption on preterm babies remain to be elucidated.

Another relevant HPT disruptor is the administration of synthetic glucocorticoids such as dexamethasone, which has been shown to affect brain development adversely [56]. Nevertheless, this drug is routinely given antenatally to pregnant mothers to improve the viability of their infants, and, until very recently, was frequently administered postnatally to reduce the severity of chronic lung disease. The administration of dexamethasone to preterm infants has been reported to cause decreased plasma thyroid hormone levels [57] but it is not known whether this is the mechanism of their abnormal brain development. Experiments on rats showed that dexamethasone caused a decrease in plasma TSH/T4 [58] and deiodinase enzyme levels were altered [59]. Direct interactions between the thyroid and cortisol axes have also been reported in animals but not in humans [60]. In non-mammalian vertebrates, corticotropin releasing hormone (CRH) has been shown to be a potent TSH releasing factor [61, 62] suggesting there may be direct interactions between these axes in humans.

Deficiency of thyroxine results in impaired neurological pathways during neurogenesis, abnormalities in myelination and alters the cytoarchitecture of specific brain structures [63]. Possible long term harmful effects of medications like dopamine and dexamethasone on thyroid hormone regulation in preterm infants may aggravate hypothyroxinaemia of prematurity already present and further understanding of their developmental stage specific-role in neurodevelopmental outcome is important. If there are disrupting effects, the development of alternative medications would be indicated.

Hypothalamic-Pituitary-Adrenal Axis in Preterm Infants

Cortisol is an important hormone during fetal maturation and it is the final product of the hypothalamic-pituitary-adrenal (HPA) axis in humans. The HPA axis is a homeostatic system which under basal conditions maintains a circadian rhythm and responds to stress. An increase in cortisol under the integrity of the HPA axis is necessary to determine appropriate behavioural reactions in response to acute stress, and resetting of the HPA axis with increased secretion of cortisol is an important adaptive response affecting the onset of inflammatory disease.

Cortisol is important for survival during illness and cortisol concentrations are expected to increase during significant stress. Extreme preterm infants may develop adrenal insufficiency in the early neonatal period requiring cortisol supplementation. The HPA axis is thought to reach adult equivalent maturity at an early age.

In premature infants, the data is conflicting with some studies reporting that sick premature infants do not release more cortisol than less severely ill infants[64] and others have demonstrated that severely ill infants under 28 weeks gestation have higher morning cortisol levels compared with premature infants of the same gestational age [65]. A randomised controlled trial of hydrocortisone treatment for prophylaxis of relative adrenal insufficiency in very low birth weight infants found that high cortisol levels were associated with severe intraventricular haemorrhage, and extremely elevated values were associated with morbidity and death [66].

In the premature infant population, the physiological significance of lower cortisol values remains unclear [67, 68]. Most studies have not consistently correlated cortisol concentrations to physiological markers of cortisol effect and outcome in preterm infants [69, 70]. In a recent study, the HPA axis was found to be unresponsive to standard stimulation tests until 11 days of age in preterm baboons indicating HPA axis immaturity [71]. Activation of the HPA axis and increased cortisol concentrations may be essential to respond to the many stressors of extra-uterine existence in the extreme preterm infants. This transient inability of the adrenals to maintain cortisol homoeostasis in premature newborns in the immediate postnatal period has been described as transient adrenocortical insufficiency of prematurity [69]. An observational study of cortisol and ACTH response of infants born at 34-37 weeks' gestational age demonstrated that inadequate response to critical illness in these infants were not due to adrenal dysfunction but were thought to be a result of a secondary insufficiency arising from inadequate stimulation of the adrenal gland [72].

Published studies have been generally been consistent with basal morning salivary cortisol ranges higher in preterm and term infants compared with older children suggesting that circadian basal HPA axis exhibits hypervariability in the first few years of life before settling into adult-equivalent rhythm [65, 66]. Whether this represent early developmental process in the neuroendocrine system, ongoing programming of adaptation to stress responsiveness remains to be elucidated. There are limited data on adrenal function of extremely premature infants during the early days after birth when a diminished cortisol response to Corticotropin Releasing Factor (CRF) has been reported. The relationship between plasma ACTH and cortisol is central to the integrity of the HPA axis; yet, there are no studies examining this in prematurity. Premature infants have been reported to have lower stimulated cortisol responses ACTH compared to normal ranges in the early neonatal period. The aetiology, diagnostic criteria and optimal treatment are under debate.

The HPA axis is thought to reach adult equivalent maturity at an early age. Published studies have been generally consistent with basal morning salivary cortisol ranges higher in preterm and term infants compared with older children [73-75] suggesting that circadian basal HPA axis exhibits hypervariability in the first few years of life before settling into adult-equivalent rhythm. Whether this represents early developmental process in the neuroendocrine system, ongoing programming of adaptation to stress responsiveness or a consequence of daytime sleeping in young children remains to be elucidated. Koupi et al found that early morning salivary cortisol showed a negative correlation with length of gestation and no real relationship to birth weight or systolic and diastolic blood pressure[76]. Santiago et al[77]'s data showed that the HPA axis and the circadian maturation occur between 2 and 8 weeks after birth, while Price et al [78] described the appearance of the circadian cycle occurred at age 3 months and 6 months.

Many of the sick preterm infants are also exposed to pharmacological doses of glucocorticoids in utero and postnatally and little is known about the physiological exposure of glucocorticoids before early preterm birth. Glucocorticoids are regulated by placental enzyme 11 beta hydroxysteroid dehydrogenase-2 (11 beta-HSD2) which converts excess cortisol to inactive cortisone and 11 beta HSD-2 activity have been shown to be inversely related to gestational age[79]. Impaired activity of this enzyme is commonly found in intrauterine growth restriction and preeclampsia, conditions which are frequently present in preterm births. It is unclear whether early morning cortisol and ACTH concentrations are correlated in the absence of stimulation in these infants. Studies have also reported that sicker infants, those who had intrauterine growth restriction and those who subsequently developed bronchopulmonary dysplasia (BPD) had decreased adrenal response to stimulation [64, 65, 67] suggesting that adrenal reserve in premature infants may be inadequate or immature.

The use of antenatal corticosteroids have been shown to reduce the incidence and severity of respiratory distress syndrome, decrease the incidence of bronchopulmonary dysplasia, intraventricular haemorrhage, necrotising enterocolitis and mortality in preterm infants [80]. PC Ng et al. [81] found that antenatal dexamethasone doses nor the time intervals between drug and delivery significantly affected HPT responsiveness in 61 preterm infants. Previous studies have found increase cortisol levels in vaginally delivered infants most likely due to intense stress induced during parturition as well as increase in maternal circulating cortisol levels after active labour as opposed to caesarean section deliveries [82]. This suggested that a continuing maturational process was occurring at the adrenal level as infant matures with increasing gestation and birth weight. In PC Ng's study [81], the lack of association between plasma ACTH and plasma cortisol in the first week of postnatal life suggest that a maturational process was also occurring at the level of the pituitary gland. Other factors may play a role such as high endothelin levels that may exert a positive drive at the level of the adrenal glands, while secretion of the atrial natriuretic hormone has an inhibitory effect on the hypothalamic and pituitary centres.

Premature infants who develop chronic lung disease have been shown to have lower plasma cortisol levels compared with similar infants who recover without developing CLD [83]. In addition, plasma cortisol was inversely related with several cytokines and proteins in the airways of intubated infants. Therefore, it is likely that some infants have a decreased capacity to synthesize cortisol resulting in adrenal insufficiency due to illness and stress, leading to a variety of physiological disruption such as increased inflammatory response resulting in development of chronic lung disease. Postnatal dexamethasone treatment have been used in the treatment of chronic lung disease. Kari et al. showed that in a randomized controlled trial of postnatal dexamethasone treatment for 1 week versus placebo, the treated group showed a decrease in both the basal and ACTH stimulated cortisol levels. One week after discontinuation of therapy, basal cortisol levels were similar between the treated group and the placebo group. A decrease in CBG levels and DHEAS levels were also seen in the treated group. This suggests that very preterm infants requiring intensive care have a reduced cortisol secretion ability and may suffer form hypocortisolism.

Maturation of fetal adrenal cortex may also be modulated by maternal cortisol. Early in gestation, the HPA axis is exposed to negative feedback from maternal cortisol which freely crosses the placenta. Later in gestation, placental metabolism occurs and the enzyme 11 beta hydroxysteroid dehydrogenase increasingly oxidises maternal cortisol to inactive metabolite cortisone. Therefore, the negative feedback from maternal cortisol that was present in early gestation gradually decreases in the later half of gestation and fetal cortisol synthesis increases gradually[84].

In extreme premature birth, the normal maturational process is disrupted and the infant's immature gland lacks the capacity to synthesize sufficient quantities of cortisol to respond to the many stressors of extra uterine life such as respiratory distress and mechanical ventilation. Similarly, the presence of accumulation of cortisol precursors like 17-OH pregnenolone, 17 OH progesterone and 11-deoxycortisol, and the increased ratios of precursor to product also supports the hypothesis that premature infants have a decreased capacity to synthesize cortisol resulting in relative adrenal insufficiency in the face of acute illness and stress after birth. In previous studies, cortisol and 17-OH progesterone levels were high on the first day of life in preterm infants, while cortisol levels decrease immediately and tend to increase at day 4, while 17-OH progesterone then declines after the first day and remains stable from Day 2 until Day 7. Cortisone levels declined within the first 2 hours after birth and very gradually thereafter through the first week of life while corticosterone levels are much lower than cortisol levels, increases in the first 2 hours, decrease until 6 hours and decreases again at 24 hours before remaining stable[64].

Endogenous glucocorticoid and synthetic glucocorticoid exposure results in modification of neurotransmitter systems and nuclear transcriptional mechanisms. Fetal exposure permanently alters HPA function in prepubertal, postpubertal and ageing offspring, in a gender-dependent manner [5, 9, 85]. Exogenous glucocorticoid manipulation may also lead to the modification of behaviour, brain and organ morphology, as well as altered regulation of other endocrine systems. There is increasing evidence that the timing of exposure to synthetic glucocorticoids antenatally and postnatally may have effects on the nature of the phenotypic outcome. Dysfunctional HPA axis has also been reported in diseases prevalent in childhood such as autism, a neurodevelopmental condition characterized by inability to interact with the social environment[86] and fragile X syndrome [87], a genetic disease associated with behavioural and physical abnormalities. Both conditions reported elevated diurnal cortisol levels compared with controls. Interestingly, preterm infants have a significantly increased risk of behavioural, language and attention problems, not unlike autistic spectrum disorders[88]. Further information about the HPA dysfunction in early childhood and effects of onset of diseases in later childhood need to be investigated. It is possible that fetal programming due to abnormal HPA axis may predispose these infants to onset of pathologies described and consequences in later life of anomalous cortisol responses to stressors.

CONCLUSION

The transition of the developing fetus to newborn life is associated with marked changes in the function of major organ systems. The complex regulation and physiopathology of HPT and HPA regulation in preterm infants remain poorly understood. Endocrine disruptors are also known to interfere with mechanisms of normal hormonal regulation. A mutifactorial model of factors affecting neurodevelopmental outcome, behaviour and growth in the extreme preterm infant is shown in Figure 1. Certain factors such as infection and medications like dopamine and dexamethasone are capable of disrupting the HPT and HPA axis, and may further exacerbate endocrine consequences of premature birth leading to an adverse outcome.

Further understanding of their role in neurodevelopmental outcome during the developmental stages is important to potentially impact on the clinical care of premature infants in future.

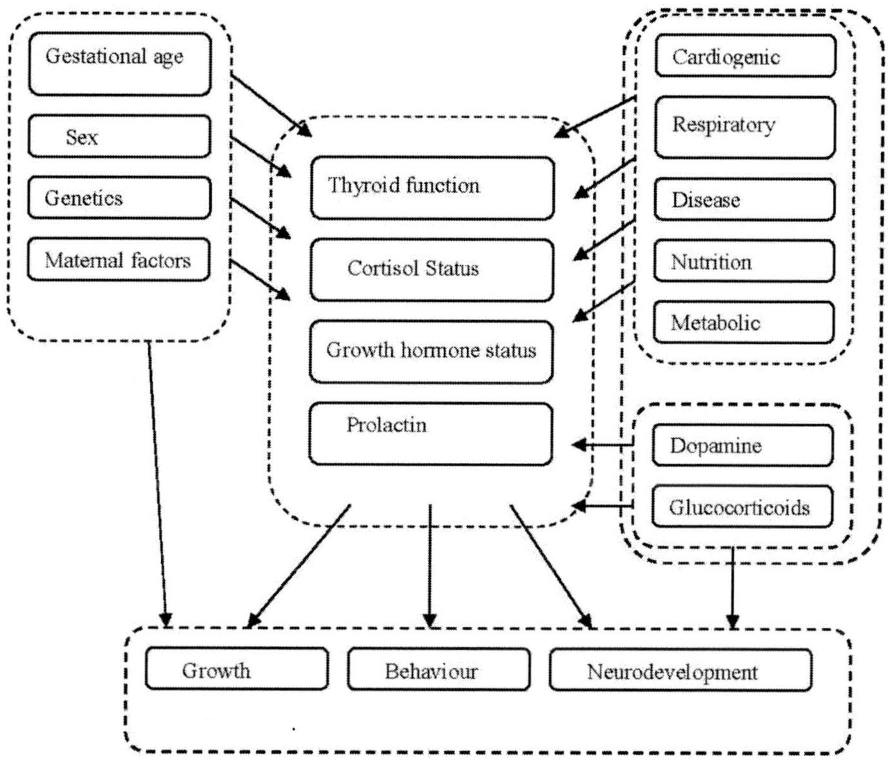

Figure 1. Mutifactorial model of factors affecting growth and neurodevelopmental outcome on the extremely premature infant.

References

[1] Wood NS, Costeloe K, Gibson AT, Hennessy EM, Marlow N, Wilkinson AR. The EPICure study: associations and antecedents of neurological and developmental disability at 30 months of age following extremely preterm birth. *Arch Dis Child Fetal Neonatal Ed* 2005;90:F134-40.

[2] Wood NS, Costeloe K, Gibson AT, et al. The EPICure study: growth and associated problems in children born at 25 weeks of gestational age or less. Neurologic and developmental disability after extremely preterm birth. EPICure Study Group. *Arch Dis Child Fetal Neonatal Ed* 2003;88:F492-500.

[3] Barker DJ. The origins of the developmental origins theory. *J Intern Med* 2007;261:412-7.

[4] Barker DJ. The developmental origins of insulin resistance. *Horm Res* 2005;64 Suppl 3:2-7.

[5] Kajantie E, Phillips DI, Andersson S, et al. Size at birth, gestational age and cortisol secretion in adult life: foetal programming of both hyper- and hypocortisolism? *Clin Endocrinol* (Oxf) 2002;57:635-41.

[6] Robinson S, Walton RJ, Clark PM, Barker DJ, Hales CN, Osmond C. The relation of fetal growth to plasma glucose in young men. *Diabetologia* 1992;35:444-6.

[7] Barker DJ, Hales CN, Fall CH, Osmond C, Phipps K, Clark PM. Type 2 (non-insulin-dependent) diabetes mellitus, hypertension and hyperlipidaemia (syndrome X): relation to reduced fetal growth. *Diabetologia* 1993;36:62-7.

[8] Hofman PL, Cutfield WS, Robinson EM, et al. Insulin resistance in short children with intrauterine growth retardation. *J Clin Endocrinol Metab* 1997;82:402-6.

[9] Kapoor A, Dunn E, Kostaki A, Andrews MH, Matthews SG. Fetal programming of hypothalamo-pituitary-adrenal function: prenatal stress and glucocorticoids. *J Physiol* 2006;572:31-44.

[10] Kooistra L, Crawford S, van Baar AL, Brouwers EP, Pop VJ. Neonatal effects of maternal hypothyroxinemia during early pregnancy. *Pediatrics* 2006;117:161-7.

[11] Salerno M, Militerni R, Bravaccio C, et al. Effect of different starting doses of levothyroxine on growth and intellectual outcome at four years of age in congenital hypothyroidism. *Thyroid* 2002;12:45-52.

[12] Mercado M, Yu VY, Francis I, Szymonowicz W, Gold H. Thyroid function in very preterm infants. Early Hum Dev 1988;16:131-41.

[13] Cuestas RA. Thyroid function in healthy premature infants. *J Pediatr* 1978;92:963-7.

[14] Delange F, Dodion J, Wolter R, et al. Transient hypothyroidism in the newborn infant. *J Pediatr* 1978;92:974-6.

[15] Reuss ML, Paneth N, Pinto-Martin JA, Lorenz JM, Susser M. The relation of transient hypothyroxinemia in preterm infants to neurologic development at two years of age. *N Engl J Med* 1996;334:821-7.

[16] Den Ouden AL, Kok JH, Verkerk PH, Brand R, Verloove-Vanhorick SP. The relation between neonatal thyroxine levels and neurodevelopmental outcome at age 5 and 9 years in a national cohort of very preterm and/or very low birth weight infants. *Pediatr Res* 1996;39:142-5.

[17] Leviton A, Paneth N, Reuss ML, et al. Hypothyroxinemia of prematurity and the risk of cerebral white matter damage. *J Pediatr* 1999;134:706-11.

[18] Paul DA, Leef KH, Stefano JL, Bartoshesky L. Low serum thyroxine on initial newborn screening is associated with intraventricular hemorrhage and death in very low birth weight infants. *Pediatrics* 1998;101:903-7.

[19] Lucas A, Morley R, Fewtrell MS. Low triiodothyronine concentration in preterm infants and subsequent intelligence quotient (IQ) at 8 year follow up. *Bmj* 1996;312:1132-3; discussion 3-4.

[20] Meijer WJ, Verloove-Vanhorick SP, Brand R, van den Brande JL. Transient hypothyroxinaemia associated with developmental delay in very preterm infants. *Arch Dis Child* 1992;67:944-7.

[21] Cai D, Su Q, Chen Y, Luo M. Effect of thyroid hormone deficiency on developmental expression of goalpha gene in the brain of neonatal rats by competitive RT-PCR and in situ hybridization histochemistry. *Brain Res* 2000;864:195-204.

[22] Bernal J. Thyroid hormone receptors in brain development and function. *Nat Clin Pract Endocrinol Metab* 2007;3:249-59.

[23] Iniguez MA, De Lecea L, Guadano-Ferraz A, et al. Cell-specific effects of thyroid hormone on RC3/neurogranin expression in rat brain. *Endocrinology* 1996;137:1032-41.

[24] Auso E, Lavado-Autric R, Cuevas E, Del Rey FE, Morreale De Escobar G, Berbel P. A moderate and transient deficiency of maternal thyroid function at the beginning of fetal neocorticogenesis alters neuronal migration. *Endocrinology* 2004;145:4037-47.

[25] Lavado-Autric R, Auso E, Garcia-Velasco JV, et al. Early maternal hypothyroxinemia alters histogenesis and cerebral cortex cytoarchitecture of the progeny. *J Clin Invest* 2003;111:1073-82.

[26] Eayrs JT, Horn G. The development of cerebral cortex in hypothyroid and starved rats. *Anat Rec* 1955;121:53-61.

[27] Eayrs JT. Thyroid hypofunction and the development of the central nervous system. *Nature* 1953;172:403-4.

[28] Berbel P, Auso E, Garcia-Velasco JV, Molina ML, Camacho M. Role of thyroid hormones in the maturation and organisation of rat barrel cortex. *Neuroscience* 2001;107:383-94.

[29] Berbel P, Guadano-Ferraz A, Angulo A, Ramon Cerezo J. Role of thyroid hormones in the maturation of interhemispheric connections in rats. *Behav Brain Res* 1994;64:9-14.

[30] Nicholson JL, Altman J. The effects of early hypo- and hyperthyroidism on the development of the rat cerebellar cortex. II. Synaptogenesis in the molecular layer. *Brain Res* 1972;44:25-36.

[31] Xiao Q, Nikodem VM. Apoptosis in the developing cerebellum of the thyroid hormone deficient rat. *Fron Biosci* 1998;3:A52-A7.

[32] Balazs R, Kovacs S, Cocks WA, Johnson AL, Eayrs JT. Effect of thyroid hormone on the biochemical maturation of rat brain: postnatal cell formation. *Brain Res* 1971;25:555-70.

[33] Balazs R, Brooksbank BW, Davison AN, Eayrs JT, Wilson DA. The effect of neonatal thyroidectomy on myelination in the rat brain. *Brain Res* 1969;15:219-32.

[34] Morreale de Escobar G, Obregon MJ, Escobar del Rey F. Role of thyroid hormone during early brain development. *Eur J Endocrinol* 2004;151 Suppl 3:U25-37.

[35] Yen PM, Ando S, Feng X, Liu Y, Maruvada P, Xia X. Thyroid hormone action at the cellular, genomic and target gene levels. *Mol Cell Endocrinol* 2006;246:121-7.

[36] Williams FL, Simpson J, Delahunty C, et al. Developmental trends in cord and postpartum serum thyroid hormones in preterm infants. *J Clin Endocrinol Metab* 2004;89:5314-20.

[37] LaFranchi S. Thyroid function in the preterm infant. *Thyroid* 1999;9:71-8.

[38] La Gamma EF, van Wassenaer AG, Golombek SG, et al. Neonatal Thyroxine Supplementation for Transient Hypothyroxinemia of Prematurity : Beneficial or Detrimental? *Treat Endocrinol* 2006;5:335-46.

[39] Williams FL, Visser TJ, Hume R. Transient hypothyroxinaemia in preterm infants. *Early Hum Dev* 2006;82:797-802.

[40] Klein AH, Oddie TH, Parslow M, Foley TP, Jr. , Fisher DA. Developmental changes in pituitary-thyroid function in the human fetus and newborn. *Early Hum Dev* 1982;6:321-30.

[41] Roti E, Gnudi A, Braverman LE, et al. Human cord blood concentrations of thyrotropin, thyroglobulin, and iodothyronines after maternal administration of thyrotropin-releasing hormone. *J Clin Endocrinol Metab* 1981;53:813-7.

[42] Uhrmann S, Marks KH, Maisels MJ, et al. Thyroid function in the preterm infant: a longitudinal assessment. *J Pediatr* 1978;92:968-73.

[43] LaFranchi SH, Haddow JE, Hollowell JG. Is thyroid inadequacy during gestation a risk factor for adverse pregnancy and developmental outcomes? *Thyroid* 2005;15:60-71.

[44] Fisher DA, Klein AH. Thyroid development and disorders of thyroid function in the newborn. *N Engl J Med* 1981;304:702-12.

[45] Klein RZ, Carlton EL, Faix JD, et al. Thyroid function in very low birth weight infants. *Clin Endocrinol* (Oxf) 1997;47:411-7.

[46] Fisher DA. Euthyroid low thyroxine (T4) and triiodothyronine (T3) states in prematures and sick neonates. *Pediatr Clin North Am* 1990;37:1297-312.

[47] Yeung MY, Smyth JP. Hormonal factors in the morbidities associated with extreme prematurity and the potential benefits of hormonal supplement. *Biol Neonate* 2002;81:1-15.

[48] DeGroot LJ. "Non-thyroidal illness syndrome" is functional central hypothyroidism, and if severe, hormone replacement is appropriate in light of present knowledge. *J Endocrinol Invest* 2003;26:1163-70.

[49] Adler SM, Wartofsky L. The nonthyroidal illness syndrome. *Endocrinol Metab Clin North Am* 2007;36:657-72, vi.

[50] Filippi L, Pezzati M, Poggi C, Rossi S, Cecchi A, Santoro C. Dopamine versus dobutamine in very low birthweight infants: endocrine effects. *Arch Dis Child Fetal Neonatal Ed* 2007;92:F367-71.

[51] Cooper DS, Klibanski A, Ridgway EC. Dopaminergic modulation of TSH and its subunits: in vivo and in vitro studies. *Clin Endocrinol (Oxf)* 1983;18:265-75.

[52] De Zegher F, Van Den Berghe G, Devlieger H, Eggermont E, Veldhuis JD. Dopamine inhibits growth hormone and prolactin secretion in the human newborn. *Pediatr Res* 1993;34:642-5.

[53] Dieguez C, Foord SM, Newman GR, et al. Rat anterior pituitary cells maintained on artificial capillaries: responses of thyrotrophs and lactotrophs to depolarization, TRH and dopamine. *Mol Cell Endocrinol* 1984;37:73-82.

[54] De Felice C, Bagnoli F, Toti P, et al. Transient hypothyroxinemia of prematurity and histological chorioamnionitis. J Perinat Med 2005;33:514-8.

[55] Kondo K, Harbuz MS, Levy A, Lightman SL. Inhibition of the hypothalamic-pituitary-thyroid axis in response to lipopolysaccharide is independent of changes in circulating corticosteroids. Neuroimmunomodulation 1997;4:188-94.

[56] Shinwell ES, Karplus M, Reich D, et al. Early postnatal dexamethasone treatment and increased incidence of cerebral palsy. *Arch Dis Child Fetal Neonatal Ed* 2000;83:F177-81.

[57] Buimer M, van Wassenaer AG, Kok JH. Postnatal administration of dexamethasone for weaning off the ventilator affects thyroid function. *Neonatology* 2008;94:164-9.

[58] Ahlquist JA, Franklyn JA, Ramsden DB, Sheppard MC. The influence of dexamethasone on serum thyrotrophin and thyrotrophin synthesis in the rat. *Mol Cell Endocrinol* 1989;64:55-61.

[59] Van der Geyten S, Darras VM. Developmentally defined regulation of thyroid hormone metabolism by glucocorticoids in the rat. *J Endocrinol* 2005;185:327-36.
[60] Geris KL, Kotanen SP, Berghman LR, Kuhn ER, Darras VM. Evidence of a thyrotropin-releasing activity of ovine corticotropin-releasing factor in the domestic fowl (Gallus domesticus). *Gen Comp Endocrinol* 1996;104:139-46.
[61] De Groef B, Goris N, Arckens L, Kuhn ER, Darras VM. Corticotropin-releasing hormone (CRH)-induced thyrotropin release is directly mediated through CRH receptor type 2 on thyrotropes. *Endocrinology* 2003;144:5537-44.
[62] Okada R, Miller MF, Yamamoto K, De Groef B, Denver RJ, Kikuyama S. Involvement of the corticotropin-releasing factor (CRF) type 2 receptor in CRF-induced thyrotropin release by the amphibian pituitary gland. *Gen Comp Endocrinol* 2007;150:437-44.
[63] Anderson GW. Thyroid hormone and cerebellar development. *Cerebellum* 2007:1-15.
[64] Huysman MW, Hokken-Koelega AC, De Ridder MA, Sauer PJ. Adrenal function in sick very preterm infants. *Pediatr Res* 2000;48:629-33.
[65] Scott SM, Watterberg KL. Effect of gestational age, postnatal age, and illness on plasma cortisol concentrations in premature infants. *Pediatr Res* 1995;37:112-6.
[66] Aucott SW, Watterberg KL, Shaffer ML, Donohue PK. Do cortisol concentrations predict short-term outcomes in extremely low birth weight infants? *Pediatrics* 2008;122:775-81.
[67] Watterberg KL, Gerdes JS, Cole CH, et al. Prophylaxis of early adrenal insufficiency to prevent bronchopulmonary dysplasia: a multicenter trial. *Pediatrics* 2004;114:1649-57.
[68] Watterberg KL. Adrenocortical function and dysfunction in the fetus and neonate. *Semin Neonatol* 2004;9:13-21.
[69] Ng PC, Lee CH, Lam CW, et al. Transient adrenocortical insufficiency of prematurity and systemic hypotension in very low birthweight infants. *Arch Dis Child Fetal Neonatal* Ed 2004;89:F119-26.
[70] Scott SM, Cimino DF. Evidence for developmental hypopituitarism in ill preterm infants. *J Perinatol* 2004;24:429-34.
71] Jobe AH, Scott SM, Polk DH, Seidner SR. Adrenal and thyroid axis function in preterm ventilated baboons. *Biol Neonate* 2003;83:208-16.
[72] Fernandez EF, Montman R, Watterberg KL. ACTH and cortisol response to critical illness in term and late preterm newborns. *J Perinatol* 2008;28:797-802.
[73] Calixto C, Martinez FE, Jorge SM, Moreira AC, Martinelli CE, Jr. Correlation between plasma and salivary cortisol levels in preterm infants. *J Pediatr* 2002;140:116-8.
[74] Bettendorf M, Albers N, Bauer J, Heinrich UE, Linderkamp O, Maser-Gluth C. Longitudinal evaluation of salivary cortisol levels in full-term and preterm neonates. *Horm Res* 1998;50:303-8.
[75] Silva ML, Mallozi MC, Ferrari GF. Salivary cortisol to assess the hypothalamic-pituitary-adrenal axis in healthy children under 3 years old. *J Pediatr* (Rio J) 2007;83:121-6.
[76] Koupil I, Mann V, Leon DA, Lundberg U, Byberg L, Vagero D. Morning cortisol does not mediate the association of size at birth with blood pressure in children born from full-term pregnancies. *Clin Endocrinol* (Oxf) 2005;62:661-6.
[77] Santiago LB, Jorge SM, Moreira AC. Longitudinal evaluation of the development of salivary cortisol circadian rhythm in infancy. *Clin Endocrinol* (Oxf) 1996;44:157-61.

[78] Price DA, Close GC, Fielding BA. Age of appearance of circadian rhythm in salivary cortisol values in infancy. *Arch Dis Child* 1983;58:454-6.

[79] Kajantie E, Dunkel L, Turpeinen U, et al. Placental 11 beta-hydroxysteroid dehydrogenase-2 and fetal cortisol/cortisone shuttle in small preterm infants. *J Clin Endocrinol Metab* 2003;88:493-500.

[80] Yeh TF, Lin YJ, Huang CC, et al. Early dexamethasone therapy in preterm infants: a follow-up study. *Pediatrics* 1998;101:E7.

[81] Ng PC, Wong GW, Lam CW, et al. Pituitary-adrenal response in preterm very low birth weight infants after treatment with antenatal corticosteroids. *J Clin Endocrinol Metab* 1997;82:3548-52.

[82] Lao TT, Panesar NS. The effect of labour on prolactin and cortisol concentrations in the mother and the fetus. *Eur J Obstet Gynecol Reprod Biol* 1989;30:233-8.

[83] Watterberg KL, Gerdes JS, Cook KL. Impaired glucocorticoid synthesis in premature infants developing chronic lung disease. *Pediatr Res* 2001;50:190-5.

[84] Pepe GJ, Albrecht ED. Actions of placental and fetal adrenal steroid hormones in primate pregnancy. *Endocr Rev* 1995;16:608-48.

[85] Sondeijker FE, Ferdinand RF, Oldehinkel AJ, Tiemeier H, Ormel J, Verhulst FC. HPA-axis activity as a predictor of future disruptive behaviors in young adolescents. *Psychophysiology* 2008;45:398-404.

[86] Jansen LM, Gispen-de Wied CC, van der Gaag RJ, van Engeland H. Differentiation between autism and multiple complex developmental disorder in response to psychosocial stress. *Neuropsychopharmacology* 2003;28:582-90.

[87] Hessl D, Glaser B, Dyer-Friedman J, et al. Cortisol and behavior in fragile X syndrome. *Psychoneuroendocrinology* 2002;27:855-72.

[88] Wolke D, Samara M, Bracewell M, Marlow N. Specific language difficulties and school achievement in children born at 25 weeks of gestation or less. *J Pediatr* 2008;152:256-62.

In: Preterm Infants
Editors: Diogo Contreiras and Johann Sampaio

ISBN 978-1-62081-819-0

Chapter 5

INFANTS PREMATURELY BORN: SOCIO-EMOTIONAL DEVELOPMENT AND EARLY INTERVENTION

***Marina Fuertes*[1,2,7,*]*, João Justo*[3]*, Miguel Barbosa*[4]*, Leopoldo Leitão*[5]*, Joana Gonçalves*[2]*, Gomes Pedro*[6]*, and Joshua Sparrow*[7]**

[1]Escola Superior de Educação de Lisboa, Portugal
[2]Centro de Psicologia, University of Porto, Portugal
[3]Faculdade de Psicologia, University of Lisbon, Portugal
[4]Faculdade de Medicina, University of Lisbon, Portugal
[5]Universidade Lusófona, Lisbon, Portugal
[6]Fundação Brazelton/Gomes-Pedro, Lisbon, Portugal
[7]Harvard Medical School, Boston, Massachusets, US

ABSTRACT

Prematurely born infants tend to be less alert, less attentive, less active and less responsive than infants born at full term, and their mothers tend to have greater difficulty knowing when and how to modulate their interactions. Although premature birth alone is not necessarily a risk factor for the parent-infant relationship or attachment, the prevalence of insecure attachment is higher in preterm infant-mother dyads. It does become a risk factor for attachment and parent-infant interactions in the presence of low socio-economic status, low maternal education, co-morbid infant health problems, or maternal depression. The primary focus of this chapter is the mother-infant relationship in the context of prematurity. We propose a literature review of three domains: a) mothers' experience and representations of premature delivery and infant development; b) mothers' interactions with preterm infants and c) the quality of mother-infant attachment. Since insecure attachment can be prevented, we include a brief review on practices promoting secure relationships and supporting mothers.

Keywords: Prematurity, preterm infants, parent-infant interaction; attachment and early intervention

[*] Corresponding author: Marina Fuertes (marinaf@eselx.ipl.pt).

Commonly in the third trimester of pregnancy, most women develop a clear and rich representation of their infants (e.g., Ammaniti, Baumgartner, Candelori, Perucchini, Pola, Tambelli et al., 1992; Bruschweiler Stern, 1998), that is influenced by a mother′s early attachment, as well as the movements and levels of fetal activity, which are organized in cycles and patterns that are interpreted by the mother (Brazelton and Cramer, 1990; Korja, Savonlahti, Haataja, Lapinleimu, Manninen, Piha, Lehtonen, and Grp, 2009). Those representations generated during the perinatal period seem to affect the mother-infant relationship (e.g., Benoit, Parker and Zeanah, 1997; Zeanah, Benoit, Hirshberg, Barton, and Regan, 1994). Yet birth reveals the 'real' baby, in contrast to the idealized baby. Prenatal representations are subject to change as a result of interactions with the 'real' baby (Stern, 1977; Fava-Vizziello, Antonioli, Cocci, and Invernizzi, 1993). Shortly after birth, parents form new and more accurate representations of their 'real' newborn (Benoit et al., 1997). For mothers who experience a premature birth, this process is interrupted before it is complete and they have to nurture a fragile baby whose survival is at risk (Bruschweiler Stern, 1998; Redshaw, 1997).

Aims: The quality of the early mother-infant interaction has been considered an important mediating factor between perinatal events and the later developmental outcome of the infant in the areas of socialization, cognition and communication (Schermann-Eizirik, Hagekull, Bohlin, Persson, and Sedin, 1997). However, mother-preterm infant dyads are at risk for disturbed patterns of interaction. Risk and protective factors for infants' development and relationships are reviewed in this chapter, as well as pre-and postnatal interventions that enhance the mother-child relationship and support parents of preterm infants.

Prematurity and Developmental Risks

Over the last decades, great advances in perinatal and neonatal medical care have significantly increased survival rates of preterm infants. Yet premature birth is still associated with higher rates of neonatal and infant mortality, health problems and development delays, especially for very low birth weight (less than 1500 g) newborns, and for preterm infants born at less than 32 weeks of gestation or with medical complications (Barnard, Osofsky, Beckwith, Hammond, and Appelbaum,1998; Escalona, 1982; Minde, 1993, Sandén Eriksson and Pehrsson, 2002; Spiker, Ferguson, and Brooks-Gunn, 1993).

From birth, infants prematurely born behave differently. Compared to full-term infants, preterm infants struggle with neurobehavioral difficulties including autonomic, motor and state modulation, arousal regulation and affective responsiveness (Mouradian, Als, and Coster, 2000). Some studies indicate long-term effects of prematurity on development (e.g., Largo, Graf, Kundu, Hunziker, and Molinari, 1990; Sticker, Brandt, and Höckey, 1998). The range of developmental challenges and delays may be manifested in physical growth (DeWitt, Sparks, Swank, and Smith, 1997), motor skills (Greenberg and Crnic, 1988; van Beek, Hopkins, Hoeksma, and Samsom, 1994), attention (Landry, 1995), cognition (Ment, Vohr, Allan, Katz, Schneider, et al., 2003), language, social communicative skills (van Beek, Hopkins, and Hoeksma, 1994) and academic performance (van Baar, van Wassenaer, Briet, Dekker, and Kok, 2005). Moreover, very low weight and extreme preterm infants with medical complications are at significantly higher risk than full term ones for later neurological impairment (such as cerebral palsy) and severe behavioral problems (Hille, den Ouden, Saigal, Wolke, Lambert, Whitaker, et al., 2001; Sajaniemi, Hakamies-Blomqvist, Mäkelä, Avellan, Rita, and von Wendt, 2001; Stewart, Rifkin, Maess, and Kirkbride, 1999; Waber and McCormick, 1995; Weisglas-Kuperus, Koot, Baerts, Fetter, and Sauer, 1993; Wolke, Ratschinski, Orth, and Riegel, 1994). There are numerous factors that contribute to such risks, including family socioeconomic disadvantage, parents' educational status and social support (Fuertes, Faria, Soares and Crittenden, 2008; Laucht, Esser, and Schmidt, 1997). In a follow-up study of preterm infants and their families, Gross, Mettelman, Dye, and Slagle, (2000) found that family stability, parents' marital status and parents' educational levels were major determinants in children's academic outcomes and behavioral problems presented at school by the age of 10. Other studies indicate that gender may increase the odds of survival, with preterm girls more likely to survive than boys (e.g., Morse, Whu Ma, Ariet, Resnick, and Roth, 2006; Shankaran, Fanaroff, Wright, et al., 2002).

Yet if early supportive and preventive intervention is provided for infants and their families, many children recover from their difficult start (e.g., Brisch, Bechinger, Betzler, Heinemann, Kächele, Pohlandt, et al., 2005; Bonnier, 2008; Koldewijn, van, Wolf, Meijssen, Houtzager, Beelen, et al., 2010; Koldewijn, Wolf, Wassenaer, Meijssen, Sonderen, Baar, et al., 2009; Meijssen, Wolf, Koldewijn, Houtzager, Wassenaer, Tronick, et al., 2010; Vanderveen, Bassler, Robertson, and Kirpalani, 2009).

Prematurity Impact on Infant-Parent Relationship

Parent-infant attachment begins during pregnancy through physiological mechanisms as well as parental representations. It evolves postpartum through complex neurohormonal and behavioral interactions between infants and parents (e.g., Bowlby, 1988; Brazelton, 1998; Brazelton and Cramer, 1990; *Kennell, Klaus, and Klaus, 1996).*

The quality of parent-infant attachment depends on multiple factors (including infant and parent interactive behaviors, as well as contextual variables) that act on parent-infant relational experience. While fathers' attachment to their infants is also significantly affected by premature birth, since this literature is far more limited, the focus here is on mother-infant attachment and interactions.

Maternal sensitivity and warm responsiveness play a crucial role in promoting secure attachment (Ainsworth, Blehar, Waters, and Wall, 1978; De Wolff and van IJzendoorn, 1997, Grossmann, Grossmann, Spangler, Suess, and Unzner, 1985; Isabella, 1993), together with positive maternal representations about infant temperament and attachment (Benoit, Parker, and Zeanah, 1997; Bretherton, Biringen, Ridgeway, Maslin, and Sherman, 1989; Cox, Hopkins, and Hans, 2000; Izard, Haynes, Chisholm, and Baak, 1991; Kochanska, 1998; Zeanah, Benoit, Hirshberg, Barton, and Regan, 1994). Each infant's individual behavior also make a major contribution to the mother-infant attachment process, particularly, the infant's capacity for and style of self-regulation (Braungart-Rieker, Garwood, Powers, and Wang, 2001; Cohn, Campbell, and Ross, 1991; Goldsmith and Alansky, 1987; Kagan, 1984; Kochanska and Coy,2002; Tronick, Als, Adamson, Wise, and Brazelton, 1978, Tronick and Cohn, 1989; Tronick, Ricks, M., and Cohn, 1982).

Taken together, maternal and infant contributions predict attachment security (Fuertes, Lopes-dos-Santos, Beeghly and Tronick, 2006; 2009). Presently, most developmental theorists propose a transactional and multi-contextual approach to explain attachment quality (e.g., Belsky, 2005; Cicchetti and Barnett, 1991; Crittenden, 2000; Grossmann et al., 1985; Rutter, 1991; Sroufe, 1996, van den Boom, 1994; see also Cassidy and Shaver, 1999 for a review). *But how then does attachment develop in dyads with infants born prematurely?*

The NICU is a structured, highly sophisticated and technological environment that aims to ensure infant survival, and recovery from the range of predictable medical problems that threaten it. Although much has been done to promote parent-newborn proximity in NICUs, this environment still limits mothers' opportunities to establish intimate contact with their newborns. For example, depending on their medical condition, babies may need life support in incubators that prevent mothers from having long and regular physical contact with them.

The preterm delivery of an infant that necessitates hospitalization in a neonatal intensive care unit (NICU) is a traumatic event for parents (Affleck, Tennen, and Rowe, 1991; Easterbrooks, 1989; Miles, Funk and Carlson., 1993; Robson, 1997) and challenges the emerging parent-infant relationship (Talmi and Harmon, 2003; Muller-Nix et al., 2004). This experience is usually accompanied by feelings of helpless and a lack of control over the infant´s health and survival (Olshtain-Mann and Auslander, 2008). An impressive study performed by Singer, Davillier Bruening Hawkins and Yamashita, (1996) revealed that mothers of preterm infants with low birth weight experienced a significantly higher incidence of psychological distress during the neonatal period, marked by anxiety about their babies' survival, future development and health. Miles et al. (1992) reported that parents rated sights and sounds of the NICU as being extremely stressful, along with their infants' behavior and appearance (consistent with infants' illness and vulnerability). Moreover, mothers of preterm infants with medical complications and of very low birth weight infants were less confident in parenting their infants and in initiating social exchanges with their baby (Singer et al., 1996; Goldberg and DiVitto, 1995).

Maternal Representations and Prematurity

Balanced and positive maternal representations, as measured pre- and postnatally, have been associated with secure attachment (Benoit, et al, 1997; Bretherton, et al.,1989; Cox, et al., 2000; Fuertes, et al., 2006; 2009; Izard, et al., 1991; Kochanska, 1998; Korja et al., 2009; Zeanah et al. 1994). Few studies regarding maternal representations include dyads with preterm infants.

As expected for full term infants, Fuertes et al. (2006; 2009) found that healthy prematurely born infants (from 31 to 36 weeks of gestation, 1500 to 2550g) classified as securely attached were perceived as being less difficult by their mothers.

Later, a comparative study with preterm and full term infants, found that attachment security was associated with maternal representations of their infant's temperament (Fuertes, Faria, Barbosa, and Fink, 2011).

However, some relevant differences were found in maternal representations of full-term and preterm infant. The early separation of mothers from their preterm newborns is potentially traumatic for mothers, causing stress reactions, with symptoms anxiety and depression (Kersting, Dorsch, Wesselmann, Ludorff, Witthaut, Ohrmann, et al., 2004;

Kersting, Kroker, Steinhard, Hoernig-Franz, Wesselmann, Luedorff, et al. 2009; Singer, Salvator, Guo, Collin, Lilien, and Baley, 1999).

These symptoms may affect maternal feelings and responses (Feldman, Weller, Leckman, Kuint, and Eidelman, 1999). Meijssen, Wolf, Koldewijn, Wassenaer, Kok, and van Baar (2011) found that mothers of very preterm infants are less likely to development balanced maternal representation. According to the authors, *"balanced attachment representations are characterized by narratives that convey coherence, openness to change, richness of detail, and a sense of the mother as engrossed in her relationship with her infant. These mothers value and enjoy their relationship with their infant and are aware that this relationship affects their child's behavior and development*" (p.74).

Others have found that mothers that delivered prematurely had more negative perceptions about their pregnancy and labor than other women (Fuertes et al., 2011). These mothers were more preoccupied with their infants' health and development than full-term infants' mothers. Nonetheless, in the context of the absence of early intervention, they were as confident as mothers of full-term infants about their ability to engage in positive relationships with their infants.

Mother-Infant Quality of Interaction

Prematurity directly affects infants' development, and their ability to engage socially, as well as parental interactive behavior. Preterm infants struggle to maintain stable physiological rhythms, to self-regulate, and to organize responses into coherent affective configurations that affect parent–infant synchrony during normal interactions (Malatesta, Culver, Tesman, and Shepard, 1989; Minde, 2000). Preterm infants tend to be easily stressed (even by low levels of stimulation), and often display negative affect. Their facial signals are less clear, and they have difficulty tolerating shifts in affective behavior. They are less able to maintain attention, and their social gaze is less frequent and more intermittent (Brachfeld, Goldberg, and Sloman, 1980; Eckerman, Oehler, Hannan, and Molitor 1995; Eckerman, Hsu, Molitor, Leung, and Goldstein, 1999; Harel Oppenheim, Tirosh, and Gini., 1999; Greene, Fox, and Lewis, 1983; McGehee and Eckerman, 1983). These difficulties affect parents' ability to read and respond to their premature infant's social cues.

Several studies have indicated that mother–infant interactive behavior processes differ in dyads with preterm or very preterm infants compared with dyads with full terms (e.g., Bozzette, 2007; Eckerman, et al. 1999; Holditch-Davis, Schwartz, Black, and Scher, 2007; Swartz, 2005). Comparative studies of full term infants, low-risk preterm infants and high-risk preterm infants indicate that very preterm infants are significantly more limited in maintaining attention and show higher negative affect during social interactions than the other two groups (Eckerman et al., 1999; Garner and Landry, 1992; van Beek et al., 1994). The mothers of these infants tend to initiate interactions without clear cues from their infants, or interactions that are less clearly adjusted to infant cues. They appear to express less positive affect, and to experience less pleasure in interacting with their babies. Some authors have also characterized them as tending to be either more overstimulating or less involved in these interactions than other mothers (Barnard and Kelly, 2000; Forcada-Guex, Pierrehumbert, Borghini, Moessinger, and Muller-Nix, 2006; Goldberg and DiVitto, 1995; Malatesta, Grigoryev, Lamb, Albin, and Culver, 1986; Muller-Nix et al., 2004).

Nevertheless, some studies emphasize that parents may compensate for the preterm's difficulties when they are responsive, emotionally involved and able to support the infant's cognitive and socio-affective development (e.g., Greenberg and Crnic, 1988; Singer, Fulton, Davillier, Koshy, Salvator, and Baley, 2003). "Low" risk preterms improve their socially and emotionally competent by six months of corrected age and their mothers improve their sensitivity to infant cues (Schermann-Eizirik, et al., 1997). However, health status, birth weight, and length of gestation are key factors in shaping infants' and mothers' responsiveness.

Schermann-Eizirik, et al. (1997) compared mother - full term infant pairs (born at a gestational age of 37-42 weeks) who needed neonatal intensive care with mother – full term infant pairs who did not need neonatal intensive care. The criterion for neonatal intensive care was one or more of the following: respirator therapy or continuous positive airway pressure (CPAP), total parenteral nutrition, monitoring and treatment of severe asphyxia (Apgar score of 4 or below 5 min after birth) and/or treatment of neonatal convulsions. Dyads with full-term infants in neonatal intensive care, as compared with the other group, consistently showed less optimal interactional behaviors, including lower scores in maternal sensitivity and involvement, and less stable infant behavior. In this study, although infants were born at term, the neonatal intensive care variable was a major factor shaping mother-infant interaction. Other research indicates that mother–child synchrony depends largely on infant medical risk at birth (Landry, Smith, Miller-Loncar, and Swank, 1998) rather than preterm status alone, suggesting that the degree of CNS insult plays an important role in the development of mother–infant reciprocity (review in Feldman, 2007).

Mother-Infant Attachment

Infant medical risk factors such as premature birth may influence attachment quality, although specific findings vary depending on whether or not other risk factors were present in the samples under investigation. In samples of relatively healthy infants from well-educated middle class samples, premature birth is not typically associated with a higher rate of attachment insecurity (e.g., Easterbrooks, 1989; Frodi and Thompson, 1985; Minde, Corter, and Goldberg, 1985; Rode, Chang, Nian, Fisch, and Sroufe, 1981). When samples are characterized by additional risk factors such as low socio-economic status (SES; Wille, 1991), low maternal education (Pederson and Moran, 1996), co-morbid infant health problems (Coppola, Cassibba, and Costantini, 2007; Mangelsdorf et al., 1996; Minde, 2000; Plunkett, Meisels, Stiefel, Pasick, and Roloff, 1986; Schmucker, Heinz-Bisch, Kohntop, Betzler, Osterle, Pohlandt, et al., 2005; Singer et al., 2003), or maternal depression (Poehlmann and Fiese, 2001), premature birth is associated with a higher prevalence of insecure attachment (see also Belsky, 2005, for a review). (Attachment constructs and assessment measures developed using well-educated middle class samples may not be universally applicable or appropriate for use with samples from other educational and socioeconomic levels.) Very low birth-weight preterm infants more often develop an insecure quality of attachment (Forcada-Guex, Borghini, Pierrehumbert, Ansermet and Muller-Nix, 2011).

The Prediction of Preterm Labor, Delivery and Birth Based on Psychosocial Variables

Since the beginning of psychological studies of pregnancy, associations between psychometric data and preterm delivery incidence have suggested the possibility that psychosocial variables may an important role (Gunter, 1963). Such associations have always been fairly weak, consistent with the view that the etiology of preterm delivery is multifactorial. A very important step in the progression of these explorations was the study of Teichmann and Breull (1989). In their sample of women recruited during the first trimester of gestation, 90% of the subjects were correctly classified in a prospective study about preterm labor. This achievement was achieved by using 19 items divided among four categories: a) adequate strategies to cope with stress, b) motivation for having a child, c) occupational stress and d) family situation. Since that study, it has become very clear that the way women experience and cope with stress plays an important role in pregnancy outcomes.

Published evidence shows several important conclusions about the interplay among etiological factors for premature delivery: a) low socioeconomic status (SES) raises the risk for preterm birth within specific ethnic populations, b) in association with SES,' educational attainment plays a remarkable role in the prediction of reproductive health outcomes, c) behavioral and psychological factors and medical ones that may be associated with those (smoking, genitourinary infections, drug addiction and excessive physical activity at work). However, a very significant number of preterm births occurs in the absence of any known etiological factor (Kramer, Séguin, Lydon, and Goulet, 2000). The large number of preterm births without a clear etiology is an opportunity window to raises the possibility that, in some instances, unidentified psychological factors, and associated may be involved. At first, attention was drawn to anxiety, depression and stressful life events (Blau, Slaff, Easton, Welkowitz, Springarn, and Cohen, 1963; Newton, Webster, Binu, Maskrey and Phillips, 1979; Omer, Elizur, Barnea, Friedlander and Palti, 1986; Omer, Friedlander, and Palti, 1986; Molfese, Bricker, Manion, Beadnell, Yaple, et al., 1996). More recently, maternal stress perception has been implicated, along with chronic stressors including poor housing, lack of employment, economic insecurity and problematic family relations such as like low quality partnership and violence (Kramer, et al., 2000). In addition, it is well known that lower levels of social support perception may stimulate higher levels of stress perception. A kind of vicious cycle may result in which negative emotions induce specific endocrine responses (Conneely and Hughes, 2010). For example, placental secretion of corticotrophin releasing hormone, which may result from increased maternal stress is capable of stimulating uterine contractions, possibly by potentiating oxytocin effects or by the resulting increase in the synthesis of other hormones like fetal cortisol or androgen-induced oestriol (Kramer, et al., 2000).

Over the last few years, new investigations into the association between stress and - preterm birth have reconfirmed the importance of the psychological functioning during pregnancy for the determination of gestational age at birth as well as for newborn health status (Wadhwa, Sandman, Porto, Dunkel-Schetter and Garite, 1993). As early as 1997, available data were very clear about the association between maternal stress by the third trimester of gestation and gestational age at birth as well as with infant birthweight (Sandman, Wadhwa, Chicz-DeMet, Dunkel-Schetter, and Porto, 1997). These conclusions are further supported by a study showing that, when compared with healthy pregnant women, women with threatened preterm labor are more likely to have lower formal educational attainment, greater difficulty accepting the pregnancy and poorer relationships with others, including the expectant father (Facchinetti, Ottolini, Fazzio, Rigatelli, and Volpe, 2007).

In order to understand how different etiological factors for preterm labor and delivery work together, it is necessary to take in account the complexity of psycho-neuro-immunological interactions. Pearce, Grove, Bonney, Bliwise, Dudley, Schendel and Thorsen (2010) have found that the macrophage migration inhibitory factor (MIF), interlukin-10 (IL-10), C-reactive protein (CRP) and tumor necrosis factor-α are good predictors of preterm birth. When immunological variables were tested together with psychosocial variables, the best predictive model included MIF, CRP, risk taking behavior and low educational level. Because IL-10 is a cytokine involved in the inhibition of inflammatory processes triggered by other cytokines, and because pro-inflammatory cytokines have recently been shown to have very specific relationships with psychological conditions (Kiecolt-Glaser, Gouin, and Hantsoo, 2010) these factors should be the focus of future research on preterm delivery. Psychological variables can influence cytokine secretion through pathways that involve neuro-immunological-behavioral factors or by amplifying negative emotional states and risk health behaviors (Kiecolt-Glaser, et al., 2010).

Finally, vast research has investigated the extent of prenatal stress effects on newborn health as well as later stages of development. According to Davis and Sandman (2010), cortisol and psychological data gathered during pregnancy provide explanations for several aspects of child progress development after birth: a) high levels of maternal cortisol early in pregnancy do predict lower levels of development by the end of the first year of life and a slower progress of the infant development during that period, b) on the contrary, high levels of cortisol late in pregnancy are good predictors of faster cognitive development during the first twelve months of age and of higher developmental levels at the end of that period and c) early in gestation, high scores of anxiety specific to pregnancy are associated with levels of infant mental development at twelve months. Consequences of prenatal exposure to maternal cortisol are observable during baby's first day of life: 1) higher newborn cortisol levels, via the heel-stick blood draw procedure (HSBDP) are associated with higher levels of maternal cortisol late in pregnancy, 2) slower reduction of the infant´s distress following the HSBDP is associated with higher levels of maternal cortisol early in pregnancy and 3) slower stabilizing of newborn behavior after the HSPBDP is also associated with maternal psychosocial stress over the course of pregnancy (Davis, Glynn, Waffarn, and Sandman, 2011).

Parent-Infant Interaction Interventions during NICU Hospitalizations

Although prematurity remains a risk for infants' survival and development, there is growing evidence that family centered, relationship based and developmentally supportive approaches are effective in reducing neonatal morbidity and improving preterm infants' behavioral and cognitive development (e.g., de Vonderweid and Leonessa, 2009, Kaaresen, Ronning, Tunby, Nordhov, Ulvund, and Dahl, 2008; Nordhov, Kaaresen, Ronning, Ulvund, and Dahl, 2010; Nordhov, Ronning Dahl, Ulvund, Tunby, and Kaarensen, 2010; Nordhov,

Ronning, Ulvund, et al., 2012; Vanderveen, et al., 2009). A meta-analysis by Vanderveen et al. (2009) indicates that, a range of interventions can significantly alter developmental paths, improving health, educational and social outcomes through 36 months. Vanderveen′s meta-analysis included 25 developmental interventions, such as NIDCAP and Kangaroo Care.

Trials of these interventions were conducted with heterogeneous groups of families and premature infants born at 25 to 26 weeks of gestation and weighing 785 to 2606 gms at birth. The results indicate that despite the diversity of clinical and families conditions, early intervention plays a crucial role in supporting parents and enhancing infant development. The most challenging target for preventive intervention is the effect of prematurity on the parent-child relationship (Bakermans-Kranenburg, Bakermans-Kranenburg and Juffer, 2003). A meta-analytic study carried out by van IJzendoorn, Bakermans-Kranenburg, and Juffer (2005) suggested that *less is more* i.e., the short-term interventions aiming at changing or preventing problematic parental behavior reviewed were more effective than the long-term interventions considered in this study. We present some short-term interventions that have shown benefits for infant health and development and for parent-infant relationships.

NIDCAP

When health care professionals first designed intensive care for preterm infants, the focus was increasing their chances for survival. Believing that handling and sensory stimulation could overwhelm preemies` physiologic stability and that raised the risk of infections, NICU staff ‘protected’ babies from ‘stressful’ interactions – including those with parents (Talmi, and Harmon, 2003), although little or no protection was provided against the bright lights, loud sounds, routine handling and medical instrumentation of NICU care.

During 80s, researchers hypothesized that preterm newborns in NICUs needed tactile, kinesthetic, auditory, and visual stimulation for adequate brain growth during human interaction. Although weight gain and early discharge have been documented as a result of these sensory enhancement first approaches, that approach did not typically address the individual strengths and challenges of either the baby or the baby`s relationship with his parents (Browne, 2000).

Presently, many researchers and clinicians have focused their attention on developmentally appropriate care for preterm infants that include parents as caregivers (Byers, 2003; Robison, 2003). One of the most influential and best studied comprehensive interventions is the Newborn Individualized Developmental Care and Assessment Program (NIDCAP).

The NIDCAP is an individualized developmental approach to environmental support and care based on reading preterm infant`s behavioral cues to formulate a care plan that enhances and builds upon the infant`s strengths, and supports the infant in areas of sensitivity and vulnerability (Als, 1982, 1986, 1991).

Its framework is applied in the delivery room, during the NICU admission, stay and discharge, and the first few months at home.

The NIDCAP methodology relies on recording detailed observations of an infant`s naturalistically occurring behaviors in the NICU, and these are understood as the infant`s continuous communication (Als, 2008). Seeing infants as able to communicate their strengths and needs and to participate in pursuing their own developmental agenda, the NIDCAP approach provides assessment, attention to the infant`s developmental goals, and recommendations for ongoing, comprehensive support for the infant in the context of the family (Als and Gilkerson, 1997).

The effectiveness of NIDCAP has been studied in several research trials. Two randomized controlled trials (Als, Lawhon, Duffy, McAnulty, Gibes-Grossman, and Blickman, 1994; Fleisher, VandenBerg, Constantinou, Heller, Benitz, Johnson, Rosenthal, and Stevenson, 1995) (RCTs) involving extremely low birth weight, medically high risk infants (□ 29 weeks PMA at birth) found that developmental care resulted in decreased time on endotracheal and continuous positive airway pressure (CPAP) ventilation, reduction in intraventricular hemorrhage and in severity of chronic lung disease, better oral feeding, decreased length of hospital stay, and reduction in hospital charges (Fleisher et al., 1995).

Additional studies, found that others improvements were achieved in medical outcomes included less time on mechanical ventilation, less supplemental oxygen, reduction in the incidence of intraventricular hemorrhage and pneumothorax, reduced severity of chronic lung disease, improved daily weight gain, shorter length of hospital stay, younger ages at discharge, and lower hospital costs (Als, Gilkerson, Duffy, McAnulty, Buehler, VandenBerg, Sweet, Sell, Parad, Ringer, Butler, Blickman, and Jones, 2003). Some studies have indicated better neurobehavioral outcome in the NIDCAP experimental group (Als et al., 1994; Als, Duffy, McAnulty, Rivkin, Vajapeyam, Mulkern, Warfield, Huppi, Butler, Conneman, Fischer, and Eichenwald, 2004). Also, NIDCAP (Als, et al., 2003) helps parents by lowering parental stress and enhancing parental competence.

Given these encouraging findings, preterm infants and their families benefit when those responsible for NICU care can provide individualized developmental care.

Kangaroo Method

Recognizing the role of parents as providers of physiological stability for the growing premature infant (Browne, 2003), many NICUs use the kangaroo method wherein infants are directly placed on parents' chests. Kangaroo care benefits newborns by promoting more organized sleep patterns, better regulated body temperature, stabilizing the respiratory and circulatory systems, improving other physiological functions (e.g,. higher oxygen levels, less apnea and periodic breathing) and weight gain (Feldman, Weller, Sirota and Eidelman, 2002; Bosque, Brady, Affonso and Wahlberg, 1995; Messmer, Rodriguez, Adams, Wells-Gentry, Washburn, Zabaleta and Abreu, 1997; Bauer, Sontheimer, Fischer and Linderkamp, 1996). In addition, Ohgi, Fukuda, Moriuchi, Kusumoto, Akiyama, Nugent, Brazelton, et al., (2002) reported that infants exposed to the kangaroo method had significantly higher scores in orientation, state regulation and supplementary items on the Brazelton and Nugent´s Neonatal Behavioral Assessment Scale (2011). Moreover, other studies have shown that mothers who provided kangaroo care maintained breastfeeding for longer periods and with more milk, and experienced less psychological and physiological stress (Hurst, Valentine, Renfro, Burns and Ferlic, 1997).

The skin to skin contact has physiological effects on mothers, increasing their levels of oxytocin that may predispose mothers to engage and to seek proximity with their infants (Tessier, Cristo, Velez, Giron, Calume, Ruiz-Palaez, Charpak and Charpak, 1998; Tessier, Cristo, Velez, Giron, Calume, Ruiz-Palaez, et al., 1998). It is also likely to provide a sense of self-efficacy, providing parents' with tangible experiences of their own importance in promoting their infants' health and development that counters the sense of helplessness and powerlessness that the NICU inevitably engenders in parents (Bruschweiler Stern, 1998).

TAC-TIC Intervention

In order to compensate for the detrimental effects of limited and stressful touch in NUCI, Elvidina Adamson-Macedo designed a program to provide positive touching experiences for preterm babies (Macedo, 1984). This program, Touching And Caressing – Tender In Caring, (TAC-TIC) prescribes a sequence of "touches" that starts with the baby's head and ends at his or her feet: first the crown of the head, after the face, the upper limbs (arms, palms of the hands and fingers), trunk and lower limbs (legs, feet and toes). Each kind of "touch" is performed three times. For the face, touches are performed at the forehead, around the eyes and around the mouth. The implementation of this touch sequence is based on four principles: delicacy, rhythm, balance and continuity.

TAC-TIC intervention was used in several experimental trials and showed that: a) during and after the TAC-TIC intervention with high-risk ventilated preterm babies there are no significant falls in transcutaneously measured oxygen saturation (TcPO2) (Adamson-Macedo, 1994); b) during the intervention, a slight increase in transcutaneously measured oxygen saturation is observable which is the opposite of results obtained with maternal random touching(Adamson-Macedo, Róiste, Wilson, Hayes, Eaton, and De Carvalho, 1997); c) after the intervention, low and very low birth weight infants during their first week of life showed less weight loss than similar babies who received no intervention (Adamson-Macedo, 1985-1986) and results are especially relevant when the intervention was started within the first 48 hours of babies life; d) three minutes after the intervention the concentration of secretory immunoglobulin A was higher, and significantly more organized behaviors were observed (Hayes, Adamson-Macedo, and Perera, 1999). Moreover, TIC-TAC method may help infant adaptation to breast feeding (de Róiste and Bushnell, 1996). Long term results include the finding that at 7 years old, children who had received the intervention had better cognitive and academic outcomes (Adamson-Macedo, Dattani, Wilson, and De Carvalho, 1993).

The cause of the global positive effects obtained by TAC-TIC with preterm babies remains unclear. However, Adamson-Macedo (2004) suggests that the intervention may trigger an opioid activation (i.e., beta-endorphins released by the pituitary).

As the author recalls, beta-endorphins are associated with social behavior in several species and there is broad agreement that endogenous endorphins participate in pain reduction pathways.

Touchpoints Approach

Touchpoints is a developmental, relational and strengths-based approach based on Brazelton's infant research and his model of child development involving periods of disorganization in children's behavior and the family system followed by reorganization in both of these at higher levels (Brazelton, 1990).

It has been used in a wide range of services for infants, young children and their families, including in NICU settings, although it has not been rigorously studied there.

However, its core elements are aligned with a range of effective evidence-based interventions aimed at enhancing interactions between parents and their infants born preterm (Brazelton, 1998; Gomes-Pedro, Patrício, Carvalho, Goldschmidt, Torgal-Garcia, and Monteiro, M.A. 1995; Sparrow, 2010a, 2010b; Sparrow and Brazelton, 2008; Stadtler, Novak, and Sparrow, 2010).

These include careful observation of infant behavior and parent-infant interactions, interpretation of infant behavior as purposeful and elicitation of its meaning to parents, active efforts to provide opportunities for parental mastery, a focus on parental strengths and expertise, and attention to the relationship between healthcare providers and parents as a parallel process supporting positive parent-infant interaction (Sparrow, 2010a, 2010b; Sparrow and Brazelton, 2008; Stadtler, Novak, and Sparrow, 2010).

In the context of the Touchpoints approach, the administration of the NBAS (Neonatal Behavioral Assessment Scale) provides an opportunity to identify the infant's competencies and individuality and to give parents a better understanding of their preterm baby's behavior, thereby enhancing the parent-infant relationship, and parental self-efficacy and self-confidence (Brazelton and Nugent, 2011; Widmayer, and Field, 1980; Widmayer, and Field, 1981; Lowman, Stone, and Gardner-Cole, 2006). The hospital discharge usually causes anxiety and stress for parents. They often lack confidence in their ability to care for their vulnerable infants who, until very recently required a highly technological environment and highly specialized medical staff to survive.

Considering the impact of the NBAS in improving parents′ confidence in their roles, increasing parental involvement in caretaking (Belsky, 1986) and enhancing parents′ knowledge of their infant, performing the NBAS once the infant is more robust and before hospital discharge can have a positive effect on subsequent parent-infant interactions.

Discussion

This chapter concerns the impact of prematurity on child development and mother-infant relationships. Overall, several studies indicate that preterm infants of extreme low birth weight (less than 1500g) and born before 32 weeks of pregnancy are at risk for persistent developmental delay (e.g., Largo, et al., 1990; Sticker, et al., 1998). These infants commonly present difficulties in early interactions because they are less attentive, less organized, and less clear in their responses (Brachfeld, ct al., 1980; Eckerman, et al., 1995; Eckerman, et al., 1999; Harel, et al., 1999; Greene, et al., 1983; McGehee and Eckerman, 1983). In the transactional model, parent-infant relationships depend on both infant and parent contributions to their interactions (Sameroff and Fiese, 2000). The combination of a fragile baby with interactive difficulties and anxious parents may lead to disturbed patterns of interaction (e.g., Bozzette, 2007; Eckerman, et al. 1999; Holditch-Davis, et al., 2007, Swartz, 2005). In dyads with clinical healthy and not very young preterm infants, only in presence of others risk factors mother-infant attachments tend to be less secure factors (e.g., Easterbrooks,

1989; Frodi and Thompson, 1985; Minde, et al., 1985; Rode, et al., 1981), but very low birth weight and very young preterm infants are at risk of insecure attachments even in the absence of psychosocial risk factors (e.g., Forcada-Guex et al., 2011).

Together, adversely affected parent-infant interactions and infant medical condition (e.g., health problems, neurological insult, feeding problems) are major influences on preterm infant development.

However, not all preterm infants are at risk for long term developmental delays and insecure relationships. In fact, healthy preterm infants born at more than 32 weeks gestation, weighing more than 1500 gms, and without social risk factors are likely to be spared. In fact, "low-risk" prematurity only affects development and attachment when other social factors are present, such as low maternal education, low socio-economic status, or maternal depression (e.g., Fuertes, et al., 2008; Feeley, Gottlieb, and Zelkowitz, 2005; Gerner, 1999, Gross, et al. 2000; Laucht, et al., 1997, Pederson and Moran, 1996, Poehlmann and Fiese, 2001, Schermann-Eizirik, et al., 1997, Wille, 1990).

Several studies indicate that post-natal intervention in the NICU (e.g., NIDCAP, Kangaroo, TIC-TAC and Touchpoints) can be effective in enhancing infant neurodevelopment and parent-infant relationships (Vanderveen et al.,2009). Yet none of these methods can reverse the impact of prematurity. This is a traumatic experience for parents who often feel powerless over their babies' threatened survival (Stern, 1998; Redshaw, 1997). Moreover, visiting their baby at the NICU is often an impersonal and unwelcoming experience for parents.

Nevertheless, the approaches presented show promising results in promoting parent-infant relationships and supporting parents during this experience. The best interventions may combine different strategies. We speculate that better results may also depend on professionals' training, their awareness of the critical impact of early experience on brain development, their understanding of the effects of prematurity on parent-infant interactions and parents' need for involvement in their infant's care, and institutional support for corresponding improvements in practice.

ACKNOWLEDGMENTS

This article was supported by a Grant from the Portuguese Science Foundation – Fundação para a Ciência e Tecnologia (PTDC/PSI-EDD/110682/2009).

REFERENCES

Adamson-Macedo, E. N. (1985-1986). Effects of tactile stimulation on low and very low birthweight infants during the first week of life. *Current Psychological Research and Reviews, 4*, 305-308.

Adamson-Macedo, E. N. (1994). TAC-TIC therapy with high-risk, distressed, ventilated preterms. *Journal of Reproductive and Infant Psychology, 12*, 249-252.

Adamson-Macedo, E. N., Dattani, I., Wilson, A., and De Carvalho, F. A. (1993). A small sample follow-up study of children who received tactile stimulation after preterm birth:

intelligence and achievements. *Journal of Reproductive and Infant Psychology, 11*, 165-168.

Adamson-Macedo, E. N., de Róiste, A., Wilson, A., Hayes, J. A, Eaton, B., and de Carvalho, F. A. (1997). Systematic gentle/light stroking and maternal random touching of ventilated preterms: a preliminary study. *International Journal of Prenatal and Perinatal Psychology and Medicine, 9*, 17-31.

Adamson-Macedo, N. E. (2004). Neonatal health psychology: theories and practice. *Neuroendocrinology, Letters, 25 (S1)*, 9-34.

Affleck, G., Tennen, H., and Rowe, J. (1991). *Infants in crisis. How parents cope with newborn intensive care and its aftermath.* New York: Springer.

Ainsworth, M. D., Blehar, M., Waters, E., and Wall, S. (1978). *Patterns of attachment: A psychological study of the Strange Situation*. New Jersey: Lawrence Erlbaum Associates.

Allen, E. C., Manuel, J. C., Legault, C., Naughton, M. J., Pivor, C., and O'Shea, T. M. (2004). Perception of child vulnerability among mothers of former premature infants. *Pediatrics*, 113, 267–273.

Als, H. (1982). Toward a synactive theory of development: Promise for the assessment and support of infant individuality. *Infant Mental Health Journal, 3*(4), 229-243.

Als, H. (1986). A synactive model of neonatal behavioral organization: Framework for the assessment of neurobehavioral development in the premature infant and for support of infants and parents in the neonatal intensive care environment. In J.K. Sweeney (Ed.). *The high-risk neonate: Developmentaltherapy perspectives* (pp. 3-53). New York: The Haworth Press.

Als, H. (1991). Neurobehavioral organization of the newborn: Opportunity for assessment and intervention. *National Institute on Drug Abuse Research Monograph, 114*, 106-116.

Als, H. (2008). Program Guide – Newborn Individualized Developmental Care and Assessment Program (NIDCAP): An Education and Training Program for Health Care Professionals. Boston: Copyright, NIDCAP Federation International.

Als, H. (2009). Newborn individualized developmental care and assessement program (NIDCAP): new frontier for neonatal and perinatal medicine. *Journal of Neonatal Perinatal Medicine, 2*, 135-147.

Als, H., and Gilkerson, L. (1997). The role of relationship-baseddevelopmentally supportive newborn intensive care in strengthening outcome of preterm infants. *Seminars in Perinatology, 21*(3), 178-189.

Als, H., Duffy, F., McAnulty, G.B., Rivkin, M.J., Vajapeyam, S., Mulkern, R.V., Warfield, S., Huppi, P.S., Butler, S., Conneman, N., Fischer, C., and Eichenwald, E. (2004). Early experience alters brain function and structure. *Pediatrics, 113*, 846-857.

Als, H., Gilkerson, L., Duffy, F.H., McAnulty, G.B., Buehler, D.M., VandenBerg, K.A., Sweet, N., Sell, E., Parad, R.B., Ringer, S.A., Butler, S., Blickman, J.G., and Jones, K.J. (2003). A three-center randomized controlled trial of individualized developmental care for very low birth weight preterm infants: Medical, neurodevelopmental, parenting and caregiving effects. *J. Dev. Behav. Pediatr., 24*, 399-408.

Als, H., Lawhon, F.H., Duffy, G.B., McAnulty, R., Gibes-Grossman, and Blickman, J.G. (1994). Individualized developmental care for the very low birthweight preterm infant: Medical and neurofunctional effects. *JAMA, 272*, 853-858.

Ammaniti, M., Baumgartner, E., Candelori, C., Perucchini, P., Pola, M., Tambelli, R., et al., (1992). Representation and narratives during pregancy. *Infant Mental Health Journal, 13*(2), 167-182.

Bakermans-Kranenburg, M. J., van Ijzendoorn, M. H., and Juffer, F. (2005). Disorganized infant attachment and preventive interventions: A review and meta-analysis. *Infant Mental Health Journal, 26*, 3, 191-216.

Bakermans-Kranenburg, M. J., van, Ijzendoorn. M. H., and Juffer, F. (2003). Less is more: meta-analyses of sensitivity and attachment interventions in early childhood. *Psychological Bulletin, 129*, 2, 195-215.

Barnard, K. E., and Brazelton, T. B. (1990). Touch: The foundation of experience. *Clinical Infant Reports, Series of the National Center for Clinical Infant Programs.* Madison CT: International Universities Press, Inc.

Barnard, K. E., and Kelly, J. F. (2000). Assessment of Parent-Child Interaction: Implications for Early intervention In S. J. Meisels and J. P. Shonkoff (Eds.), *Handbook of early childhood intervention* (pp. 258-289). New York: Cambridge University.

Barnard, K., Osofsky, J., Beckwith, L., Hammond, M., and Appelbaum, M. (1998). A collaborative effort to study mother-child interaction in three risk groups: Social risk mother, adolescent mother, preterm infant. *Infant Mental Health Journal, 17,* 293–301.

Bauer, J., Sontheimer, D., Fischer, C. and Linderkamp, O. (1996). Metabolic rate and energy balance in very low birth weight infants during kangaroo holding by their mothers and fathers. *The Journal of Pediatrics*, *129*, 608–11.

Belsky, J. (1986). A tale of two variances: between and within. *Child Development, 57*, 1301–1305.

Belsky, J. (2005). Attachment theory and research in ecological perspective. In Klaus Grossmann, Karin Grossmann and E. Waters (Eds.), *Attachment From Infancy to Adulthood: The Major Longitudinal Studies* (pp. 71-97). New York: Guilford Press.

Benoit, D., Parker, K. C., and Zeanah, C. H. (1997). Mothers' representations of their infants assessed prenatally: stability and association with infants' attachment classifications. *Journal of Child Psychology and Psychiatry, 38*(3), 307-313.

Blau, A., Slaff, B., Easton, K., Welkowitz, J., Springarn, J., and Cohen, J. (1963). The psychogenic etiology of premature births: a preliminary study. *Psychosomatic Medicine, 25, 3*, 201-211.

Bonnier, C. (2008). Evaluation of early stimulation programs for enhancing brain development. *Acta Paediatrica*, *97*, 853–858.

Borghini, A., Pierrehumbert, B., Miljkovitch, R., Muller-Nix, C., Forcada-Guex, M. and Ansermet, F. (2006). Mother's representation of their premature infant at 6 and 18 months after birth. *Infant Mental Health Journal, 10*(3), 203-221.

Bosque, E.M., Brady, J.P., Affonso, D.D., and Wahlberg, V. (1995). Physiologic measures of kangaroo versus incubator care in a tertiary-level nursery. *Journal of Obstetrical Gynecological and Neonatal Nursing 24*(3), 219-226.

Bowlby, J. (1988). *A secure base. Clinical implications of attachment theory.* London: Routledge.

Bozzette, M. (2007). A review of research on premature infant–mother interaction. *Newborn and Infant Nursing Reviews*, 7, 49–55.

Brachfeld, S., Goldberg, S., and Sloman, J. (1980). Parent–infant interaction in free play at 8 and 12 months: Effects of prematurity and immaturity. *Infant Behavior and Development*, 3, 289–305.

Braungart-Rieker, J. M., Garwood, M. M., Powers, B. P., and Wang, X. (2001). Parental sensitivity, infant affect, and affect regulation: predictors of later attachment. *Child Development, 72*(1), 252-270.

Brazelton, T. B. (1998). How to help parents on young children: The Touchpoints model. *Clinical Child Psychology and Psychiatry,* 3(3), Special issue: Parenting, 481-483.

Brazelton, B. and Cramer, B. (1990). *The Earliest Relationship.* Reading. MA: Addison-Wesley/Lawrence.

Brazelton, B. and Nugent, K. (2011). The Neonatal Behavioral Assessment Scale (4th ed.). London: Mac Keith Press.

Bretherton, I., Biringen, Z., Ridgeway, D., Maslin, C., and Sherman, M. (1989). Attachment - the Parental Perspective. *Infant Mental Health Journal, 10*(3), 203-221.

Brisch, K. H., Bechinger, D., Betzler, S., Heinemann, H., Kächele, H., Pohlandt, F., et al. (2005). Attachment quality in very low-birthweight premature infants in relation to maternal attachment representations and neurological development. *Parenting: Science and Practice, 5, 11–31.*

Browne, J. (2003). New perspectives on premature infants and their parents. *Zero to Three, 24(2)*, 4-12.

Browne, J. V. (2000). Considerations for touch and massage in the neonatal intensive care unit. *Neonatal Network, 19*(1), 61-64.

Bruschweiler Stern, N. (1998). Early Emotional Care for Mothers and Infants, *Pediatrics*, 102, Supplement E1, 1278 -1281.

Butler, S., and Als, H. (2008). Individualized developmental care improves the lives of infants born preterm. *Acta Paediatric, 97*(9), 1173-1175.

Byers, J. F. (2003). Components of developmental care and the evidence for their use in the NICU. MCN: *American Journal of Maternal Child Nursing, 28*(3), 174-180.

Cassidy, J. and Shaver, P.R. (Eds.) (1999). *Handbook of attachment: Theory, research, and clinical applications*. NY: Guilford.

Cicchetti, D., and Barnett, D. (1991). Attachment organization in maltreated preschoolers. *Development and Psychopathology, 3*, 397-411.

Cohn, J. F., Campbell, S. B., and Ross, S. (1991). Infant responses in the still-face paradigm at 6 months predicts avoidant and secure attachment at 12 months. *Development and Psychopathology, 3*, 367-376.

Conneely, S., and Hughes, B. (2010). Test anxiety and sensitivity to social support among college students: effects on salivary cortisol. *Cognition, Brain and Behavior, 14, 4*, 295-310.

Cooper, R. L., Goldenberg, R. L., Das, A., Elder, N., Swain, M., Norman, G., Ramsey, R., Cotroneo, P., Collins, B. A., Johnson, F., Jones, P., Meier, A., and the NICHHDMFMUN (1996). The preterm prediction study: maternal stress is associated wit spontaneous preterm birth at less than thirty five weeks' gestation. *American Journal of Obstetrics and Gynecology, 175, 5*, 1286-1292.

Coppola, G., Cassibba, R., and Costantini, A. (2007). What can make the difference? Premature birth and maternal sensitivity at 3 months of age: The role of attachment organization, traumatic reaction and baby's medical risk. *Infant Behavior and Development, 30*, 679–684.

Cox, S. M., Hopkins, J., and Hans, S. L. (2000). Attachment in preterm infants and their mothers: Neonatal risk status and maternal representations. *Infant Mental Health Journal, 21*, 464-480.

Crittenden, P. M. (2000). A dynamic-maturational exploration of the meaning of security and adaptation: empirical, cultural and theoretical considerations. In P. M. C. A. Claussen (Ed.), *The organization of attachment relationships: Maturation, Culture and Context* (pp. 358-384). NY: Cambridge University Press.

Davis, E. P., and Sandman, C. A. (2010). The timing of prenatal exposure to maternal cortisol and psychosocial stress is associated with human infant cognitive development. *Child Development, 81*, 131-148.

Davis, E. P., Glynn, L. M., Waffarn, F., and Sandman, C. A. (2011). Prenatal maternal stress programs infant stress regulation. *Journal of Child Psychology and Psychiatry, 52*, 119-129.

de Róiste, A. and Bushnell, I. W. R. (1996). Tactile stimulation: short- and long-term benefits for pre-term infants. *British Journal of Developmental Psychology, 14*, 41-53.

de Róiste, A. and Bushnell, I. W. R. (2000). Cardiorespiratory and transcutaneous oxygen monitoring of high risk preterms receiving systematic stroking. *International Journal of Prenatal and Perinatal Psychology and Medicine, 12*, 89-95.

de Róiste, A., and Bushnell, I. W. R. (1993). Tactile stimulation and pre-term infant performance on an instrumental conditioning task. *Journal of Reproductive and Infant Psychology, 11*, 155-163.

de Róiste, A., and Bushnell, I. W. R. (1995). The immediate gastric effects of a tactile stimulation programme on premature infants. *Journal of Reproductive and Infant Psychology, 13*, 57-62.

de Róiste, A., Bushnell, I., and Burns, J. (1995). Behavioral reactions of preterm and low-birthweight infants to a program of tactile stimulation. *Journal of Prenatal and Perinatal Psychology and Health, 9*, 295-315.

de Vonderweid, U., and Leonessa, M. (2009). Family centered neonatal care. *Early Human Development, 85*, 10, S37-S38.

De Wolff, M. S., and van IJzendoorn, M. H. (1997). Sensitivity and attachment: a meta-analysis on parental antecedents of infant attachment. *Child Development, 68*, 571–591.

DeWitt, S. J., Sparks, J. W., Swank, P. B., and Smith, K. (1997). Physical growth of low birther-weight infants in the first year of life: Impact of maternal behavior. *Early Human Development, 47*, 19–34.

Easterbrooks, M. A. (1989). Quality of Attachment to Mother and to Father - Effects of Perinatal Risk Status. *Child Development, 60*(4), 825-830.

Eckerman, C. O., Hsu, H., Molitor, A., Leung, E. H. L., and Goldstein, R. F. (1999). Infant arousal in an en-face exchange with a new partner: Effects of prematurity and perinatal biological risk. *Developmental Psychology, 35*, 282–293.

Eckerman, C.O., Oehler, J.M., Hannan, T.E., and Molitor, A. (1995). The development prior to term age of very prematurely born newborns' responsiveness in *en face* exchanges. *Infant Behavior and Development*, 18, 283–297.

Escalona, S. K. (1982). Babies at double hazard: Early development of infants at biologic and social risk. *Journal of Pediatrics, 70,* 670–676.

Facchinetti, F., Ottolini, F., Fazzio, M., Rigatelli, M. and Volpe, A. (2007). Psychosocial factors associated with preterm uterine contractions. *Psychotherapy and Psychosomatics, 76*, 391-394.

Fava-Vizziello, G., Antonioli, M., Cocci, V. and Invernizzi, R. (1993). From pregnancy to motherhood: the structure of representative and narrative change. *Infant Mental Health Journal, 14*(1), 4-16.

Feeley, N., Gottlieb, L. and Zelkowitz, P. (2005). Infant, Mother, and Contextual Predictors of Mother–Very Low Birth Weight Infant Interaction at 9 Months of Age. *Developmental and Behavioral Pediatrics, 26,* 1, 24-33.

Feldman, R. (2007). Parent-infant synchrony: Biological foundations and developmental outcomes. *Current Directions in Psychological Science, 16*, 6, 340-345.

Feldman, R., Weller, A., Leckman, J.F., Kuint, J., and Eidelman, A.I. (1999). The nature of the mother's tie to her infant: Maternal bonding under conditions of proximity, separation, and potential loss. *Journal of Child Psychology and Psychiatry*, 40(6), 929–939.

Feldman, R., Weller, A., Sirota, L., and Eidelman, A. I. (2002). Skin-to-skin contact (kangaroo care) promotes self-regulation in premature infants: Sleep-wake cyclicity, arousal modulation, and sustained exploration. *Developmental Psychology, 38*, 2, 194-207.

Fleisher, B. F., VandenBerg, K.A., Constantinou, J., Heller, C., Benitz, W.E., Johnson, A., Rosenthal, A., and Stevenson, D.K. (1995). Individualized developmental care for very-low-birth-weight premature infants. *Clinic Pediatr, 34*, 523-529.

Forcada-Guex, M., Borghini, A., Pierrehumbert, B., Ansermet, F. and Muller-Nix, C. (2011). Prematurity, maternal posttraumatic stress and consequences on the mother–infant relationship. *Early Human Development*, 87, 21–26.

Forcada-Guex, M., Pierrehumbert, B., Borghini, A., Moessinger, A. and Muller-Nix, C. (2006). Early dyadic patterns of mother-infant interactions and outcomes of prematurity at 18 months. *Pediatrics*, *118*, 1, 107-114.

Frodi, A., and Thompson, R. (1985). Infants' affective responses in the strange situation: effects of prematurity and of quality of attachment. *Child Development, 56*(5), 1280-1290.

Fuertes, M., Faria, A., Fink, N. and Barbosa, M. (2011). Associations among maternal representation at birth and attachment in Portuguese dyads with preterm and full term infant. *International Journal of Development and Educational Psychology, 1, 76-86.*

Fuertes, M., Faria, A., Soares, H., and Crittenden, P. (2008). *Mother-child patterns of interaction: the impact of premature birth and social economical background.* Actha Ethologica, *12*, 1, 1-11.

Fuertes, M., Lopes dos Santos, P., Beeghly, M., and Tronick, E. (2009). *Infant Coping and Maternal Interactive Behaviour Predict Attachment in a Portuguese Sample of Healthy Preterm Infants*. *European Psychologist*, *4*, 320-331.

Fuertes, M., Lopes dos Santos, P., Beeghly, M., and Tronick, E. (2006). More than maternal sensitivity shapes attachment: infant coping and temperament. *Annals New York Academy of Sciences, 1094*, 292-296.

Garner, P.W., and Landry, S. H. (1992). Preterm infants' affective responses in independent versus toy-centered play with their mothers. *Infant Mental Health Journal*, *3*, 219–230.

Gerner, E. M. (1999). Emotional Interaction in a Group of Preterm Infants at 3 and 6 Months of Corrected Age *Infant and Child Development, 8*, 117-128.

Goldberg, S., and DiVitto, B. (1995). Parenting children born preterm. In M. Bronstein (Ed.), *Handbook of parenting*, vol. I. (pp. 209-231).

Gomes-Pedro, J.C., Patrício, M., Carvalho, A., Golds chmidt, T., Torgal-Garcia, F., and Monteiro, M.A. (1995). Early intervention on Portuguese Mothers: A Two Year Follow-Up. *Journal of Developmental and Behavioral Pediatrics, 16*(1), 21-28.

Greenberg, M. T., and Crnic, K. (1988). Longitudinal predictors of developmental status and social interaction in premature and full-term infants at age two. *Child Development, 59*, 554–570.

Greene, J. G., Fox, N. A., and Lewis, M. (1983). The relationship between neonatal characteristics and three-month mother–infant interaction in high-risk infants. *Child Development, 54*, 1286–1296.

Gross, S. J., Mettelman, B. B., Dye, T. D. and Slagle, T. A. (2001) Impact of family structure and stability on academic outcome in preterm children at 10 years of age. *Journal of Pediatrics,138,*2,169-175.

Grossmann, K., Grossmann, K. E., Spangler, G., Suess, G., and Unzner, L. (1985). Maternal sensitivity and newborns' orientation responses as related to quality of attachment in northern Germany. *Monographs of the Society for Research in Child Development, 50*(1-2), 233-256.

Gunter, L. M. (1963). Psychopathology and stress in the life experience of mothers of premature infants. *American Journal of Obstetrics and Gynecology, 86, 3,* 333-340.

Harel, J., Oppenheim, D., Tirosh, E., and Gini, M. (1999). Associations between mother–child interactionand children's later self and mother feature knowledge. *Infant Mental Health Journal, 20*, 123–137.

Hayes, J. A., Adamson-Macedo, E. N., Perera, S. (1999). The mediating role of cutaneous sensitivity within neonatal psychoneuroimmunology, *International Journal of Prenatal and Perinatal Psychology and Medicine, 11*, 459-468.

Hille, E. T. M., den Ouden, L. A., Saigal, S., Wolke, D., Lambert, M., Whitaker, A., et al. (2001). Behavioural problems in children who weigh 1000 g or less at birth in four countries. *The Lancet, 357,* 1641–1643.

Holditch-Davis, D., Schwartz, T., Black, B., and Scher, M. (2007). Correlates of mother–premature infant interactions. *Research in Nursing and Health, 30*, 333–346.

Hurst, N., Valentine, C., Renfro, L., Burns, P. and Ferlic, L. (1997). Skin-to-skin holding in the neonatal intensive care unit influences maternal milk volume. *Journal of Perinatology, 17*, 213-217.

Isabella, R. A. (1993). Origins of attachment: maternal interactive behavior across the first year. *Child Development, 64*(2), 605-621.

Izard, C. E., Haynes, O. M., Chisholm, G., and Baak, K. (1991). Emotional determinants of infant-mother attachment. *Child Development, 62*(5), 906-917.

Kaaresen, P. I., Ronning, J.A., Tunby, J., Nordhov, S.M., Ulvund, S.E., and Dahl, L.B. (2008). A randomized controlled trial of an early intervention program in low birth weight children: outcome at 2 years. *Early Human Development, 84*, 201-209.

Kagan, J. (1984). *The nature of the child.* Cambridge: Harvard University Press.

Kennell, H. Klaus, M.H. and Klaus, P.H. (1996). Bonding - Building the Foundations of Secure Attachment and Independence. London: Cedar.

Kersting, A., Dorsch, M., Wesselmann, U., Ludorff, K., Witthaut, J., Ohrmann, P., et al. (2004). Maternal posttraumatic stress response after the birth of a very low-birth-weight infant. *Journal of Psychosomatic Research*, 57, 473–476.

Kersting, A., Kroker, K., Steinhard, J., Hoernig-Franz, I., Wesselmann, U., Luedorff, K., et al. (2009). Psychological impact on women after second and third trimester termination of pregnancy due to fetal anomalies versus women after preterm birth-a 14-month follow up study. *Archives of Women's Mental Health*, *12*, 193–201.

Kiecolt-Glaser, J. K., Gouin, J-P., and Hantsoo, L. (2010). Close relationships, inflammation, and health. *Neuroscience and Biobehavioral Reviews, 35*, 33-8.

Kochanska, G. (1998). Mother-child relationship, child fearfulness, and emerging attachment: a short-term longitudinal study. *Developmental Psychology, 34*(3), 480-490.

Kochanska, G., and Coy, K. C. (2002). Child emotionality and maternal responsiveness as predictors of reunion behaviors in the strange situation: links mediated and unmediated by separation distress. *Child Development, 73*, 1, 228-240.

Koldewijn, K., van, W. A., Wolf, M. J., Meijssen, D., Houtzager, B., Beelen, A., et al. (2010). A neurobehavioral intervention and assessment program in very low birth weight infants: Outcome at 24 months. Journal of Pediatrics, *156*, 359–365.

Koldewijn, K., Wolf, M. J., Wassenaer, v. A., Meijssen, D., Sonderen, v. L., Baar, v. A., et al. (2009). The Infant Behavioral Assessment and Intervention Program for very low birth weight infants at 6 months corrected age. *Journal of Pediatrics*, *154*, 33–38.

Korja, R., Savonlahti, E., Ahlqvist-Bjorkroth, S., Stolt, S., Haataja, L., Lapinleimu, H., et al. (2008). Maternal depression is associated with mother–infant interaction in preterm infants. *Acta Paediatrica*, *97*, 6, 724–730.

Korja, R., Savonlahti, E., Haataja, L., Lapinleimu, H., Manninen, H., Piha, J., Lehtonen, L., and Grp, P. S. (2009). Attachment representations in mothers of preterm infants. *Infant Behavior and Development, 32*, 3, 305-311.

Kramer, M. S., Séguin, L., Lydon, J., and Goulet, L. (2000). Socio-economic disparities in pregnancy outcome: why do the poor fare so poorly? *Paediatric and Perinatal Epidemiology, 14,* 194-210.

Landry, S. H. (1995). The development of joint attention in premature low birth weight infants: Effects of early medical complications and maternal attention-directing behaviors. In C. Moore and P. Dunham (Eds.), *Joint attention: Its origins and role in development* (pp. 223–250). Hillsdale, NJ: Erlbaum.

Landry, S.H., Smith, K.E., Miller-Loncar, C.L., and Swank, P.R. (1998). The relation of change in maternal interactive style to the developing social competence of full-term and preterm children. *Child Development*, *69*, 105–123.

Largo, R. H., Graf, S., Kundu, S., Hunziker, U., and Molinari, L. (1990). Predicting developmental outcome at school age from infant tests of normal, at-risk and retarded infants. *Developmental Medicine and Child Neurology, 1990*(32), 30–45.

Laucht, M., Esser, G., and Schmidt, M. H. (1997). Developmental outcome of infants born with biological and psychosocial risks. *Journal of Child Psychology and Psychiatry and Allied Disciplines, 38*, 843–854.

Lowman, L., Stone, L. and Gardner Cole, J. (2006). Using developmental assessments in the NICU to empower parents. *Neonatal Network*, 25(3), 177-185.

Macedo, E. N. (1984). Effects of very early tactile stimulation on very-low birthweight infants: a 2 year follow-up study. *Unpublished doctoral dissertation, University of London,* Bedford College.

Malatesta, C. Z., Culver,C. Tesman, J. R. and Shepard, B. (1989). The development of emotion expression during the first two years of life. *Monographs of the Society for Research in Child Development, 54 (1-2, Serial N° 219).*

Malatesta, C. Z., Grigoryev, P., Lamb, C., Albin, M., and Culver, C. (1986). Emotion socialization and expressive development in preterm and full-term infants. *Child Development*, *57*, 316–330.

Mangelsdorf, S. C., Plunkett, J. W., Dedrick, C. F., Berlin, M., Meisels, S., McHale, J., et al. (1996). Attachment security in velow birth weight infants. *Developmental Psychology*, *32*(5), 914–920.

McGehee, L. J., and Eckerman, C. O. (1983). The preterm infant as a social partner: Responsive but unreadable. *Infant Behavior and Development*, *6*, 461–470.

Meijssen, D. E., Wolf, M. J., Koldewijn, K Wassenaer, v. A. G., Kok, J. H, and van Baar, A. L. (2011). Parenting stress in mothers after very preterm birth and the effect of the Infant Behavioural Assessment and Intervention Program. *Child: Care, Health and Development*, 37(2), 195–202.

Meijssen, D. E., Wolf, M. J., Koldewijn, K., Houtzager, B. A., Wassenaer, v. A. G., Tronick, E. Z., et al. (2010). The effect of the Infant Behavioral Assessment and Intervention Program on mother-infant interaction after very preterm birth. *Journal of Child Pyschology and Psychiatry*, *51*, 1287–1295.

Ment, L. R., Vohr, B., Allan, W., Katz, K. H., Schneider, K. C., Westerveld, M., Duncan, C. C., and Makuch, R. W. (2003). Changes in cognitive function over time in very low-birth-weight infants. *Journal of American Medical Association*, *289*(6), 705–711.

Messmer P., Rodriguez S., Adams J., Wells-Gentry, J., Washburn, K., Zabaleta, I. and Abreu, S. (1997). Effect of kangaroo care on sleep time for neonates. *Pediatric Nursing*, *23*, 408-414.

Miles, M., Funk, S. and Carlson, J. (1993). Parental stressor scale: Neonatal intensive care unit. *Nursing Research*, *42*, 148-152.

Minde, K. (1993). The social and emotional development of low-birthweight infants and their families up to age four. In S. Friedman andM. Sigman (Eds.), *The psychological development of low-birthweight children: Advances in applied developmental psychology* (pp. 157–185). Norwood, NJ: Ablex.

Minde, K. (2000). Prematurity and serious medical conditions in infancy: implications for development, behaviour and intervention. In C. H. Zeanah (Ed.), *Handbook of infant mental health, second edition* (pp. 176–194). New York: Guilford Press.

Minde, K., Perrota, M. and Marton, P. (1985). Maternal caretaking and play with full-term and premature infants. *Journal of Child Psychology and Psychiatry*, *26*(2), 231-244.

Molfese, V. J., Bricker, M. C., Manion, L. G., Beadnell, B., Yaple, K., and Moires, K. A. (1987). Anxiety, depression and stress in pregnancy: a multivariate model of intra-partum risks and pregnancy outcomes. *Journal of Psychosomatic Obstetrics and Gynaecology, 7,* 77-92.

Morse, S. B., Wu, S.S., Ma, C., Ariet, M., Resnick, M., and Roth, J. (2006). Racial and Gender Differences in the Viability of Extremely Low Birth Weight Infants: A Population-Based Study. *Pediatrics*, e106-e112.

Mouradian, L. E., Als, H., and Coster, W. J. (2000). Neurobehavioral functioning of healthy preterm infants of varying gestational ages. *Journal of Developmental and Behavioral Pediatrics*, *21*, 408–416.

Muller-Nix, C., Forcada-Guex, M., Pierrehumbert, B., Jaunin, L., Borghini, A., and Ansermet, F. (2004). Prematurity, maternal stress and mother-child interactions. *Early human Development,, 79*, 145-158.

Newton, R. W., Webster, P. A., Binu, P. S., Maskrey, N., and Phillips, A. B. (1979). Psychosocial stress in pregnancy and its relation to the onset of premature labour. *British Medical Journal, 18*, 411-413.

Nordhov, S.M., Kaaresen, P.I., Ronning, J.A., Ulvund, S.E., and Dahl, L.B. (2010). A randomized study of the impact of a sensitizing intervention on the child-rearing attitudes of parents of low birth weight preterm infants. *Scandinavian Journal of Psychology, 51*(5), 385-391.

Nordhov, S.M., Ronning, J.A., Dahl, L.B., Ulvund, S.E., Tunby, J., and Kaarensen, P.I. (2010). Early intervention improves cognitive outcomes for preterm infants: randomized controlled trial. *Pediatrics, 126*(5), 1088-1094.

Nordhov, S.M., Ronning, J.A., Ulvund, S.E., et al. (2012). Early intervention improves behavioral outcomes for preterm infants: randomized controlled trial. *Pediatrics, 129*(1), 9-16.

Ohgi, S., Fukuda, M., Moriuchi, H., Kusumoto, T., Akiyama, T., Nugent, K., Brazelton, B., Arisawa, K., Takahashi, T. and Saitoh, H. (2002). Comparison of kangaroo care and standard care: Behavioral organization, development, and temperament in healthy, low-birth-weight infants through 1 year. *Journal of Perinatology, 22,* 374-379.

Olshtain-Mann, O. and Auslander, G. (2008). Parents of preterm infants two months after discharge from the hospital: Are they still at (parental) risk? *Health and Social Work*, *33*, (4), 299-308.

Omer, H., Friedlander, D., and Palti, Z. (1986a). Life stresses and premature labor: real connection or artifactual findings. *Psychosomatic Medicine, 48,* 5, 362-369.

Pearce, B. D., Grove, J., Bonney, E. A., Bliwise, N., Dudley, D. J., Schendel, D. E., and Thorsen, P. (2010). Interrelationship of cytokines, hypothalamic-pituitary-adrenal axis hormones, and psychosocial variables in the prediction of preterm birth. *Gynecologic and Obstetric Investigation, 70,* 40-46.

Pederson, D. R., and Moran, G. (1996). Expressions of the attachment relationship outside of the strange situation. *Child Development, 67*(3), 915-927.

Plunkett, J. W., Meisels, S. J., Stiefel, G. S., Pasick, P. L., and Roloff, D. W. (1986). Patterns of attachment among preterm infants of varying biological risk. *Journal of the American Academy of Child and Adolescent Psychiatry, 25*(6), 794-800.

Poehlmann, J., and Fiese, B. H. (2001). The interaction of maternal and infant vulnerabilities on developing attachment relationships. *Development and Psychopathology, 13*(1), 1-11.

Redshaw, M. E. (1997). Mothers of babies requiring special care: Attitudes and experiences. *Journal of Reproductive and Infant Psychology*, 15, 109–120.

Robison, L. D. (2003). An organizational guide for an effective developmental program in the NICU. *Journal of Obstetric, Gynecologic, and Neonatal Nursing, 32*(3), 379-386.

Robson, A. L. (1997). Low birth weight and parenting stress during early childhood. *Journal of Pediatric Psychology, 22,* 297–311.

Rode, S., Chang, P., Fisch, R. O., and Sroufe, L. A. (1981). Attachment patterns of infants separated at birth. *Developmental Psychology,* 17(2), 188-191.

Rutter, M. (1991). Protective Factors - Independent or Interactive. *Journal of the American Academy of Child and Adolescent Psychiatry, 30*(1), 151-152.

Sajaniemi, N., Hakamies-Blomqvist, L., Mäkelä, J., Avellan, A., Rita, H., and von Wendt, L. (2001). Cognitive development, temperament and behavior at 2 years as indicative of language development at 4 years in pre-term infants. *Child Psychiatry and Human Development, 31,* 329–346.

Sameroff, A., and Fiese, B. (2000). Transactional regulation and early intervention. In S. Meisels and J. Shonkoff (Eds.), *Handbook of Early Childhood Intervention.* (pp. 135-160). Cambridge: Cambridge University Press.

Sandén Eriksson, B., and Pehrsson, G. (2002). Evaluation of psycho-social support to parent with an infant born preterm. *Journal of Child Health Care, 6*(1), 19—33.

Sandman, C. A., Wadhwa, P. D., Chicz-DeMet, A., Dunkel-Schetter, C., and Porto, M. (1997). Maternal stress, HPA activity, and fetal/infant outcome. *Annals of the New York Academy of Sciences, 24*, 266-275.

Schermann-Eizirik, B., Hagekull, G., Bohlin, K., Persson, G., and Sedin, G. (1997). Interaction between mothers and infants born at risk during the first six months of corrected age. *Acta paediatrica*, *86*(8), 864-872.

Schmucker, G., Heinz-Bisch, K., Kohntop, B., Betzler, S., Osterle, M., Pohlandt, F., et al. (2005). The influence of prematurity, maternal anxiety, and infants' neurobiological risk on mother–infant interactions. *Infant Mental Health Journal*, *26*(5), 423–441.

Shankaran, S., Fanaroff, A. A., Wright, L. L, et al. (2002) Risk factors for early death among extremely low birth-weight infants. *American Journal of Obstetrics and Gynecology, 186*, 796–802.

Singer, L., Davillier, M., Bruening, P., Hawkins, S., and Yamashita, T. (1996). Social support, psychological distress, and parenting strains in mothers of very low birthright infants. *Family Relations,* 45, 343–350.

Singer, L. T., Fulton, S., Davillier, M., Koshy, D., Salvator, A., and Baley, J. E. (2003). Effects on infant risk status and maternal psychological distress on maternal–infant interactions during the first year of life. *Journal of Developmental and Behavioral Pediatrics*, *24*(4), 233–241.

Singer, L. T., Salvator, A., Guo, S., Collin, M., Lilien, L., and Baley, J. (1999). Maternal psychological distress and parenting stress after the birth of a very low-birth-weight infant. *Journal of the American Medical Association*, *281*, 799–805.

Sizun, J., Ansquer, H., Browne, J. et al. (2002). Developmental care decreases physiologic and behavioral pain expression in preterm neonates. *Journal of Pain, 3*, 446-50.

Sparrow, J. D., and Brazelton,, T. B. (2008). A Developmental Approach to the Prevention of Common Behavioral Problems. In: McInerny TK, Adam HM, Campbell DE, Kamat DM, Kelleher KJ, editors. *American Academy of Pediatrics Textbook of Pediatric Care* 1st Ed. Elk Grove Village, IL: American Academy of Pediatrics.

Sparrow, J. D. (2010a). Aligning Systems of Care with the Relational Imperative of Development: Building Community through Collaborative Consultation. In: Lester B, Sparrow JD, editors. *Nurturing Young Children and Their Families: Building on the Legacy of T.B. Brazelton.* Oxford: Wiley-Blackwell Scientific.

Sparrow, J. D. (2010b). Improving Healthcare Service Delivery Systems and Outcomes with Relationship-based Nursing Practices In: Lester B, Sparrow JD, editors. *Nurturing Young Children and Their Families: Building on the Legacy of T.B. Brazelton.* Oxford: Wiley-Blackwell Scientific.

Spiker, D., Ferguson, J., and Brooks-Gunn, J. (1993). Enhancing maternal interactive behavior and child social competence in low birth weight, premature infants. *Child Development, 64,* 754–768.

Sroufe, L. A. (1996). Emotional development: The organization of emotional life in the early years. Cambridge: *Cambridge Studies in Social and Emotional World.*

Stadtler, A.C., Novak, J.C., and Sparrow, J.D. (2010). Improving Healthcare Service Delivery Systems and Outcomes with Relationship-based Nursing Practices In: Lester B, Sparrow JD, editors. *Nurturing Young Children and Their Families: Building on the Legacy of T.B. Brazelton.* Oxford: Wiley-Blackwell Scientific.

Stern, D. (1977). *The first relationship.* Cambridge, MA: Harvard University Press.

Stewart, A. L., Rifkin, L., Maess, P. N., and Kirkbride, V. (1999). Brain structure and neurocognitive and behavioural function in adolescents who were born very preterm. *Lancet, 353,* 1653–1657.

Swartz, M.K. (2005). Parenting preterm infants: A metasynthesis. *MCN: The American Journal of Maternal Child Nursing*, 30, 115–120.

Talmi, A. and Harmon, R. (2003). Relationships between preterm infants and their parents: disruption and development. *Zero to three,* 24(2), 13-20.

Talmi, A., and Harmon, R. J. (2003). Relationships between preterm infants and their parents disruption and development. *Zero to Three, 24*(2), 13-20.

Teichmann, A., and Breull, A. (1989). Ein neues Konzept psychosomatischer Forschung am Beispiel der vorzeitigen Wehentatigkeit. *Zeitschrift fur Psychosomatische Medizin,35,* 256-276.

Tessier, R., Cristo, M., Velez, S., Giron, M., Calume, Z., Ruiz-Palaez, J., Charpak, Y. and Charpak, N. (1998). Kangaroo mother care and the bonding hypothesis. *Pediatrics,* 102(2):e17.

Tronick, E. Z., and Cohn, J. F. (1989). Infant-mother face-to-face interaction: Age and gender differences in coordination and the occurrence of miscoordination. *Child Development, 60*, 85-92.

Tronick, E. Z., Ricks, M., and Cohn, J. F. (1982). Maternal and infant affective exchanges: Patterns of adaptation. In T. Field and A. Fogel (Eds.), *Emotion and interaction: Normal and high-risk infants* (pp. 83-100). Hillsdale, NJ: Erlbaum.

Tronick, E., Als, H., Adamson, L., Wise, S., and Brazelton, T. B. (1978). The infant's response to entrapment between contradictory messages in face-to-face interaction. *American Academy of Child Psychiatry, 17,* 1-13.

van Baar, A. L., vanWassenaer, A. G., Briet, J. M., Dekker, F.W., and Kok, J. H. (2005). Very preterm birth is associated with disabilities in multiple developmental domains. *Journal of Pediatric Psychology*, *30*, 247–255.

van Beek, Y., Hopkins, B., and Hoeksma, J. B. (1994). Development of communicative behaviors in preterm infants: The effects of birthweight status and gestational age. *Infant Behavior and Development*, *17*, 107–117.

van Beek, Y., Hopkins, B., Hoeksma, J. B., and Samsom, J. F. (1994). Prematurity, posture and the development of looking behavior during early communication. *Journal of Child Psychology and Psychiatry, 35*, 1093–1107.

van den Boom, D. (1994). The influence of temperament and mothering on attachment and exploration: An experimental manipulation of sensitive responsiveness among lower-class mothers with irritable infants. *Child Development, 65*, 1457-1477.

van IJzendoorn, M., Bakermans-Kranenburg, M. J., and Juffer, F. (2005). Why Less is More: From the Dodo Bird Verdict To Evidence-Based Interventions on Sensitivity and Early Attachment. In Berlin, L. J., Ziv, Y., Amaya-Jackson, Greenberg, M. *Enhancing Early Attachments - Theory, Research, Intervention and Policy*. (pp. 297-312). New York: Guilford.

Vanderveen, J. A., Bassler, D., Robertson, C. M., and Kirpalani, H. (2009). Early interventions involving parents to improve neurodevelopmental outcomes ofpremature infants: A meta-analysis. *Journal of Perinatology, 29*, 343–351.

Waber, D. P., and McCormick, M. C. (1995). Late neuropsychological outcomes in preterm infants of normal IQ: Selective vulnerability of the visual system. *Journal of Pediatric Psychology, 20,* 721–735.

Wadhwa, P. D., Sandman, C. A., Porto, M., Dunkel-Schetter, C., and Garite, T. J. (1993). The associations between prenatal stress and infant birth weight and gestational age at birth: a prospective investigation. *American Journal of Obstetrics and Gynecology, 169, 4*, 858-865.

Weisglas-Kuperus, N., Koot, H. M., Baerts, W., Fetter, W. P. F., and Sauer, P. J. J. (1993). Behavioral problems of very low-birthweight children. *Developmental Medicine and Child Neurology, 35,* 406–416.

Widmayer, S., and Field, T. (1980). Effects of Brazelton demonstrations on early interaction of preterm infants and their teenage mothers. *Infant Behavior and Development, 3*, 79-89.

Widmayer, S., and Field, T. (1981). Effects of Brazelton demonstrations for mothers on the development of preterm infants. *Pediatrics, 67,* 711-714.

Wille, D. E. (1991). Relation of preterm birth with quality of mother-infant attachment at one year. *Infant Behavior and Development, 14*, 227-240.

Wolke, D., Ratschinski, G., Orth, B., and Riegel, K. (1994). The cognitive outcome of very preterm infants may be poorer than often reported: An empirical investigation of how methodological issues make a big difference. *European Journal of Pediatrics, 153,* 906–915.

Zeanah, C. H. and Benoit, D. (1995). Clinical applications of a parent perception interview in infant mental health. *Child and Adolescent Psychiatric Clinic of North America*, 4, 539-554.

Zeanah, C. H., Benoit, D., Hirshberg, L., Barton, M. L., and Regan, C. (1994). Mothers′ representations of their infants are concordant with infant attachment classifications. *Developmental Issues in Psychiatry and Psychology, 1*, 1-14.

Zeanah, C. H., Boris, N. W., and Larrieu, J. A. (1997). Infant development and developmental risk: a review of the past 10 years. *Journal of American Academy of Child and Adolescent Psychiatry, 36*(2), 165-178.

In: Preterm Infants
Editors: Diogo Contreiras and Johann Sampaio

ISBN 978-1-62081-819-0

Chapter 6

EFFECT OF ADDITIONAL WEIGHT IN PROXIMAL AND DISTAL ADJUSTMENTS OF REACHING BEHAVIOR IN PRETERM INFANTS

***Aline M. Toledo**[*,1] **and Eloísa Tudella**[†,2]*
[1]Federal University of Mato Grosso do Sul, Brazil
[2]Federal University of São Carlos, São Paulo, Brazil

ABSTRACT

The use of additional weight on infant's voluntary motor skills has been a strategy used to examine how infants adjust their movements when submitted to context manipulations. The evaluation of these issues in a population at risk, such as premature infants, is extremely important since there are significant differences in their motor behavior when compared to full-term infants. Thus, the aim of this chapter was to assess the effects of additional weight on proximal and distal adjustments of the reaching behavior and whether additional weight can be use to facilitate manual reaching.

1. INTRODUCTION

The works of Thelen in the early 80's pioneered in demonstrating that changes in motor development are determined by the interaction between intrinsic and extrinsic constraints to the body (Thelen and Fisher, 1982, Thelen et al., 1983, 1984). Since then, several studies have investigated how the actions of infants adapt to changes in information provided by the external environment (Carvalho, et al., 2008; Fagard, et al., 2009; Heathcock, et al. 2008; Rochat, 1992; Van Wermeskerken et al., 2011).

Clinically, this approach allows designing intervention strategies aimed at modifying movement patterns in the attempt to facilitate their movements.

* E_mail: toledo_am@yahoo.com.br.
† E_mail: tudella@terra.com.

Studies in this context are based on the assumption that to learn to control their movements, infants should perceive the dynamic information available in the context of the movement and adapt to such conditions (Ulrich, et al., 1997). Several constraints are used in different motor skills of infants. Among them, additional weight stands out. Excess weight has important clinical relevance, since it contributes to the understanding of the complex adaptability of the infant against environmental influences, in addition to its therapeutic applicability and easy replication. The use of additional weight has been explored in various motor skills such as kicking (Chen et al., 2002; Vaal et al. 2002; Landgraf and Tudella, 2008), gaiting (Adolph and Avolio, 2000) fidgety movements (low-amplitude circular movements observed in the limbs) (Dibiase and Einspieler, 2004), and reaching (Rocha, et al., 2009; Van der Fits and Hadders-Algra, 1998; Out, et al., 1997; Toledo, 2011).

Studies assessing the influence of weight on the reaching behavior have been developed in our laboratory - NENEM (Center for Studies in Neuropediatrics and Human Movement) - since 2005. Due to the fact that manual reaching is a skill dependent on the integrity of the proprioceptive system which is influenced by the presence of weight perceived by weight receptors that monitor the gravity effects on the body segments (Massion, 1999), it is believed that weight can be a factor that influences the reaching movements. These studies we will be discussed a little more later on this work.

Besides the use of weight, studied have been also aimed at investigating how risk populations behave under different manipulations. The groups most commonly studied are: Down syndrome (Ulrich, et al., 1997), brain lesions (Kuhtz-Buschbeck, et al., 2003; Van der Heide, et al., 2004) and prematurity (Toledo and Tudella, 2008; Toledo, Soares and Tudella, 2011; Fallang, et al., 2003). The interest in the study of prematurity has increased recently due to high survival rate of this population and the high risk of presenting delays in motor development. Several studies have shown that preterm infants present changes when compared to full-term infants in relation to postural control (Van der Fits, et al., 1999; Van der Heide, et al., 2004; Fallang, et al, 2003), kicking movements (Jeng, Chen and Yau, 2002; Piek and Gasson, 1999; Fetters, et al., 2004), head control, sucking, muscle tone (Howard, et al., 1976) and manual reaching (Toledo and Tudella, 2008). In relation to manual skills, it has been found that the quality of the reaching movement is lower for preterm infants when compared to full-term infants (Plantinga, Perdock and de Groot, 1997; Gorga et al., 1988). Prematurity, more specifically with regard to the manual reaching, will also be detailed in the following subtopics.

Given the above, our research group believes that by verifying the effect of additional weight on the early reaching behavior, novel decisions may be made in the physiotherapy Intervention and in the guidance for parents of infants at risk, especially those born prematurely. Thus, this chapter aims to present the study "Using the additional weight in the proximal and distal adjustments of the manual reaching of premature infants", which proposed to assess the effects of additional weight on the proximal and distal adjustments of the manual reaching.

To this end, a brief review of studies that used additional weight in different motor skills, as well as a study on the influence of additional weight on the proximal and distal adjustments of the manual reaching will be presented. Finally, the chapter will present a brief approach on the therapeutic use of additional weight.

1.1. Use of the Additional Weight in Different Motor Abilities

Additional weight has been attached to the upper and lower limbs during the performance of different motor skills of healthy and risk infants. Despite the growing scientific interest, there is still no consensus in literature concerning the actual effect of additional weight in motor skills, since different objectives, methods, amount of weight and variables are used in each study. However, the results of these studies have important clinical relevance and should be considered in practice since the objectives of each study and the therapeutic goal specifically of physiotherapy and occupational therapy are considered.

Some studies using additional weight in the lower limbs of full-term infants showed changes in the frequency of kicking movements with the use of weight observed by the increased frequency of kicks in the leg without weight and decreased frequency in the leg with weight (Thelen, et al., 1987; Chen, et al, 2002; Vaal et al, 2000). Thelen, Kelso and Skalla (1987) inferred that the weight disturbance may have increased levels of neural activation observed by the change in kicking frequency and the in the speed and amplitude in the movement of the leg without weight.

Chen et al. (2002) attributed the learning of kicks in full-term infants to the proprioceptive information provided by the weight. Similarly, Ulrich et al. (1997) found a synergy in the frequency between limbs with and without weight, demonstrating that typical full-term infants and those with Down syndrome are able to respond to the information from the weight.

Also with respect to the lower limbs, Vaal, et al. (2002) questioned whether the use of unilateral weight on the lower limb would affect the kinematic parameters of the kicking movements in children with and without ventricular leukomalacia, with 26 weeks of corrected age. Their results showed no statistically significant difference in any of the groups in relation to the influence of weight. Thus, the authors suggested that the corticospinal influences are not involved in the regulation of the kinematic parameters.

Infants with and without Down syndrome have also been investigated in order to assess the bilateral sensitivity threshold to the increase of unilateral weight to the lower limb. Ulrich, et al. (1997) used weights corresponding to 25%, 50% and 100% the mass of the lower limb and verified that 100% of infants in both groups showed increased level of activity of the leg without weight when compared with the leg with weight. By comparing the sensitivity threshold between groups, it was found that infants with Down syndrome showed less adaptation to weight disturbances.

The study by Landgraf and Tudella developed at the NENEM in 2008 showed that adding weight to the lower limbs of infants at ages of 1 and 2 months corresponding to 1/10 the mass of the lower limb increased the kicking frequency. Furthermore, the weight corresponding to 1/3 the mass of the lower limb caused a decrease in the contact of the foot to the panel to activate the mobile at the age of 1 month and increased this contact at the age of two months. The authors concluded that the spontaneous kicking of infants aged between one and two months are influenced by the increased proprioception caused by additional weight. In 2011, in order to verify the influence of additional weight in the kinematic parameters of kicking in healthy infants during the first 4 months of life, Landgraf observed that the weight of 1/10 and 1/3 the mass of the lower limb did not change these parameters. However, in both conditions, a decreased contact of the feet to the panel was observed. The author concluded that when weight was added, infants observed the change that occurred and tried to keep the kicking pattern in a way not to change the kinematic variables. Figure 1 shows the experimental design of the aforementioned studies.

Dibiase and Einspieler (2004) in a longitudinal study with infants aged 3 to 5 months stimulated the proprioceptive system through the use of weight on the lower and upper limbs in order to study the effect of weight on the fidgety movements (low-amplitude circular movements observed in the limbs). The authors reported that the neural mechanisms responsible for the fidgety movements are not influenced by mechanical properties, such as additional weight.

With regard to the manual reaching, which topic is highlighted in this chapter, studies have found interesting findings. Out et al. (1997), investigated the influence of weight of the manual reaching of infants aged 3-5 months and concluded that the movement speed was greater and the number of reaching movement units was lower when adding weight corresponding to 20 % the mass of the upper limb, i.e., the movement became faster and with less acceleration and deceleration during the trajectory of the arm to touch the object.

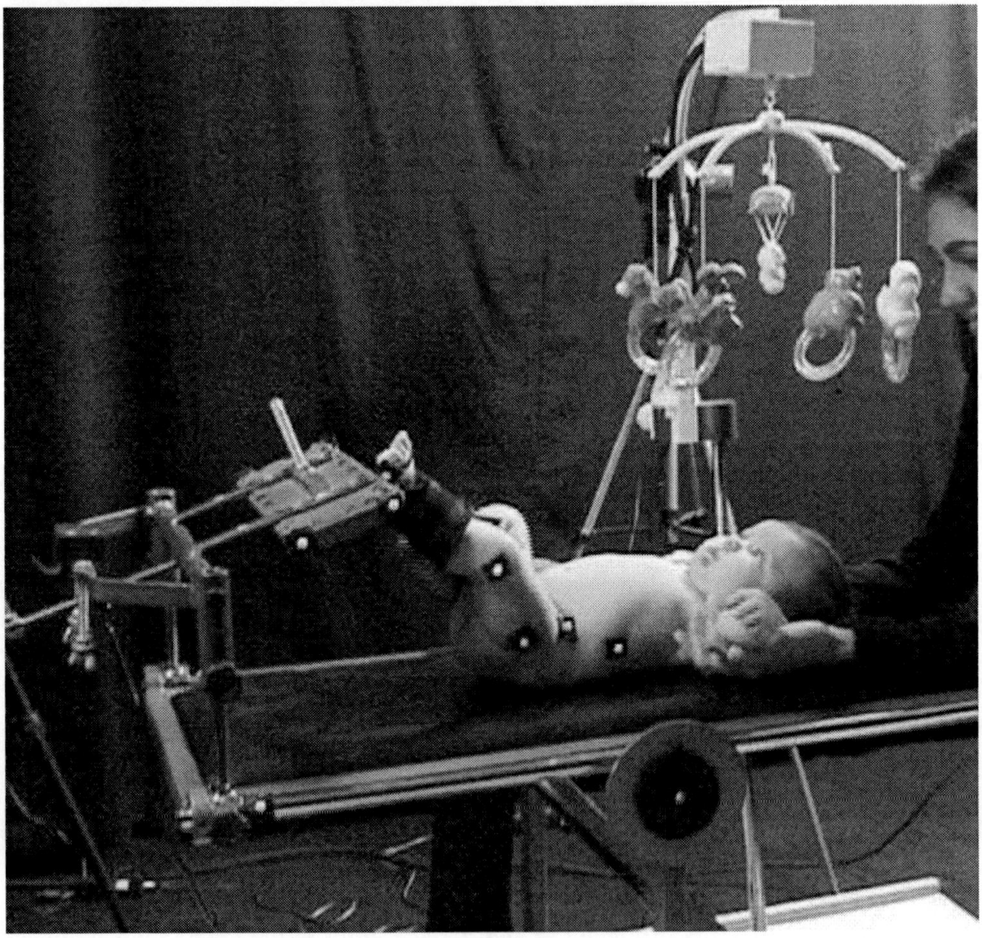

Figure 1. Positioning of the infant in the experimental condition with the use of weight corresponding to 1/3 the mass of the lower limb.

On the other hand, Van der Fits and Hadders-Algra (1998) found that the average speed of the upper limb during the reaching movement did not change by adding weight of 56 grams to the wrists of infants.

The NENEM has developed some studies assessing the influence of weight on the reaching movement of both typical infants and infants at risk. Rocha et al. (2009) assessed the influence of weight corresponding to 10% the mass of the upper limb on the qualitative characteristics typical of the reaching movement of infants aged 4-6 months. The authors found that the weight did not influence the variables related to the proximal and distal adjustments of the reaching movements; however, it caused a better coupling between the upper limbs, reducing the time between hands in bimanual reaches. In the study of Toledo (2011), it was found that adding weight corresponding to 20% the mass of the upper limb influenced the kinematic variables of the reaching movements in preterm infants aged 5-7 months. It was also observed that the addition of weight increased the average speed, decreased the movement units and decreased the successful grasping. The author inferred that the systems Involved in the reaching movements of preterm infants aged 5-7 months are likely to undergo changes due to weight disturbances.

In the next topic, the study conducted at the NENEM will be explored in order to verify how proximal and distal adjustments of the manual reaching behave against the disturbance caused by additional weight corresponding to 20% the mass of the upper limb of preterm and full-term infants. The methodology of this study is the same used in the study of Toledo, Soares and Tudella (2011). In this study, was added, however, the second procedure in which a additional weight was placed on the wrist of infants.

2. Use of the Additional Weight in Proximal and Distal Adjustments of Reaching Behavior in Preterm Infants

The accuracy in reaching for and grasping objects is known to require the performance of both proximal (uni or bimanual movements) and distal (hand orientation, hand opening) adjustments (Fagard, 2000). According to Fagard (2005), fluctuations in the choice of one-handed versus two-handed reaching have often been observed in full-term infants and reflect the variability inherent to the infant's motor behavior. The frequency of bimanual reaching is relatively high around 3-4 months of age, decreases around 5-6 months of age, and increases again around the end of the first year (Fagard and Peze, 1997). Regarding the distal adjustments, reaching movements are initially horizontally oriented and vertical orientation is elicited at about 5 months. Studies have demonstrated that hand opening is directly related to object properties. Von Hofsten and Rönnqvist (1988) showed that 5-6-month-old full-term infants closed their hands around the target before touching it, thus controlling their grasping actions visually according to the object size.

In preterm infants, the acquisition of reaching and grasping may be affected by a disturbed muscle tone regulation, which is a transient alteration typical of these infants. This alteration affects the axial muscles and may result in hyperextension of neck and trunk. Studies have demonstrated that the lack of postural control caused by the hyperextension of trunk may interfere with the development of arm and hand function (Plantinga, et al., 1997), as well as with the emergence of successful reaching (Van Beek, et al., 1994). According to

Plantinga et al. (1997), some qualitative variables of hand function, such as voluntary pronation and supination, were less satisfactory for pre-term infants when compared to full-term ones.

The study of Toledo, Soares and Tudella (2011) found that in the period of 5-7 months of age, both groups of preterm and full-term infants showed a higher frequency of unimanual reaching, increased hand vertically oriented and open hand, and higher frequency of reaching with grasp over the months. Furthermore, it was found that preterm infants had higher frequency of open hand than full-term infants, which may be partially explained by the low muscle tone present in preterm infants.

Despite the knowledge on how proximal and distal adjustments occur in preterm infants, it is important to investigate how they behave against context manipulations, since their intrinsic dynamics seems to be different from typical infants. The use of additional weight can be an important tool to determine how preterm infants adjust their movements to carry out reaching movements.

When a weight is added to the limbs of infants, they apply countervailing forces that oscillate the arms during the reaching movements. These movements may be sufficient to stimulate mechanoreceptors to detect the additional weight (Meer et al., 1996). In turn, proprioceptive information is necessary for the spatial direction of movement during changes of external weights on the upper limb (Feldman and Levin, 1995). Thus, as additional weight can add mechanical and proprioceptive information, it becomes an interesting tool to investigate the adaptability of the sensorimotor system against external disturbances.

Thus, the objective of this study was to investigate how proximal and distal adjustments behave under the disturbance of additional weight in low-risk preterm infants from 5 to 7 months of corrected age. The results may facilitate the understanding on how the sensorimotor system of typical infants adjusts to changes of external weights on the upper limbs.

2.1. Procedures and Methods

The study included 9 preterm infants, with a mean gestational age of 35.6 (± 0.5) weeks. Ten fullterm infants with a mean gestational age of 39 (± 0.73) weeks participated as control. The infants were evaluated longitudinally, in the age group of 5 to 7 months. The age was correct for prematurity for the preterm infants. The evaluations coincided with the birth date, with a tolerance of ± 5 days of the scheduled age. Both groups had adequate birth weight and Apgar score above 7 in the first and fifth minutes.

At the beginning of each evaluation, the following anthropometric measurements were assessed: body weight (grams), length (cm), arm length (distance from the acromion to the elbow joint line, in cm) and forearm (distance from the elbow joint line to the wrist, in cm), circumference of the arm and forearm proximal third (in centimeters) and hand width (transverse distance between the second and fifth metacarpal joints, in cm). These measures were used to estimate the total mass of each upper limb using the regression equation by Schneider and Zernicke (1992). The result was used to calculate the weight of 20% the total upper limb mass in each month.

After measurement of the upper limbs, the infants were placed in a baby chair with back support reclined 50° from the horizontal plane (Von Hofsten, 1984; Toledo et al., 2011). The back support had enough height to promote the headrest. A strap of 15.0 cm wide was fastened to the infant's trunk in order to provide truncal stability, while allowing freedom of movement to the upper and lower limbs. An initial 5-minute period was allowed for the infants to adapt to the position. An attractive soft rubber object, 5.0 cm diameter x 10.0 cm height, unfamiliar to the infants, was used to elicit reaching movements. The object was held by the experimenter, who was positioned in front and out of the infant's reaching distance, and was presented for 2 minutes at the infant's midline, shoulder height and arm length (Toledo et al. 2011; Van Der Fits, et al., 1999; Corbetta, et al.,, 2000). During this period, the object was taken away carefully and presented again after each reach, and a 5-second interval was allowed between reaches. Thus, the total number of trials depended on the infant. The infants remained in an either inactive or active alert state throughout the experiment (Prechtl & Beintema, 1964). The experiments were recorded by five digital cameras. One of them was positioned posterosuperiorly to the chair in a way that the infant's arms were entirely visible throughout the reaching movement. The other four cameras, two of them positioned anterolaterally (each on one of the sides) and two positioned posterolaterally (each on one of the sides) to the chair, were used in order to clarify doubts related to the visualization of the variables studied (Toledo et al., 2011)

The infants were evaluated in two experimental conditions:

a) Procedure 1 (P1): the object was shown by the examiner, who was positioned in front and out of the infant's reaching distance, during 2 minutes at the infant's midline, shoulder height, and arm length (Toledo & Tudella, 2008; Toledo et al., 2011). After reach, the object was carefully removed (or caught) and shown again in order to elicit a new reaching movement, with an interval between them of approximately 5 seconds. Thus, the total number of reaches depended on the infant.
b) Procedure 2 (P2) - Additional Weight: The experimental conditions of this procedure were similar to Procedure 1; however, a bracelet with weight corresponding to 20% the total mass of the infant's upper limb was added to both wrists. This percentage was obtained by regression equation (Schneider & Zernicke, 1992). The mean weight of the bracelet was 78,56 (± 8,4) grams in the preterm and 80,43 (± 8.2) grams in fullterm group.

System of Analysis

The images were picked up by an image capture board. Adobe Premier 6.3 was used to obtain files in AVI format. The files were opened in the Dvideow 5.0 image analysis system (Barros, et al., 1999), which was used for identifying, frame by frame, the beginning and the end of the reaches.

A reaching movement was considered as the hand movement towards the object resulting in touching it, whether or not followed by grasping. The beginning of a reach was defined as the first frame when the infant's arm began an uninterrupted movement towards the object. The end of a reach was defined as the first frame when the infant's hand touched the object (Toledo, Soares e Tudella, 2011; Thelen, et al., 1996; Fallang et al., 2000; Carvalho, et al., 2007).

Description of Variables and Measurements

Proximal Adjustments

The adjustment was considered *unimanual* when the infant moved only one hand towards the object managing to touch it (Cobertta et al. , 2000) or when both hands were moved from the initial position with a difference of more than 20 frames (7.2 ms) between them and also managing to touch the object (Toledo et al. , 2011) (Figure 2a).

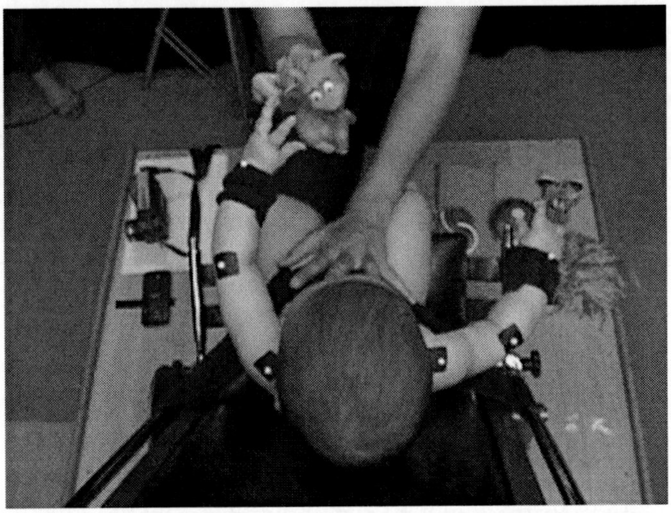

a

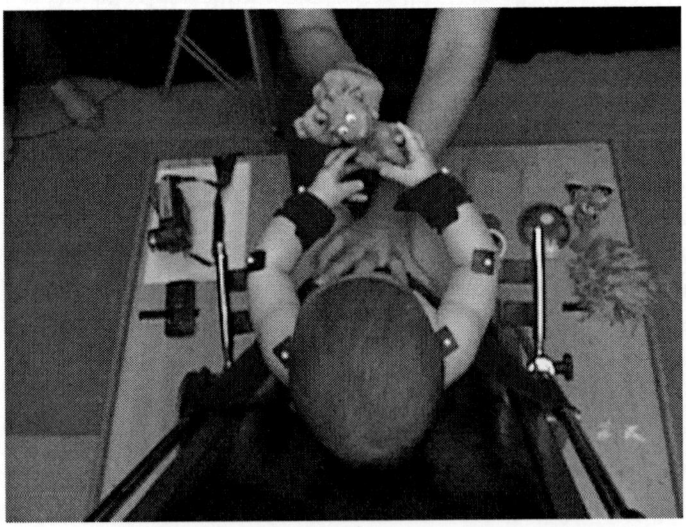

b

Figure 2. Proximal Adjusments: (a) Unimanual reaching; (b) bimanual reaching.

The adjustment was considered as *bimanual* when the infant moved both hands simultaneously towards the object and touched it (Cobertta et al., 2000), or when both hands were moved from the initial position with a difference of less than or equal to 20 frames between them and managing to touch the object (Toledo et al., 2011) (Figure 2b). In this case, hands should move simultaneously for at least 50% of the movement arch (i.e. 50% of the trajectory), and the object could be touched with both hands at the same time or initially with only one of them (Cobertta et al., 2000; Toledo et al, 2011).

Distal Adjustments

Distal adjustments were analyzed at the end of the reaching movement, that is, when the infant touched the object.

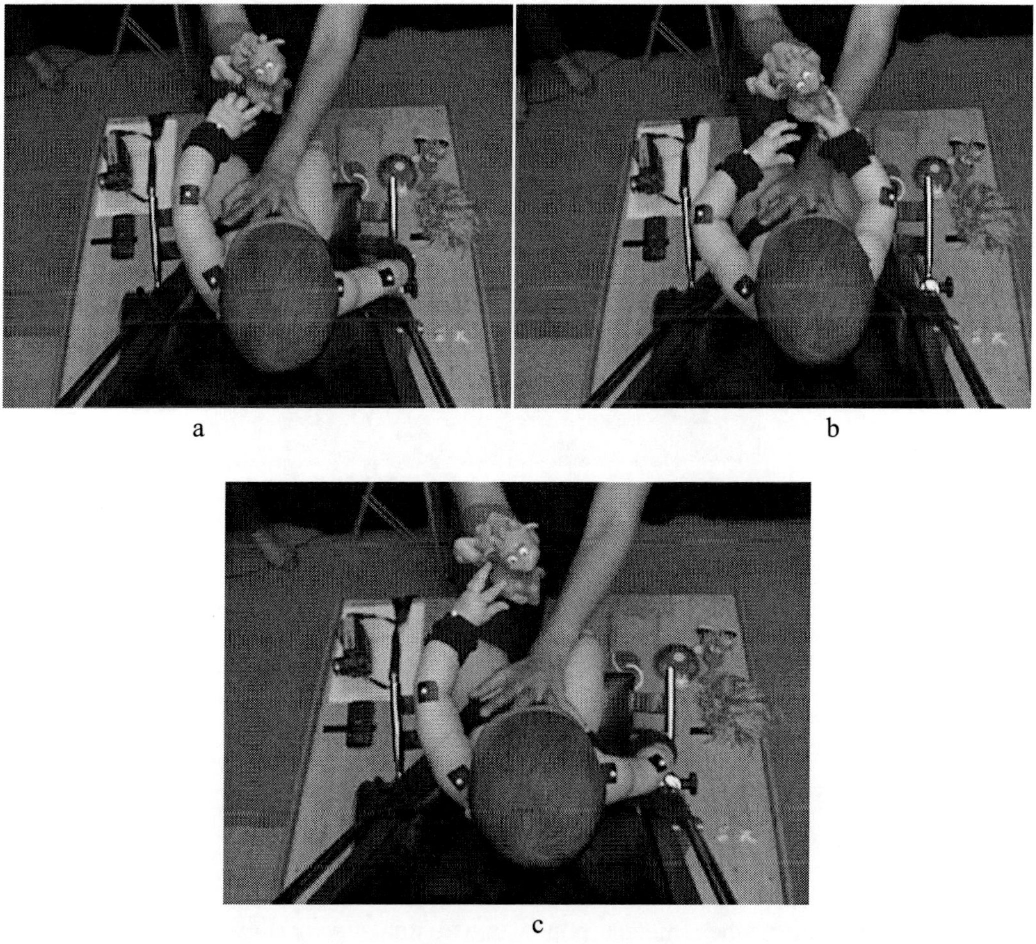

Figure 3. Hand orientation: (a) horizontal hand; (b) vertical hand; (c) oblique hand.

Hand orientation was coded as:

a) horizontal – when the palm of the hand was faced downwards (Figure 3a);
b) vertical – when the palm of the hand was oriented towards the infant's midline (neutral position) (Figure 3b)
c) oblique – when the hand was in an intermediary position in relation to the two aforementioned positions (Figure 3c).

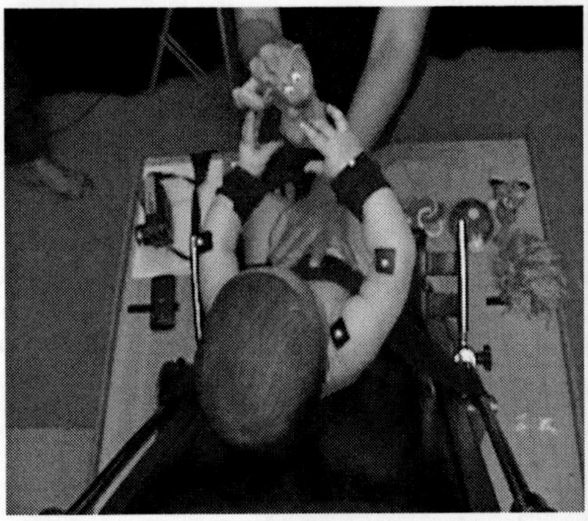

a

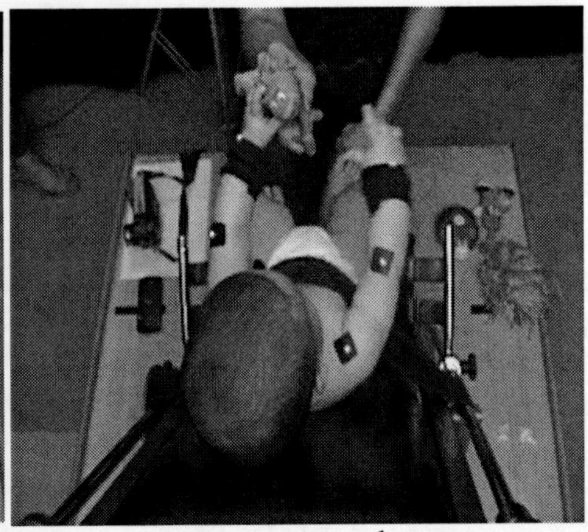

b

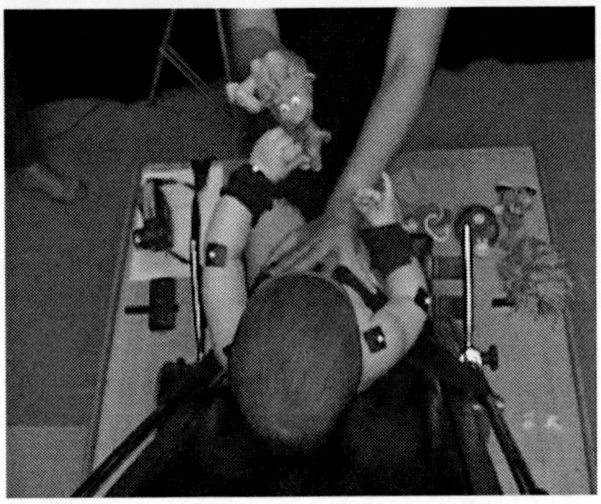

c

Figure 4. Hand opening: (a) open hand, (b) closed hand, (c) semi-open hand.

Hand opening was coded as:

a) open - when metacarpophalangeal and interphalangeal joints were fully extended (Figure 4a);
b) closed - when metacarpophalangeal and interphalangeal joints were fully flexed (Figure 4b);
c) semi-open - when metacarpophalangeal joints were flexed (regardless of the degree of flexion) and interphalangeal joints were extended, or when metacarpophalanges were extended and interphalanges were flexed (regardless of thc degree of flexion) (Figure 4c).

Data Analysis

The Statistical Package for Social Sciences (SPSS, Version 10.0) was used for statistical analysis. A significance level of $p \leq 0.05$ was used for all analyses. The variables were analyzed by frequencies of their occurrence. Data were analyzed using the chi-square test (χ^2) and frequency tables were used to verify the existence of association between variables. The significance (α) was set at 5% ($p<0.05$).

3. RESULTS

Overall, 1071 reaches were collected, from these, 931 were analyzed and 140 were excluded. The reaching frequency analyzed in each group, as well as those excluded from the analyses, is shown in Table 1.

Table 1. Number of reaches analyzed and excluded in each group and each procedure

Group	Reaches analyzed		Reaches excluded	
	P1	P2	P1	P2
Preterm	231	224	42	32
Full-term	229	247	36	30
Total	460	471	78	62

Proximal Adjustments

It was found that at 5 and 7 months and in the preterm group, there was a increased frequency of unimanuall reaches ((x2 (2)=8.0418; p=0.0179) ; (x2 (2)=8.1861; p=0.0167)) in the procedure 2, respectively (Table 2). There was no influence of weight on the proximal adjustments of full-term infants in the age group analyzed.

Table 2. Frequency (%) of the uni and bimanual reaches in each procedure in each age

Group	5 months				6 months				7 months			
	Uni		Bi		Uni		Bi		Uni		Bi	
	P1	P2	P1	P2	P1	P2	P1	P2	P1	P2	P1	P2
Preterm	78.4	89.7	21.6	10.3	96.9	97.4	3.1	2.6	82.8	92.3	17.2	7.7
Full-term	84.7	86.0	15.3	14.0	81.6	89.6	18.4	10.4	92.1	91.8	7.9	8.2

Distal Adjustments

In the preterm group, the addition of weight decreased the frequency of open hand in preterm infants at 6 months of age (x2 (2) = 45.5740, p <0.0001) and 7 (x2 (2) = 38.6596, p <0.0001) (Table 3). For the full-term group, there was an decreased frequency of reaches with vertical-oriented hand movement at 5 (x2 (4)=12.9732; p=0.0114), decreased frequency of reaches with vertical-oriented hand movement and increased frequency of reaches with horizontal-oriented hand movement at 7 (x2 (2)=28.2144; p <0.0001) months (Table 4); there was decreased frequency of open hand at 6 (x2 (2)=7.1996; p=0.0273) and 7 (x2 (2)=7.7400; p=0.0208) months (Table 3).

Em ambos os grupos não foram observados alcances com a mão fechada. Desta forma, não foi apresentado esta categoria na tabela 3.

Table 3. Frequency (%) of the open and semi-open hand in each procedure in each age

Group	5 months				6 months				7 months			
	Open		Semi-Open		Open		Semi-Open		Open		Semi-Open	
	P1	P2	P1	P2	P1	P2	P1	P2	P1	P2	P1	P2
Preterm	10.2	7.6	89.8	92.4	50.7	12.6	49.3	87.4	51.4	16.6	48.6	83.4
Full-term	5.6	11.4	94.4	88.6	6.8	17.2	93.2	82.8	43.4	26.7	56.6	73.3

Table 4. Frequency (%) of the oblique, horizontal and vertical position of the hand in each procedure in each age

Group	5 months						6 months						7 months					
	Oblique		Horizontal		Vertical		Oblique		Horizontal		Vertical		Oblique		Horizontal		Vertical	
	P1	P2	P1	P2	P1	P2	P1	P2	P1	P2	P1	P2	P1	P2	P1	P2	P1	P2
Preterm	76.1	75.6	13.6	19.2	10.3	5.2	72.3	79.7	23	18.9	4.7	1.4	51.4	61.5	15.7	12.8	32.9	25.7
Full-Term	63.8	68.5	23.4	27.2	12.8	4.3	75.8	75.8	14.9	17.2	9.3	7	48.6	68.6	6.5	15.2	44.9	16.2

CONCLUSION

With the presented results it can be stated that a weight of 20% disturbed the reaching of preterm and fullterm infants, in the age of 5 to 7 months.

It can be observed that the weight restricted the reaching movement, because it reduced hand opening in both groups; decreased vertical hand position in fullterm infants and increased unimanual reaching frequencies in preterm ones. It can also be observed that a movement disturbance occurred, considering that along with the reaching development, both the frequency of the hand vertical orientation and hand opening frequency had increased significantly through months, besides the increase in successfully grasping frequencies (Toledo et al., 2011 ; Fagard, 2000). This movement disturbance was also observed in our previous study (Toledo, 2011), in which the additional weight caused an increase in unsuccessfully grasping. This finding may be explained by the fact that an additional weight may have imposed difficulties during reaching movement, because it requires different types of muscle contractions of different muscle groups. In this sense, when performing the elbow extension with a load on the distal forearm, the infant needs to perform an eccentric contraction of the biceps in order to keep the arm extended against gravity, while intrinsic hand muscles and wrist flexors are contracting concentrically (Smith, et al., 1997), in addition to a stabilizing action of flexors and extensors of wrist and hand muscles. We believe that this difficulty may also have affected hand opening.

For the infant adopt finger opening, it is necessary fingers' extensor muscles contraction, and also an adequate control of intrinsic muscles of the hand. However, the weight may have led to an overload on the wrist joint, and thus, some difficulties during the opening of the phalanges during grasping and the reduction of vertical hand position.

Thus, results from categorical variables demonstrate that the additional weight disturbs reaching movements and impose difficulties for infants to achieve their goal, i.e, to grasp the object. However, during clinical decision making process, we must consider other issues such as weight effects on kinematic variables of reaching (for example, mean velocity and movement units). It can be seen in the literature that the weight of 20% of the upper limb mass leads to an increase of the mean velocity and a decreased number of movement units (Out et al., 1997; Toledo, 2011), which leads to a more fluent and faster movement. Therefore, it is important to highlight that the decision of using an additional weight as a therapeutic strategy in preterm infants must be taken based on well-defined therapeutic goals.

REFERENCES

Adolph, K.E.; Avolio, A.M. Walking infants adapt locomotion to changing body dimensions. *Journal Experimental Psychology Human Percept Performance,* v. 26, p. 1148-1166, 2000.

Barros, R. M. L., Brenzikofer, R., Leite, N. J., Figueiroa, P. J. Development and evaluation of a system for three-dimensional kinematic analysis of human movements. *Revista Brasileira de Engenharia Biomédica*, v. 15, p. 79–86, 1999.

Carvalho, R. P., Tudella, E., Caljouw, S. A., & Savelsbergh, G. J. P. Early control of reaching: Effects of experience and body orientation. *Infant Behavior and Development,* 31, 23–33, 2008.

Carvalho, R. P., Tudella, E., Savelsbergh, G. J. P. Spatio-temporal parameters in infant's reaching movements are influenced by body orientation. *Infant Behavior and Development,* v. 30, p. 23–35, 2007.

Chen, Y.P. ; Fetters, L. ; Holt, K.G. ; Saltzman, E. Making the mobile move: constraining task and environment. *Infant Behavior and Development*, v. 25, p. 195-220, 2002.

Corbetta, D.; Thelen, E.; Johnson, K. Motor constraints on the development of perception-action matching in infant reaching. *Infant Behavior and Development,* v.23, p.351-374, 2000.

Dibiasi, J; Einspieler, C. Load perturbation does not influence spontaneous movements in 3-month-old infants. *Early Human Development*, v.77, p. 37-46, 2004.

Fallang, B., Saugstad, O. D., Hadders-Algra, M. Goal directed reaching and postural control in supine position in healthy infants. *Behavioral Brain Research,* v.115, p. 8–18, 2000.

Fallang, B., Saugstad, O. D., Grogaard, J., Hadders-Algra. Kinematic quality of reaching movements in preterm infants. *Pediatric Research*, v. 53, p. 836–842, 2003.

Fagard, J. (2000). Linked proximal and distal changes in the reaching behavior of 5-to 12-month-old human infants grasping objects of different sizes. *Infant Behavior and Development*, 23, 317-329.

Fagard, J.; Lockman, J. J. The effect of task constraints on infants' (bi)manual strategy for grasping and exploring objects. *Infant Behavior and Development,* v. 28, n. 3, p. 305-315, 2005.

Fagard, J.;Pezé, A. Age changes in interlimb coupling and the development of bimanual coordination. *Journal of Motor Behavior*, 29(3), 199–208, 1997.

Fagard, J., Spelke, E., & Von Hofsten C. Reaching and grasping a moving object in 6-, 8-, and 10-month-old infants: laterality and performance. *Infant Behavior and Development*, 32(2), 137-146, 2009.

Fetters, L. Chen, Y.P.; Jonsdottir, J.; Tronick, E.Z. Kicking coordination captures differences between full term and premature infants with white matter disorder. *Human Movement Science*, v. 22, p. 729-748, 2004.

Gorga, D.; Stern, F.M.; Ross, G.; Nagler, W. Neuromotor development of preterm and full-term infants. *Early Human Development*, v. 18, p.137-149, 1988.

Feldman, A. G.; Levin, M. F. The origen and use of positional frames of reference in motor control. *Behavior Brain and Science*, 18 : 723-806, 1995.

Heathcock, J. C., Lobo, M., Galloway J. C. Movement training advances the emergence of reaching in infants born at less than 33 weeks of gestational age. *Physical Therapy*, 88, 310–22, 2008.

Howard, J; Parmelee, A.H; Kopp, C.B.; Littman, B. A neurologic comparison of pre-term and full-term infants at term conceptional age. *Journal Pediatrics*, v. 88, p. 995-1002, 1976.

Jeng, S. F.; Chen, L. C.; Yau, K.I.T. Kinematic analysis of kicking movements in preterm infants with low birth weight and full term infants. *Physical Therapy*, v. 82, p. 148-159, 2002.

Kuhtz-Buschbeck, J.P.; Stolze, H.; Golge, M.; Ritz, A. Analyses of Gait, Reaching, and Grasping in Children After Traumatic Brain Injury. *Archives Physiology Medicine Rehabilitation,* v.4, 2003.

Landgraf. (2011). *Influence of Additional Weight on spontaneous kicking in the first four months of life*. Thesis (Ph.D.) – Federal University of Sao Carlos, Sao Carlos - Brazil

Landraf, J.F.; Tudella, E. Effects of external load on spontaneous kicking by one and two-month-old infants. *Brazilian Journal of Phisiotherapy*, v.12, p.468-475, 2008.

Massion, J. Postural Control Systems in Developmental Perspective. *Neuroscience and Biobehavioral Reviews*, v. 22, n 4, p. 465–472, 1999.

Mathew, A., Cook, M. The control of reaching movements by young infants. *Child Development*, v.61, p.1238-1257, 1990.

Meer, A. L. H. van der, Weel, F. R. van der & Lee, D. N. Lifting weights in neonates: Developing visual control of reaching. *Scandinavian Journal of Psychology, 37,* 424 – 436, 1996.

Plantinga, Y.; Perdock, J.; De Groot, M. Hand function in low-risk preterm infants: its relation to muscle power regulation. *Development Medicine and Child Neurology*, v. 38, p.6-11, 1997.

Piek, J. P; Gasson, N. Spontaneous kicking in full term and preterm infants: are there leg asymmetries? *Human Movement Science*, v. 18, p. 377-395, 1999.

Prechtl, H. F. R.; Beintema, D. J. The neurological examination of the full-term newborn infant. *Clinics in Developmental Medicine*. v. 12, p. 1-73, 1964.

Rocha, N. A. C. F., Costa, C. S. N., Savelsbergh, G., Tudella, E. The effect of additional weight load on infant reaching. *Infant Behavior and Development*, v. 32, p. 234-237, 2009

Schneider, K.; Zernicke, R. F. Biomechanics and developmental neuromotor control. *Child Development*, 64,982–1004, 1992.

Smith, L.K.; Weiss, E.L.; Lehmkuhl, L.D.. *Cinesiologia Clínica de Brunnstrom*. Editora Manole. 1th ed, 1997.

Thelen, E., & Fisher, D. M. Newborn stepping: an explanation for a "disappearing reflex". *Developmental Psychology*, 8, 769-775, 1982.

Thelen, E., Fisher, D. M., & Ridley-Johnson, R. The relationship between physical growth and a newborn reflex. *Infant Behavior and Development*, 7, 479-498, 1984.

Thelen, E., Ridley Johnson, R. & Fisher, D. Shifting patterns of bilateral coordination and lateral dominance in the leg movements of young children. *Developmental Psychobiology*, 16, 29-46, 1983.

Thelen, E; Skala, K. D.; Kelso, J. A. S. The dynamic nature of early coordination: evidence from bilateral leg movements in young infants. *Development Psychology,* v. 23, n. 2, 179-186, 1987.

Thelen, E., Corbetta, D., Spencer, J. P. Development of reaching during the first year: role of movement speed. *Journal Experimental Psychology: Human Percept Perform,* v. 22, p. 1059-1076, 1996

Toledo, A. M., & Tudella, E. The development of reaching behavior in low-risk preterm infants. *Infant Behavior and Development*, 31, 398–407, 2008.

Toledo, A. M. *Influence of Additional Weight and Late Prematurity in the Reach of Infants.* Thesis (Ph.D.) – Federal University of Sao Carlos, Sao Carlos – Brazil, 2011

Toledo, A. M., Soares, D. A., & Tudella, E. Proximal and distal adjustments of reaching behavior in preterm infants. *Journal of Motor Behavior*, 43(2), 137-145, 2011.

Ulrich, B.D.; Ulrich, D.A.; Angulo-Kinzler, R.M. The impact of context manipulation on movement patterns during a transition period. *Human Movement Science*, v. 17, p.327-346, 1997

Vaal, J.; Van Soest, A. J., K.; Hopkins, B. Spontaneous kicking behavior in infants: age-related effects of unilateral weighting. *Developmental Psychobiology*, v. 33, p. 111-122, 2000.

Vaal, J.; Van Soest, K.; Hopkins, B.; Sie, L.T.L. Spontaneous leg movements in infants with and without periventricular leukomalacia: effects of unilateral weighting. *Behavioural Brain Research*, v. 129, p. 83-92, 2002.

Van Beek, Y., Hopkins, B., Hoeksma, J.B., & Samson, J.F. Pre-maturity, posture, and the development of looking behaviour during early communication. *Journal of Child Psychology and Psychiatry*, 35, 1093-1107, 1994.

Van Der Fits, I.B.M; Hadders-Algra, M. The development of postural responses patterns during reaching in healthy infants. *Neuroscience and Biobehavioral*, p.521-526, 1998

Van Der Fits, I.B; Flikweert, E.R.; Stremmelaar, E.F.; Martijn, A.; Hadders-Algra, M. Development of postural adjustments during reaching in preterm infants. Pediatric Research, v. 46, p. 1-7, 1999.

Van Der Heide, J.C.; Fock, J.M.; Otten, B.; Stremmelaar, E.; Van Eykern, La.; Hadders-Algra, M. Postural control during reaching in preterm children with cerebral palsy. *Developmental Medicine & Child Neurology* , v.46, p.253–266, 2004.

Van Wermeskerken, M., Van Der Kamp, J., & Savelsbergh, G. J. On the relation between action selection and movement control in 5- to 9-month-old infants. *Experimental Brain Reseach*, 211(1), 51-62, 2011.

Von Hofsten, C., & Rönnqvist, L. Preparation for grasping and object: a developmental study. *Journal of Experimental Psychology: Human Perception and Performance,* 14(4), 610-621, 1988.

Von Hofsten, C. Developmental changes in the organization of prereaching movements. *Developmental Psychology*, v.20, n.3, p.378–388, 1984.

BIBLIOGRAPHICAL NOTES

Aline Martins de Toledo has a Master's degree and PhD in Physical Therapy, Federal University of São Carlos (UFSCar). Currently, is Professor at the School of Physical Therapy, Federal University of Mato Grosso do Sul (UFMS) in the discipline of Children and Adolescents' health.

Eloisa Tudella has a Master's degree in Physical Education, Universidade Gama Filho (1989) and a PhD in Psychology (Experimental Psychology), University of São Paulo (1996). Currently, is Associate Professor at the Department of Physical Therapy and at the undergraduate program in Physical Therapy, Federal University of São Carlos (UFSCar). Develops research in the area of Physiotherapy in Neuropediatrics.

In: Preterm Infants
Editors: Diogo Contreiras and Johann Sampaio

ISBN 978-1-62081-819-0

Chapter 7

COGNITIVE, MOTOR AND COMMUNICATIVE-LINGUISTIC DEVELOPMENTAL TRAJECTORIES OF EXTREMELY LOW GESTATIONAL AGE PRETERMS COMPARED TO FULL-TERMS: A LONGITUDINAL STUDY IN THE FIRST YEAR OF LIFE

Alessandra Sansavini*[*]*, Silvia Savini, and Annalisa Guarini
Department of Psychology, University of Bologna, Bologna, Italy

ABSTRACT

We tested the hypothesis that extremely low gestational age (ELGA) preterm birth without major cerebral damage impacts developmental outcomes and trajectories in the first year, expecting poorer developmental outcomes, a higher rate of impairments and different developmental trajectories in ELGA with respect to full term (FT) infants. Direct tools and a parental questionnaire with four assessments in the first year were employed.

Method. Seventeen monolingual Italian ELGA (≤28 weeks) preterms without major cerebral damage and 11 monolingual Italian full terms, comparable for biological and social characteristics, were evaluated at 3, 6, 9 and 12 months (corrected age for preterms) through the Griffiths Mental Development Scales (GMDS-R), providing a general developmental quotient (DQ) and five sub-quotients (SQ). The "Primo Vocabolario del Bambino" -PVB- (Italian form of the MB-CDI) was administered to the parents at 9 and 12 months.

Results. Use of repeated measure multivariate analyses of variance showed that, compared to FTs, ELGA infants exhibited significantly lower DQ and SQ scores (personal and social skills, eye and hand coordination, performance, tendency in locomotor and hearing and language) in the GMDS-R, with mild or moderate impairments in some ELGA at 6 (6%), 9 (12%) and 12 months (24%), while not in FT

[*] Corresponding author: Alessandra Sansavini, PhD, Department of Psychology, University of Bologna, viale Berti Pichat 5, 40127 Bologna, Italy. Phone: +39 051 2091879. Fax: +39 051 243086. e-mail: alessandra.sansavini@unibo.it.

infants. ELGA compared to FT infants showed also significantly lower gesture/action production and word comprehension scores in the PVB. Differences between the two samples became larger toward the end of the first year of life.

Conclusions. Our findings highlight that several domains are impacted by ELGA preterm birth in the first year with poorer developmental outcomes, evidence of impairment in some infants and different developmental trajectories between ELGAs and FTs. Relevance of repeated assessments by employing both developmental scales assessing specific cognitive, motor, and linguistic competences and a parental questionnaire providing deeper information for communicative-linguistic competences observed in natural daily contexts was shown.

Keywords: Extremely preterm birth, cognitive development, communicative-linguistic development, developmental trajectories, Griffiths Scales, MacArthur-Bates CDI

INTRODUCTION

Preterm birth, defined by the World Health Organization as a birth occurring before 37 weeks (259 days) of gestational age -GA-, has become a quite common and increasing phenomenon in recent years, i.e. about 12% in the US and between 5 and 9% in European countries (Goldenberg, Culhane, Iams, and Romero, 2008; Sansavini and Guarini, 2010). In fact, medical and technological advances in the last two decades have led to an increasing survival of children born with severe neonatal immaturity (extremely low gestational age and birthweight) and consequently with more neonatal complications and diseases (Rees and Inder, 2005; Riley, Roth, Sellwood, and Wyatt, 2008). In particular, with regard to the respiratory system, the use of surfactant and mechanical ventilation have highly increased the survival rate of babies born before 28 weeks of gestation so that even babies born at 25-26 weeks have reached a survival rate of about 70-80% in several European, Australian and US neonatal units (Saigal and Doyle, 2008). Among all babies born preterm, about 5% are extremely low gestational age -ELGA- (i.e., GA <28 weeks) and 15% are very low gestational age -VLGA- (i.e., GA >28 and <32 weeks), while the other 80% are mildly preterm (20% between 32 and 33 weeks and 60% between 34 and 36 weeks of GA) (Goldenberg et al., 2008). The increasing of ELGA and VLGA preterms and consequently the higher frequency of neonatal complications with or without neurological damages and developmental problems, has determined a growing effort to shift from focussing only on the newborn's physical health to setting up diagnostic and therapeutic programs increasing the overall welfare of the baby within his/her environment both during the recovery in the Neonatal Intensive Care Unit (NICU) and, after discharge, during the child's growth and development.

Until about 10 years ago most studies have considered birth weight, while not gestational age, as the main criterion of neonatal immaturity. In fact, many studies were run on very low birth weight -VLBW- infants (i.e., < 1500 g) and a few specifically on extremely low birth weight -ELBW- (i.e., < 1000 g) showing, for instance, a mean difference of about 10 standard score points at school-age between LBW and VLBW preterms and full terms on measures of general intellect (i.e., IQ) (Bhutta, Cleves, Casey, Cradock, and Anand, 2002; Sansavini, Rizzardi, Alessandroni, and Giovanelli, 1996), the presence of at least one identified neurodevelopmental disability in about one-half of VLBW infants (Cole, Binney, Casey,

Fiascone, Hagadorn, and Kim, 2002), cognitive and linguistic difficulties in VLBW at preschool and school age (Jansson-Verkasalo, Valkama, Vainionpää, Pääkkö, Llkko, and Lehtihalmes, 2004; Wolke and Meyer, 1999), cognitive delays in ELBW infants in the second year of life (Vohr, Wright, Dusick, Mele, Verter, Steichen, et al., 2000) and school difficulties in ELBW children (Anderson, Doyle, and The Victorian Infant Collaborative Study Group, 2003; Hack, Wilson-Costello, Friedman, Taylor, Schluchter, and Fanaroff, 2000; Saigal, den Ouden, Wolke, Hoult, Paneth, Streiner, Whitaker, and Pinto-Martin, 2003; Whitfield, Grunau, and Holsti, 1997).

In the last decade some studies have begun to consider gestational age as the main criterion of immaturity, since it has recently been discovered that very relevant and extensive changes occur in the development of the nervous system and the motor and sensory systems between 23 and 40 weeks of gestational age (Als, Duffy, McAnulty, Rivkin, Vajapeyan, Mulkern, et al., 2004; Counsell, Rutherford, Cowan, and Edwards, 2003; Rakic, 2006). Recent studies, have shown that preterms exhibit an elevated rate of significant developmental difficulties and disabilities as compared to full terms (Pritchard, Clark, Liberty, Champion, Wilson, and Woodward, 2009). Among these studies a few have focused specifically on ELGA infants. In particular, the EPICure study run in England on children born of less than 26 weeks has shown that ELGA preterms present cognitive delays at 2½ years (Wood, Marlow, Costeloe, Gibson, Wilkinson, for The EPICure Study Group, 2000) and cognitive and linguistic delays at 6 years in about 40% of the sample compared to full term children (Marlow, Wolke, Bracewell, and Samara, 2005; Wolke, Samara, Bracewell, and Marlow, 2008). Similar results were found by another study run on ELGA infants at preschool age (Doyle and The Victorian Infant Collaborative Study Group, 2001).

Recent neuro-imaging studies have found in preterms an altered brain development with respect to full term infants from the first weeks of life (Ajayi-Obe, Saeed, Cowan, Rutherford, and Edwards, 2000) until adolescence (Schafer, Lacadie, Vohr, Kesler, Katz, Schneider, et al., 2009). Following a neuroconstructivist approach which describes how neural development and mental representations depend on the mutual and continuous interaction among genes, brain development, body and physical and social environment (Karmiloff-Smith, 2006; Westermann, Mareschal, Johnson, Sirois, Spartling, and Thomas, 2007), in our recent papers on preterms' language and cognitive development, we have made the hypothesis that this complex interaction in preterms is characterised by atypical constraints occurring in a period of rapid changes for the neural system and that the premature transition from intrauterine to extrauterine life is associated with a different cortical organization during development which impacts on psychological development in the medium and long term (Guarini and Sansavini, 2010; Guarini and Sansavini, 2011; Sansavini and Guarini, 2010). According to our hypothesis, this impact should be stronger in function of the time in which atypical constraints occur; therefore, higher is the immaturity of the brain and longer the exposure of the immature nervous system to the often stressful, painful and mostly artificial stimuli of NICU, stronger and longer will be the impact on development. Recent neurological studies support this hypothesis showing that preterm birth can result in subtle cerebral neuropathologies because of the fragility of the immature central nervous system (CNS) (Volpe, 1995; Rees and Inder, 2005) and the impact of the NICU's environment and frequent poor nutritional status becomes more critical as gestational age decreases (Als, 1992; Maalouf, Duggan, Rutherford, Counsell, Fletcher, Battin, Cowan and Edwards, 1999; Volpe 2008). These conditions make more difficult also the beginning of mother-infant communication and relationship (Goldberg and DiVitto, 2002; Salerni, Suttora, and D'Odorico, 2007).

The impact of an extremely low gestational age (ELGA) on development has been investigated mainly after two years of life, while early abilities of ELGA preterms have received less attention except for a very few studies which have evaluated ELGA infants at a single age point after 18 months (Dezoete, MacArthur, and Tuck, 2003; Hintz, Kendrick, Vohr, Poole, and Higgins, 2005). Furthermore, most of the existing studies on ELGAs' outcomes include infants with cerebral damages, are mainly focused at single points of development, and have not described the developmental trajectories of ELGA infants through repeated assessments in the first two years of life nor have compared their trajectories with those of full terms (FT). A very recent longitudinal study has shown how ELGAs' developmental trajectories begin to deflect from those of typical development in the first two years of life (Sansavini, Savini, Guarini, Broccoli, Alessandroni, and Faldella, 2010). These authors examined the psychomotor development of 88 infants, without major cerebral damage, divided into three GA groups (ELGA: ≤ 28 weeks; VLGA: 29-32 weeks; FT: ≥ 37 weeks) assessed longitudinally at 6, 12, 18, and 24 months showing that GA impacts developmental outcomes and trajectories of preterms, with poorer developmental outcomes and higher rate of impairment at the decreasing of GA and with increasing differences between the ELGA and the FT sample from the first to the second year. In particular, ELGA preterms exhibited lower developmental quotients with major difficulties in cognitive, visuo-motor and motor abilities compared to the VLGA and FT groups. Furthermore, mild, moderate or severe cognitive impairments was found in some ELGAs, mild impairments in a few VLGAs, while no impairment in the FT infants.

With regard specifically to communicative-linguistic development, several studies have been run on VLBW and VLGA infants and children, while few studies specifically on ELGA children, and most of them concern development after the second year of life (for a review see Guarini and Sansavini, 2010; Guarini and Sansavini, 2011). Difficulties in lexicon production and grammar were found starting from 2-2 ½ years (Foster-Cohen, Edgin, Champion, and Woodward, 2007; Gayraud and Kern, 2007; Sansavini, Guarini, Alessandroni, Faldella, Giovanelli, and Salvioli, 2006; Sansavini, Guarini, Alessandroni, Faldella, Giovanelli, and Salvioli, 2007), becoming more evident in the third year of life in terms of lower scores (Fasolo, D'Odorico, Costantini, and Cassibba, 2010; Grunau, Kearney, and Whitfield, 1990; Van Lierde, Roeyers, Boerjan, and De Groote, 2009) and of a higher percentage of language delays (Sansavini Guarini, Justice, Savini, Broccoli, Alessandroni, and Faldella, 2010), persisting at preschool and school age (Guarini, Sansavini, Fabbri, Alessandroni, Faldella, and Karmiloff-Smith, 2009; Sansavini, Guarini, Savini, Alessandroni, and Faldella, 2008; Woodward, Moor, Hood, Champion, Foster-Cohen, Inder, and Austin, 2009) and affecting school attainment and the acquisition and consolidation of reading and writing processes (Anderson et al., 2003; Guarini et al., 2010). Among the above studies, some of them have shown that lower lexical and grammatical scores were found in those newborns characterised by a higher neonatal immaturity because of an extremely low gestational age with respect to a very low gestational age and a full term birth (Foster-Cohen et al., 2007; Gayraud and Kern, 2007) or an extremely low birth weight (Grunau et al., 1990; Sansavini et al., 2006; Van Lierde et al., 2009).

Few studies, however, have been run on communicative-linguistic development in the first two years of life and they are not fully concordant in their results (Casiro, Moddemann,

Stanwick, Panikkar-Thiessen, Cowan and Cheang, 1990; Cattani, Bonifacio, Fertz, Iverson, Zocconi, and Caselli, 2010; Sansavini et al., submitted; Smith, Landry, Swank, Baldwin, Denson and Wildin, 1996; Stolt, Haataja, Lapinleimu, and Lehtonen, 2009). In fact, some of them, employing corrected age, found lower scores in word comprehension and production at 12 months (Casiro et al., 1990), in word comprehension from 9 to 15 months and in word production at 24 months (Stolt et al., 2009), in word comprehension from 12 to 18 months and in word production from 12 to 24 months (Sansavini et al., submitted), while others did not (Smith et al., 1996) or found lower scores in word comprehension from 12 to 18 months and in word production from 12 to 24 months only when employing chronological age, but not when corrected age was used (Cattani et al., 2010). Furthermore, the above studies were not specifically focused on extreme preterm infants and did not consider both infants' linguistic and cognitive profiles.

Aims of the Study

In the present study we tested the hypothesis that ELGA without major cerebral damage impacts developmental outcomes and trajectories in several domains; i.e. cognitive, motor and communicative-linguistic, already in the first year of life. In particular, we expected poorer developmental outcomes and frequent and severe impairments in ELGA infants with respect to full terms and the ELGAs' developmental trajectory deflecting from that of full terms. Infants were longitudinally evaluated at four relevant developmental times, i.e. 3, 6, 9, and 12 months, in order to deeply understand ELGAs' developmental trajectory. At 9 and 12 months also the emergence of specific communicative-linguistic abilities was analysed. A further aim was to understand whether children showing impairment were delayed in all abilities or only in some of them. Both direct tools and parental questionnaires were employed in order to have a wide comprehension of ELGAs' early development.

METHOD

Participants

Seventeen monolingual Italian preterms infants characterized by an extremely low gestational age (ELGA, ≤28 weeks), without major cerebral damage (periventricular leukomalacia, intra-ventricular haemorrhage > II grade, hydrocephalus, retinopathy of prematurity > II grade), congenital malformations, or visual or hearing impairment were recruited, during the hospitalization period, at the Unit of Neonatology of Bologna University. The ELGA infants were examined longitudinally in the first year of life (at corrected age within two weeks of their 3, 6, 9, and 12 month-birthday). Birth dates ranged from January 2007 to July 2008. Their mean gestational age at birth was 25.7 weeks (SD = 1.4; range from 23 to 28 weeks), and their mean birth weight was 800 grams (SD = 196.7; range from 509 to 1093 grams). Seven were males and 10 females. Twelve were first-born and 5 were second-born. Gestational age was determined by the date of the mother's last menstrual period and confirmed by first-trimester early ultrasonography (US). For all participants these two criteria were concordant, as gestational age estimated through the ultrasonography assessment never differed by more than 14 days from that estimated from menstrual date. Cerebral echography had been routinely carried out at birth, after 15 days, at the predicted date of birth, and at 3 months (corrected age). Contact between mothers and their preterm neonates in the incubators had been strongly encouraged. We allowed for some degree of medical complication related to their premature birth: 17 (100%) had had respiratory distress with (n. 8, 47%) or without (n. 9, 53%) mechanical ventilation, 10 (59%) broncho-pulmonary dysplasia defined as need of supplemental oxygen at 36 weeks of post-conceptional age, 5 (29%) apnoea, 1 (6%) intra-ventricular haemorrhage of grade I detected by US,,12 (71%) retinopathy of prematurity of grade I or II, 14 (82%) persistent hyperechogenicity of white matter (≥ 14 days) as indicated by US, 13 (77%) hyperbilirubinemia treated with phototherapy, 2 (12%) were small for gestational age. Their mean days of hospitalization was 93.4 (*SD* = 33.9; range from 49 to 152 days). By contrast, any infant had, periventricular leukomalacia nor significant motor and sensory impairments, at birth or at subsequent medical assessments. With respect to social factors, maternal levels of education were described using two categories: a low-middle level of education (mother had completed the basic education or the high-school) and a high level of education (mother had completed the University/Master's degree or beyond). Ten (59%) mothers had a low-middle level of education and 7 (41%) had a high level of education.

A comparison control group of 11 monolingual Italian full term infants (FT) was recruited at birth from the neonatal ward of the same Hospital of Bologna University and examined longitudinally in the first year of life (at chronological age within two weeks of their 3, 6, 9, and 12 month-birthday). Their mean gestational age at birth was 39.1 weeks (*SD* = 0.9; range from 38 to 41 weeks), and their mean birthweight was 3379 grams (*SD* = 429.8; range from 2430 to 4120 grams). Six were males and 5 were females. Nine were first-born and 2 were second-born. All full term infants had experienced normal birth and absence of neonatal complications. Their mean days of hospitalization was 2.4 (*SD* = 0.7; range from 2 to 4 days). With respect to social factors, maternal levels of education were distributed as follows: six (54%) mothers had a low-middle level of education and 5 (45%) had a high level of education. The ELGA and FT samples had a similar distribution of biological and social factors. The Chi-square test revealed that the preterm and the control samples did not differ significantly on gender and the Fisher's exact test revealed that the preterm and the control samples did not differ significantly on the maternal level of education. The study met ethical guidelines for human subjects protections, including adherence to the legal requirements of the study country, and received a formal approval by the Research Ethical Committee of the Department of Psychology at the University of Bologna. Moreover, all parents of the preterm and full term infants gave informed written consent for participation to the study, data analysis, and data publication.

Measures

To evaluate psychomotor development the revised Griffiths Mental Development Scales 0-2 years (GMDS-R, Griffiths, 1996) were used. These scales were administered in an approximately 45-min. session and assessed infant development across five main areas (locomotor, personal and social skills, hearing and language, eye and hand coordination, and performance), providing a general developmental quotient (DQ) of infant's abilities and five sub-quotients (SQ). The DQ and SQ scores were calculated both for preterms and full terms using the tables of standardized scores for the English population (Griffiths, 1996), since an Italian standardization of these scales is not available yet. Furthermore, by using the standard deviation (*SD*) scores of the English normative sample (mean DQ = 100.5, *SD* = 11.8) and following the criteria used in the studies investigating developmental outcomes (The Victorian Infant Collaborative Study Group, 1997; Vohr et al., 2000; Wood et al., 2000; Marlow et al., 2005; Johnson and Marlow 2006; Sansavini, Savini, et al., 2010), impairment was defined as: mild (-1 to -2 SD, corresponding to 88.6 – 76.9 DQ), moderate (-2 to -3 SD, corresponding to 76.8 – 65.1 DQ), and severe (< -3 SD, corresponding to ≤ 65 DQ).

To evaluate specific communicative and linguistic competences parents were requested to fill the questionnaire "Primo Vocabolario del Bambino" Gestures and Words- PVB, which is the Italian long form of the MacArthur-Bates Communicative Development Inventory (MB-CDI) -Gestures and Words (Caselli and Casadio, 1995), in the week corresponding to the infant's month-birthday at 9 and 12 months (corrected age for the preterm infants). The PVB Gestures and Words assess the onset of communication skills in infants between 8 and 18 months of age. The first part of this form consists of a checklist of 408 words; next to each word, the parent is asked to check whether the infant understands (word comprehension) or understands and says (word production) the word. The second part consists of a checklist of 63 gestures/actions divided into five categories, and the parent is asked to indicate those that the infant produces. The 408 lexical items consists of 51 social words (i.e., onomatopoeia, routine words and personal names), 209 nouns (i.e., animals, vehicles, toys, food and drink, clothing, body parts, furniture and rooms, small household items and outside things), 92 predicates (i.e., verbs and adjectives), 17 adverbs, and 39 function words (i.e., pronouns, question words, prepositions and locations, quantifiers and articles). The list of 63 gestures/actions consists of five categories. The first two categories, include 12 first communicative gestures (i.e., deictic and conventional gestures) and 6 games and routines gestures. The last three categories include 17 items concerning actions with objects of the infant's daily use (familiar functional actions), 13 items concerning actions in which the infant pretends to be a parent using a puppet (pretending actions), and 15 items concerning imitations of adult's actions with objects (imitating actions). With regard to gesture/action production, data were analyzed both keeping all gestures/actions together and separating the first two categories (identified by us as gestures) and the second three categories (identified by us as actions) (for this distinction see Sansavini, Bello, Guarini, Savini, Stefanini, and Caselli, 2010).

A score of 1 was given for each item (word comprehended, word produced, gesture/action produced) checked. Furthermore, in order to identify children at risk for lexical comprehension and gesture/action production at 12 months, we referred to the mean values (*M*) and standard deviation (*SD*) of the lexical comprehension (*M*= 109, *SD*= 57) and of the gesture/action production (*M*= 29, *SD*= 8) of the Italian normative sample (Caselli and Casadio, 1995; Cattani et al., 2010) and we applied the cut-point of -1.5 SD from the mean (i.e., risk for lexical comprehension: < 24 words, risk for gesture/action production: <17 gestures/actions).

Procedure

All infants were tested individually at 3 (ELGAs: $M = 3.09$, $SD = 0.19$; FTs: $M = 3.07$, $SD = 0.38$), 6 (ELGAs: $M = 6.05$, $SD = 0.25$; FTs: $M = 6.12$, $SD = 0.38$), 9 (ELGAs: $M = 9.13$, $SD = 0.24$; FTs: $M = 9.06$, $SD = 0.21$) and 12 months (ELGAs: $M = 12.17$, $SD = 0.35$; FTs: $M = 12.03$, $SD = 0.27$) with the GMDS-R. Assessments were conducted in a quiet room of the Day Hospital of the Unit of Neonatology of Bologna University. The GMDS-R were administered by one professional trained psychologist over the duration of the study and were implemented in the presence of the infant's parent.

The PVB questionnaire was given to the parents about ten days before the 9- and 12-month infant's assessment by a psychologist, who provided basic instructions for completing the inventory. Parents completed the inventory at home within a few days before each infant's assessment.

As in many studies on preterms' development in the first years of life, the age was corrected for the preterms in order to take into account their level of neurobiological maturation (Johnson and Marlow, 2006; Pietz et al., 2004; Riley et al., 2008; Sansavini et al., 1996; Sansavini, Savini, et al., 2010; The Victorian Infant Collaborative Study Group, 1997; Vohr et al., 2000; Wood et al., 2000).

Table 1. Mean, standard deviation and range of GMDS-R scores of ELGA and FT groups at 3, 6, 9, and 12 months

GMDS-R scores		ELGA			FT		
	Months	Mean	(SD)	Range	Mean	(SD)	Range
Developmental quotient	3	116.1	(8.7)	93-129	119.5	(6.2)	111-133
	6	104.9	(12.1)	80-130	115.7	(8.1)	106-133
	9	104.3	(15.8)	76-135	115.5	(9.6)	101-130
	12	94.6	(14.5)	67-118	108.1	(9.5)	96-128
Locomotor	3	112.2	(16.8)	69-132	115.1	(14.8)	90-139
	6	100.1	(18.8)	57-150	113.7	(13.1)	97-142
	9	94.4	(19.1)	68-134	106.4	(20.3)	79-146
	12	85.2	(20.3)	50-117	97.5	(17.7)	65-125
Personal and social skills	3	118.3	(10.3)	96-131	122.0	(10.9)	108-150
	6	106.8	(12.1)	92-132	121.8	(14.1)	106-150
	9	107.6	(23.7)	67-150	120.7	(14.3)	100-145
	12	97.7	(15.7)	60-130	109.5	(8.9)	93-122
Hearing and language	3	118.4	(10.6)	98-146	126.0	(6.9)	114-138
	6	119.9	(11.0)	102-140	126.4	(5.1)	121-135
	9	110.7	(14.1)	91-149	115.8	(7.7)	106-130
	12	104.5	(17.9)	74-150	110.2	(14.7)	92-129
Eye and hand coordination	3	115.5	(10.8)	88-134	110.4	(9.5)	88-119
	6	98.8	(16.5)	63-123	106.7	(13.5)	88-128
	9	106.4	(22.1)	65-139	121.4	(4.9)	113-129
	12	94.9	(18.9)	63-138	112.5	(8.0)	106-128
Performance	3	107.3	(11.1)	76-125	117.5	(6.7)	104-125
	6	97.7	(15.1)	64-117	107.1	(9.5)	91-126
	9	101.8	(17.8)	68-133	113.5	(21.1)	80-150
	12	91.8	(13.5)	68-118	110.5	(16.5)	93-148

Data Analysis

All statistical analyses were carried out using SPSS 17.0 for Windows. The significance level was set at 5%. The effects of gestational age (coded as ELGA and FT) and of the age of evaluation (3, 6, 9, and 12 months) on the GMDS-R and on the PVB scores were assessed using repeated measure multivariate analyses of variance (RM-MANOVAs). Multivariate differences were estimated through Pillai's trace.

RESULTS

Descriptive analyses showed that the mean DQ and SQ scores of the GMDS-R of both groups were in the normal range of the English normative sample (Griffiths, 1996) at all four ages of evaluation, except for the ELGAs' locomotor SQ score at 12 months (see Table 1).

The RM-MANOVAs revealed a significant effect of gestational age, with lower scores in ELGAs than in FTs [test of between-subjects effect: $p = 0.012$; see Figure 1 and Table 2], and of age of evaluation [multivariate test: $p < 0.001$, see Figure 1 and Table 2] on the DQ score, while the interaction between these variables was not significant.

By referring to the mean and SD scores of the English normative sample (mean DQ = 100.5, *SD* = 11.8), four infants of the ELGA group resulted to have impairments at 12 months (24%). Among these infants, one presented a (mild) delay at 12 months, one a delay (mild) at 9 and (moderate) at 12 months, one a delay (moderate) at 9 and (mild) at 12 months and the last one a delay (mild) at 6 and (moderate) at 12 months. For the FT group, none infant presented impairments at any age.

Table 2. Effects of gestational age (ELGA and FT groups) and age of evaluation (3, 6, 9 and 12 months) on GMDS-R scores

GMDS-R	Developmental quotient	Loco-motor	Personal and social skills	Hearing and language	Eye and hand coordination	Performance
Gestational Age (A)	$F_{(1,26)}$= 7.25 p=0.012	$F_{(1,26)}$= 3.28 p=0.082	$F_{(1,26)}$= 7.18 p=0.013	$F_{(1,26)}$= 3.01 p=0.095	$F_{(1,26)}$= 4.63 p=0.041	$F_{(1,26)}$= 9.39 p=0.005
Age of evaluation (B)	$F_{(3,24)}$= 14.45* p<0.001	$F_{(3,24)}$= 13.77* p<0.001	$F_{(3,24)}$= 8.34* p=0.001	$F_{(3,24)}$= 9.27* p<0.001	$F_{(3,24)}$= 9.67* p<0.001	$F_{(3,24)}$= 5.87* p=0.004
(A) x (B)	$F_{(3,24)}$=1.14* p=0.354	$F_{(3,24)}$=0.59* p=0.627	$F_{(3,24)}$= 1.19* p=0.336	$F_{(3,24)}$=0.09* p=0.964	$F_{(3,24)}$=3.41* p=0.034	$F_{(3,24)}$=0.78* p=0.519

*Multivariate test.

Results of repeated measure multivariate analyses of variance (RM-MANOVAs).

With regard to the SQ scores (see Table 2), the RM-MANOVAs indicated an effect of gestational age, with lower scores in ELGAs than in FTs, on the scores of the following subscales: locomotor [test of between-subjects effect: $p = 0.082$, tendency], personal and social skills [test of between-subjects effect: $p = 0.013$], hearing and language [test of between-subjects effect: $p = 0.095$, tendency], eye and hand coordination [test of between-subjects effect: $p = 0.041$], and performance [test of between-subjects effect: $p = 0.005$]. Moreover, a significant effect of age of evaluation was found in all subscales: locomotor [multivariate test: $p < 0.001$], personal and social skills [multivariate test: $p < 0.001$], hearing and language [multivariate test: $p < 0.001$], eye and hand coordination [multivariate test: $p < 0.001$], performance [multivariate test: $p = 0.004$]. A significant interaction between gestational age and age of evaluation was found on eye and hand coordination subscale scores [multivariate test: $p = 0.034$] with a decreasing trajectory in ELGAs while not in full terms.

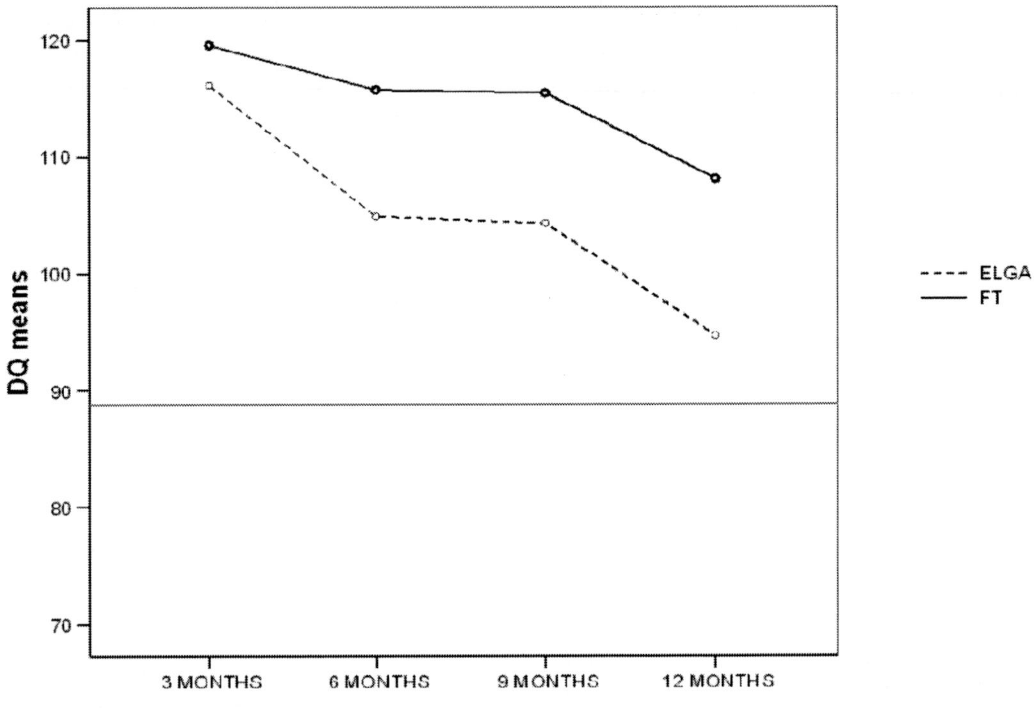

Figure 1. Developmental trajectories of the DQ scores (GMDS-R) of the ELGA and FT groups at 3, 6, 9, and 12 months.

With regard to specific communicative-linguistic abilities, descriptive analyses showed that means of word comprehension, word production and gesture/action production scores of the PVB of both groups were in the normal range by referring to the Italian normative sample (Caselli and Casadio, 1995) at both 9 and 12 months (see Table 3).

The RM-MANOVA revealed a significant effect of gestational age [test of between-subjects effect: $p = 0.044$] and of age of evaluation [multivariate test: $p < 0.001$] on word comprehension. In particular, lower scores in word comprehension were found in ELGAs in comparison to FTs (see Figure 2 and Table 4). By using a cut-point of < -1.5 SD from the mean of the Italian normative sample, 1 ELGA infant (6%) and none FT infant resulted at risk at 12 months. With regard to word production, the RM-MANOVA revealed a significant effect of age of evaluation [multivariate test: $p = 0.013$] (see Figure 3 and Table 4). Concerning the category of gesture/action production, the RM-MANOVA revealed a significant effect of gestational age [test of between-subjects effect: $p = 0.005$], of age of evaluation [multivariate test: $p < 0.001$] and of the interaction between these variables [multivariate test: $p = 0.034$]. In particular, lower scores in gesture/action production were found in the ELGA group as compared to the FT group with a slower rate of development in ELGAs (see Figure 4 and Table 4). By using a cut-point of < -1.5 SD from the mean of the Italian normative sample, 10 ELGAs (59%) and 1 FT (9%) resulted at risk in gesture/action production at 12 months. In details, regarding gesture production, the RM-MANOVA revealed a significant effect of age of evaluation [multivariate test: F(1, 26)=90.94; $p <$ 0.001], while with respect to action production, significant effects of gestational age [test of between-subjects effect: F (1, 26)=11.71; $p = 0.002$], of age of evaluation [multivariate test: F(1, 26)=24.87; $p < 0.001$] and a tendency of the interaction between these variables [multivariate test: F(1,26)=3.51; $p = 0.072$] were found. The RM-MANOVA showed significantly lower action production scores and a slower increasing from 9 to 12 months in the ELGA group as compared to the FT group.

Table 3. Mean, standard deviation and range of PVB scores of ELGA and FT groups at 3, 6, 9, and 12 months

		ELGA			FT		
PVB scores	Months	Mean	(SD)	Range	Mean	(SD)	Range
Word Comprehension (408 items)	9 12	38.4 83.5	(34.5) (54.1)	0-122 0-170	64.8 138.8	(46.8) (93.9)	22-183 35-297
Word Production (408 items)	9 12	1.2 3.4	(2.5) (3.6)	0-9 0-11	1.3 3.2	(1.8) (4.3)	0-5 0-14
Gestures/Actions (63 items)	9 12	8.5 15.9	(5.6) (8.0)	2-18 6-33	12.1 25.7	(4.6) (7.9)	6-18 15-39
Gestures (18 items)	9 12	5.2 9.6	(3.1) (3.4)	1-11 4-16	5.8 11.5	(2.2) (2.9)	1-8 6-15
Actions (45 items)	9 12	3.3 6.9	(2.9) (6.4)	0-10 0-24	6.3 14.2	(3.7) (5.7)	0-12 6-25

Table 4. Effects of gestational age (ELGA and FT groups) and age of evaluation (3, 6, 9 and 12 months) on PVB scores. Results of repeated measure multivariate analyses of variance (RM-MANOVAs)

PVB	Word Comprehension	Word Production	Gestures/Actions
Gestational Age (A)	$F_{(1,26)} = 4.47$ $p = 0.044$	$F_{(1,26)} = 0.05$ $p = 0.945$	$F_{(1,26)} = 9.24$ $p = 0.005$
Age of evaluation (B)	$F_{(1,26)} = 26.59^*$ $p < 0.001$	$F_{(1,26)}=7.17^*$ $p=0.013$	$F_{(1,26)}=57.47^*$ $p < 0.001$
(A) x (B)	$F_{(1,26)} = 1.57^*$ $p = 0.221$	$F_{(1,26)} = 0.02^*$ $p = 0.891$	$F_{(1,26)} = 5.03^*$ $p = 0.034$

* Multivariate test.

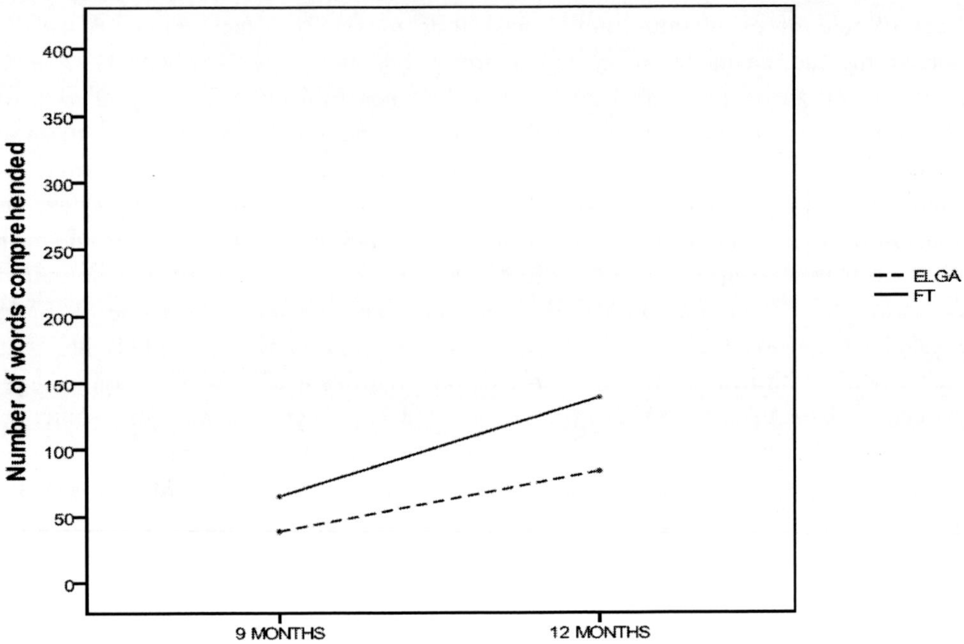

Figure 2. Developmental trajectories of word comprehension (PVB) of the ELGA and FT groups at 9 and 12 months.

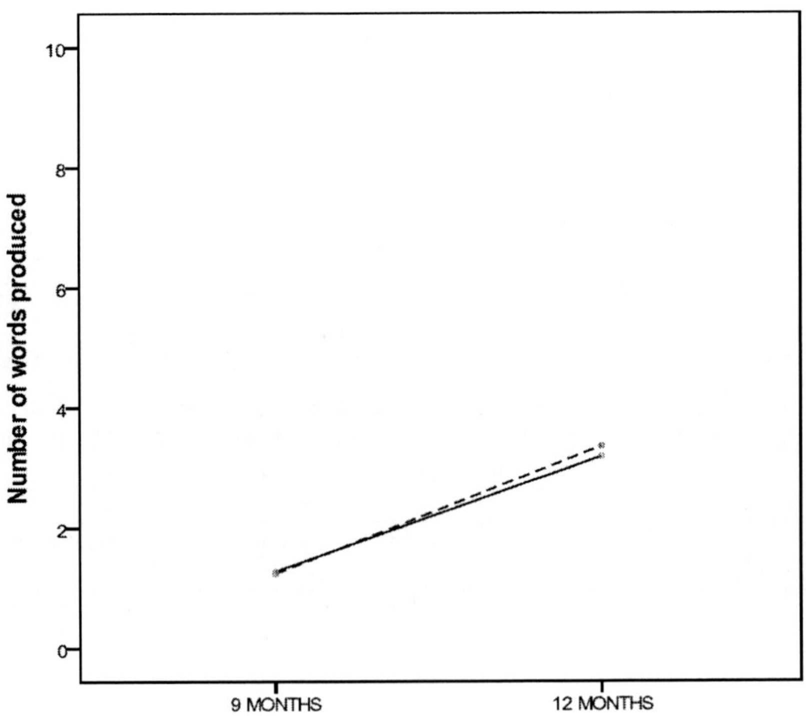

Figure 3. Developmental trajectories of word production (PVB) of the ELGA and FT groups at 9 and 12 months.

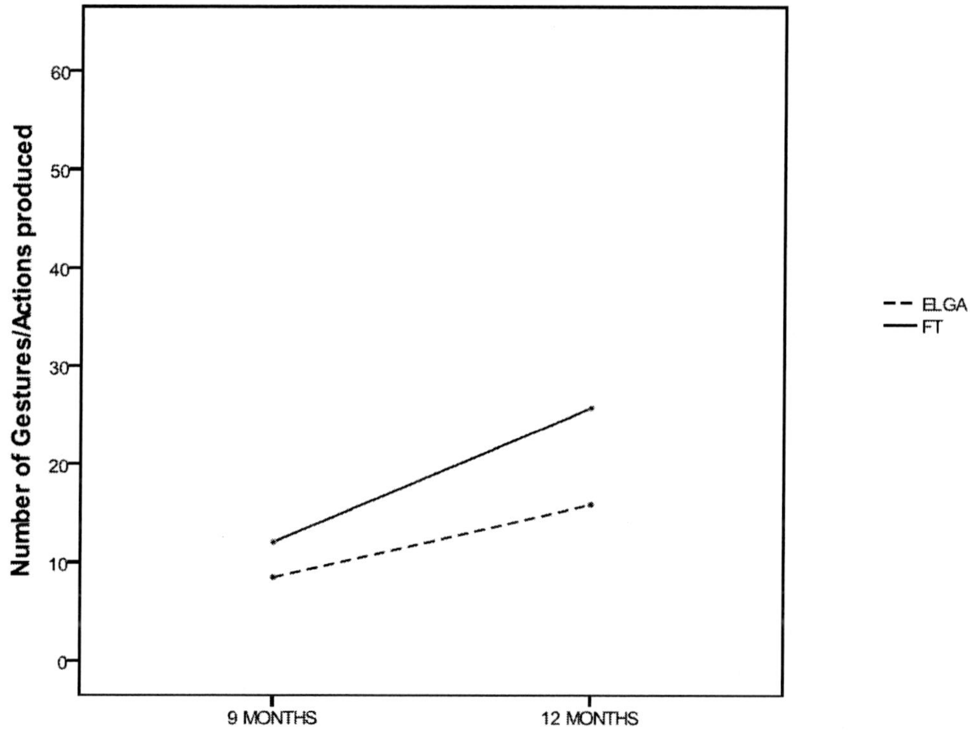

Figure 4. Developmental trajectories of gesture/action production (PVB) of the ELGA and FT groups at 9 and 12 months.

A further analysis of the presence of risk in the psychomotor and communicative-linguistic domains showed that 4 (24%) ELGA infants had a psychomotor impairment at 12 months; 3 of them (18%) had delay in the communicative-linguistic domain as well (one both in word comprehension and gesture/action production, and two only in gesture/action production), while one (6%) ELGA showed only a psychomotor impairment but no delay in the communicative-linguistic domain. Instead, 7 (41%) ELGA infants presented a specific delay in gesture/action production. With regard to the FT group, only one (9%) infant showed a specific delay in gesture/action production at 12 months.

Discussion

Several studies and reviews have highlighted how preterm birth affects cognitive, behavioral and linguistic development and school attainment from preschool to school age until adolescence (Aarnoudse-Moens, Weisglas-Kuperus, van Goudoever, and Oosterlaan, 2009; Aylward, 2005; Bhutta et al., 2002, Marlow, 2004; Guarini and Sansavini, 2010; Sansavini and Guarini, 2010). Instead, less research has been conducted on preterms' development in the first year of life, and, more specifically, scarce are the studies focused on ELGA infants, and very rare those which have adopted a longitudinal design with several points of assessments.

The present study makes a relevant contribution to the literature, as it describes the developmental trajectories of ELGA and FT infants within a longitudinal design involving four points of direct evaluation over the first year of life for cognitive, motor and communicative-linguistic development. Specific communicative-linguistic competencies have also been evaluated in this study at the last two points of assessment through the use of the Italian long form of the MacArthur-Bates CDI.

The first major finding of interest was that ELGA, even in the absence of major cerebral damage, affects developmental trajectories already in the first year of life on different aspects of development. In fact, ELGA infants showed lower developmental psychomotor outcomes (DQ scores) in the Griffiths Scales from 3 to 12 months as compared to FT infants. Furthermore, 24% of the ELGA infants, while none of the FT infants, presented a mild or moderate psychomotor delay at 12 months and 3 out of 4 delayed children showed already a mild or moderate delay in a previous assessment (at 9 or at 6 months). When considering Griffiths' subscales, significant lower scores were found in ELGA infants compared to full terms on the developmental trajectories of the visuo-motor (eye and hand coordination), cognitive (performance) and social subscales, and in motor (locomotor) and communicative-linguistic (hearing and language) subscales (tendency). Moreover, a significant interaction between gestational age and age of evaluation in the eye and hand coordination subscale was revealed, with a slower rate of development in ELGAs. Furthermore, at 12 months the mean value of the ELGA's locomotor subscale was below 1 *SD* of the normative value (Griffiths, 1996), underlining how the difficulty in the motor competence becomes more evident at the end of the first year. These results are in agreement with a previous study (Sansavini, Savini, et al. 2010) which showed increasing differences between ELGA and FT infants from the first to the second year of life and a major deficit in visuo-motor, locomotor and cognitive abilities. The further and original contribution of the present study is to show that the developmental trajectory of ELGA infants without major cerebral damage starts to deflect from those of FT infants already between 3 and 6 months and become more evident between 9 and 12 months. This deflection appears to be due in the first year of life mainly to difficulties in visuo-motor coordination, fine and gross motor and cognitive abilities. These results support our hypothesis (Sansavini, Savini, et al., 2010) that the interaction among several risk factors, biological (subtle neuropathologies, neonatal morbidity, and poor nutritional status) and environmental (prolonged hospitalization in the NICU where not optimal stimuli are available and postural constraints are experienced), associated with an extreme preterm birth, impacts development and, primarily, visuo-motor, locomotor, and cognitive abilities. This hypothesis is confirmed by findings of studies run during pre-school age which showed that motor abilities, visuo-motor integration and executive function continue to be impaired in the extreme immature preterms for a long time (Burns, O'Callaghan, McDonell, and Rogers, 2004; Hemgremm and Persson, 2004; Taylor, Minich, Klein, and Hack, 2004).

A second major finding concerns specific communicative-linguistic abilities examined at 9 and 12 months through the PVB questionnaire. Our results showed that word comprehension and gesture/action production observed by the parents in daily contexts, appear to be affected in ELGA infants who presented lower scores with respect to FT infants. Moreover, a significant interaction between gestational age and age of evaluation was also found on gesture/action production showing that on these specific abilities preterm infants presented, besides lower scores at all ages of assessment, also a significant slower rate of development from 9 to 12 months with respect to FT infants. Our findings add new information to another study comparing very preterm and full term infants (Sansavini et al., submitted) which has shown an increasing difference between 12 and 18 months in word comprehension and gesture/action production, and between 12, 18 and 24 months in word production. In fact, our findings highlight that in ELGA infants difficulties in word comprehension and gesture/action production can be observed already between 9 and 12 months. Since word comprehension is strictly related to the processing of joint attention, we make the hypothesis that ELGAs' difficulty in word comprehension could be due to a delay in the developing of joint attention, which is a competence based on visuo-motor coordination, cognition and communication. Difficulties in early communicative abilities have in fact been identified by a few studies (Reissland and Stephenson, 1999; Smith et al., 1996). Looking more in details at gestures/actions production, our results highlight that both gestures and actions are delayed in ELGA infants from 9 to 12 months, but especially actions (i.e., familiar functional actions, pretending actions, and imitating actions). This result is particularly interesting both from a theoretical and a methodological point of view. In fact, visuo-motor coordination, motor abilities and non verbal cognition appear to be the main compromised developmental aspects in preterms in the first year of life, and these deficits are pointed out both by a direct tool, the Griffiths scales, as previously discussed, and an indirect tool, the PVB questionnaire. Interestingly, these visuo-motor, motor and cognitive difficulties may affect language development in the first years of life, as other research on typical and atypical language development seems to suggest (Iverson, 2010). In fact, some authors have shown how in typical development infants first employ actions for making and representing meanings which they will later express with referential gestures and words (Capirci and Volterra, 2008). The effect of visuo-motor and cognitive abilities on language development can be observed at the end of the first year in word comprehension and mental representation, while their effect on word production and phono-articulatory ability may become evident in the following months (Sansavini et al., submitted). In fact, no differences emerged in word production which is still very scarce at 12 months in both ELGA and FT infants. This result is in agreement with the data of FT normative samples (Caselli and Casadio, 1995; Caselli, Rinaldi, Stefanini, and Volterra, 2009; Fenson, Dale, Reznick, Bates, Thal, and Pethick, 1994) and of longitudinal studies on FT infants (Reilly et al., 2009; Sansavini, Bello, et al., 2010) and on very preterm infants (Cattani et al., 2010; Sansavini et al., submitted; Stolt et al., 2009) which have shown that increase in word production can be evidentiated in the following months.

The third interesting point to be highlighted concerns the wide variability which characterises both samples, even if, as it can be seen from the results, this variability tends to be more spread toward lower values in the ELGA sample and toward higher values in the FT sample. The presence of a wide inter-individual variability makes it relevant to compare two populations, i.e. an atypically and a typically developing one, not only at a single age point, but in their developmental trajectories through a longitudinal design, taking into account the age-related inter-individual variability of both and examining how this inter-individual variability changes in the two populations when moving from the acquisition to the consolidation of an ability (Thomas, Annaz, Ansari, Scerif, Jarrold, and Karmiloff-Smith, 2009). When an increasing difference is found between the developmental trajectories of the two populations, as we have shown in the present study and in previous studies on preterms' early cognitive and linguistic development (Sansavini, Savini, et al., 2010; Sansavini,

Guarini, et al., 2010; Sansavini et al., submitted), this means that the atypically developing population, i.e. the ELGA sample in our case, not only has more difficulties with respect to the typically developing sample, but it has also a slower rate of development with infants who have difficulties in consolidating their competences. The wide inter-individual variability toward lower scores in the ELGA sample is also shown by the presence of delayed infants. But even in this case, different profiles have been highlighted. In fact, 18% of the ELGA sample showed diffuse difficulties involving both psychomotor and communicative-linguistic development, 6% had only a psychomotor delay, 41% had a specific delay in gesture/action production. By contrast, in the FT sample only one (9%) infant had a specific delay in gesture/action production. The different profiles found in the ELGA sample underline the heterogeneity of this population already at 12 months with some infants presenting more generalized delays, some infants more specific delays and some infants apparently no delay. A continuation of this longitudinal study could confirm whether children delayed at 12 months continue to show delays/difficulties at later ages. In fact, previous studies have shown that gestational age together with the developmental quotient at 12 months is predictive of the developmental quotient at 24 months (Sansavini, Savini, et al., 2010) and that a neurofunctional assessment of ELBW infants at 12 months was predictive of their cognitive performance at 3 years (Giannì, Picciolini, Vegni, Gardon, Fumagalli, and Mosca, 2007).

We recognize that this study employed small ELGA and FT samples, but we point out the relevance of comparing our ELGA sample both to a FT sample and to the normative values of the tools used, since, as shown by Marlow and colleagues (2005), only this double comparison allows to understand the severity of the difficulties of the preterm children.

CONCLUSION

The present study gives relevant theoretical, clinical and methodological contributions. First, we have described how the developmental trajectory of the ELGA infants start to deflect from that of the FT infants already between 3 and 6 months with regard to psychomotor development, with major difficulties in visuo-motor, motor and cognitive abilities, and between 9 and 12 months with regard to specific communicative-linguistic abilities, such as word comprehension and gesture/action production, with a major difficulty in the latter.

Second, the present study highlights the relevance of running a longitudinal study with several ages of assessments in the first year of life in order to understand when and which abilities start to be delayed in ELGA infants and, consequently, to identify infants at risk or delayed and support them with well-timed interventions. Third, we have shown the relevance of employing both a direct tool, such as the Griffiths scales, which allow to describe both global development and specific abilities, and an indirect tool, such as the PVB questionnaire, which allows to describe specific communicative-linguistic competences, as they are expressed in daily and contextualized uses.

ACKNOWLEDGMENTS

We are grateful to the parents and their infants for the participation in the research. We thank the neonatologists Rosina Alessandroni and Giacomo Faldella, Head of the Unit of Neonatology of Bologna University, for the organisation of the medical follow-up, the medical examination of the preterm infants and their precious collaboration for medical data collection. To Cristina Fabbri, we express our gratitude for helping in data coding and management. To Maria Cristina Caselli goes our thank for her valuable suggestions and the collaborative work with which we have engaged for several years on the Primo Vocabolario del Bambino questionnaire.

Funding: This research was supported by research grants from University of Bologna: Basic Oriented Research ex 60% 2004-2009; Strategic Project 2007-2009 "Early communicative-linguistic and cognitive abilities: risks linked to preterm birth". This research was also supported by a national research grant PRIN 2008 "Gestures and language in children with atypical and at risk developmental profiles: relationships among competences, mother-child interaction modalities and proposals of intervention".

Ethical approval: The study met the ethical guidelines, including adherence to the legal requirements of the study country, and all parents of the infants gave informed written consent for participation to the study, data analysis and data publication.

Declaration of interest: The authors report no conflicts of interest.

REFERENCES

Aarnoudse-Moens, C.S., Weisglas-Kuperus, N., van Goudoever, J.B., and Oosterlaan, J. (2009). Meta-analysis of neurobehavioral outcomes in very preterm and/or very low birth weight children. *Pediatrics, 124* (2), 717-728.

Ajayi-Obe, M., Saeed, N., Cowan, F.M., Rutherford, M.A., and Edwards, A.D. (2000). Reduced development of cerebral cortex in extremely preterm infants. *The Lancet, 356,* 1162-1163.

Als, H., (1992). Individualized, family-focused developmental care for the very-low-birthweight preterm infant in the NICU. In S. L. Friedman and M.D. Sigman (Eds.), *The psychological development of low birthweight children* (pp. 341-388). Norwood, NJ: Ablex.

Als, H., Duffy F.H., McAnulty, G.B., Rivkin, M.J., Vajapeyam, S., Mulkern, RV., Warfield, S.K., Huppi, P.S., Butler, S.C., Conneman, N., Fischer, C., and Eichenwald, E.C. (2004). Early experience alters brain function and structure. *Pediatrics*, *113,* 846-857.

Anderson, P., Doyle, L.W., and The Victorian Infant Collaborative Study Group (2003). Neurobehavioral outcomes of school-age children born extremely low birth weight of very preterm in the 1990s. *The Journal of the American Medical Association, 289,* 3264 - 3272.

Aylward, G.P. (2005). Neurodevelopmental outcomes of infants born prematurely. *Journal of Developmental Behavioral Pediatrics, 26*, 427-440.

Bhutta, A.T., Cleves, M.A., Casey, P.H., Cradock, M.M., and Anand, K.J.S. (2002). Cognitive and behavioural outcomes of school-age children who are born preterm. *The Journal of the American Medical Association, 288*, 728-237.

Burns, Y., O'Callaghan, M., McDonell, B., and Rogers, Y. (2004). Movement and motor development in ELBW infants at 1 years is related to cognitive and motor abilities at 4 years. *Early Human Development, 80* (1), 19-29.

Capirci, O., and Volterra, V. (2008). Gesture and speech. The emergence and development of a strong and changing partnership. *Gesture, 8* (1), 22-44.

Caselli, M. C., and Casadio, P. (1995). *Il primo vocabolario del bambino.* Milano: Franco Angeli.

Caselli, M.C., Rinaldi, P., Stefanini, S., and Volterra, V. (2009). Il repertorio di azioni e gesti in bambini tra 8 e 18 mesi e rapporti con la comprensione e produzione delle prime parole. *Età Evolutiva, 93*, 70-78.

Casiro, O.G., Moddemann, D.M., Stanwick, R.S., Pannikkar-Thiessen, V.K., Cowan, H., and Cheang, M.S. (1990). Language development of very low birth weight infants and fullterm controls at 12 months of age. *Early Human Development, 24,* 65-77.

Cattani, A., Bonifacio, S., Fertz, M.C., Iverson, J.M., Zocconi, E., and Caselli, M.C. (2010). Communicative and linguistic development in preterm children: a longitudinal study from 12 to 24 months. *International Journal of Language and Communication Disorders, 45*, 162-173.

Cole, C., Binney, G., Casey, P., Fiascone, J., Hagadorn, J., and Kim, C.(2002). Criteria for Determining Disability in Infants and Children: Low Birth Weight. Evidence Report/Technology Assessment No. 70 (Prepared by Tufts New England Medical Center Evidence-based Practice Center under Contract No. 290-97-0019). AHRQ Publication No. 03-E010. Rockville, MD: Agency for Healthcare Research and Quality.

Counsell, S.J., Rutherford, M.A., Cowan, F.M., and Edwards, A.D. (2003). Magnetic resonance imaging of preterm brain injury. *Archives of Disease in Childhood Fetal Neonatal Edition, 88*, F269-F274.

Dezoete, J.A., MacArthur, B.A., Tuck, B. (2003). Prediction of Bayley and Stanford-Binet scores with a group of very low birthweight children. *Child: Care, Health and Development, 29* (5), 367-372.

Doyle, L.W. and The Victorian Infant Collaborative Study Group. (2001). Outcome at 5 years of age of children 23 to 27 weeks' gestation: refining the prognosis. *Pediatrics, 108,* 134-41.

Fasolo, M., D'Odorico, L., Costantini, A., Cassibba, L (2010). The influence of biological, social, and developmental factors on language acquisition in pre-term born children. *International Journal of Speech-Language Pathology, 13* (3), 1-11.

Fenson, L., Dale, P. S., Reznick, J. S., Bates, E., Thal, D. J., and Pethick, S. (1994). Variability in early communicative development. *Monographs of the society for Research in Child Development, 59*, (5, Serial No. 242).

Foster-Cohen, S., Edgin, J.O., Champion, P.R., and Woodward, L.J. (2007). Early delayed language development in very preterm infants: evidence from the MacArthur-Bates CDI. *Journal of Child Language, 34*, 655-675.

Gayraud, F., and Kern, S. (2007). Influence of preterm birth on early lexical and grammatical acquisition. *First Language, 27*, 159-173.

Giannì, M.L., Picciolini, O., Vegni, C., Gardon, L., Fumagalli, M., and Mosca, F. (2007). Twelve-month neurofunctional assessment and cognitive performance at 36 months of age in extremely low birth weight infants. *Pediatrics, 120,* 1012-1019.

Goldberg, S., DiVitto, B. (2002). Parenting children born preterm. In M. H. Bornstein (Eds.), *Handbook of parenting, vol. 1, Children and parenting* (pp. 329-354). Mahwah, NJ: Lawrence Erlbaum Associates.

Goldenberg, R.L., Culhane, J.F., Iams, J.D., and Romero, R. (2008). Epidemiology and causes of preterm birth. Lancet, 371, 75-84.

Griffiths, R. (1996). *The Griffiths Mental Development Scales from birth to two years, manual, the 1996 revision.* Henley: Association for Research in Infant and Child Development, Test Agency.

Grunau, R.V., Kearney, S.M., Whitfield, M.F. (1990). Language development at 3 years in pre-term children of birth weight below 1000g. *British Journal of Disorders of Communication, 25,* 173-182.

Guarini, A., and Sansavini, A. (2010). Sviluppo cognitivo e competenze linguistiche orali e scritte nei nati pretermine: traiettorie evolutive a rischio o atipiche? *Psicologia Clinica dello Sviluppo, 14* (1), 3-32.

Guarini, A., and Sansavini, A. (2011). Language and literacy in preterm children. In A.M. Columbus (Ed.), *Advances in Pshychology Research, 82.* Hauppauge, NY: Nova Science Publishers, Inc.

Guarini, A., Sansavini, A., Fabbri, C., Alessandroni, R., Faldella, G., and Karmiloff-Smith, A. (2009). Reconsidering the impact of preterm birth on language out come. *Early Humam Development, 85*, 639-645.

Guarini, A., Sansavini, A., Fabbri, C., Savini, S., Alessandroni , R., Faldella, G., and Karmiloff-Smith, A. (2010). Long-term effects of preterm birth on language and literacy at eight years. *Journal of Child Language, 37* (4), 865-885.

Hack, M., Wilson-Costello, D., Friedman, H., Taylor, G.H., Schluchter, M., and Fanaroff, A.A. Neurodevelopment and predictors of outcomes of children with birth weight of less than 1000g: 1992-1995 (2000). *Archives of Pediatrics and Adolescent Medicine,154* (7),725-31.

Hemgrem, E., and Persson, K. (2004). Quality of motor performance in preterm and full-term 3-year-old children. *Child: Care, Health and Development, 30* (5), 515-527.

Hintz, S.R., Kendrick, D.E., Vohr, B.R., Poole, K., and Higgins, R.D. (2005). Changes in neurodevelopmental outcomes at 18 to 22 months' corrected age among infants of less than 25 weeks gestational age born in 1993-1999. *Pediatrics, 115* (6), 1645-1651.

Iverson, J. (2010). Developing language in a developing body: the relationship between motor development and language development. *Journal of Child Language, 37*, 229-261.

Jansson-Verkasalo, E., Valkama, M., Vainionpää, L., Pääkkö, E., Llkko, E., and Lehtihalmes, M. (2004). Language development in very low birth weight preterm children: a follow-up study. *Folia Phoniatrica et Logopaedica, 56*, 108-119.

Johnson, S., and Marlow, N. (2006). Developmental screen or developmental testing? *Early Human Development, 82*, 173-183.

Karmiloff-Smith, A. (2006). The tortuous route from genes to behavior: a neuroconstructivist approach. *Cognitive Affective and Behavioral Neuroscience, 6,* 9-17.

Maalouf, E.F., Duggan, P.J., Rutherford, M.A., Counsell, S.J., Fletcher, A.M., Battin, M., Cowan, F., and Edwards, A.D. (1999). Magnetic resonance imaging of the brain in a cohort of extremely preterm infants. *Journal of Pediatrics, 135,* 351-357.

Marlow, N. (2004). Neurocognitive outcome after very preterm birth. *Archives of Disease Childhood- Fetal and Neonatal Edition, 89*, F224-F228.

Marlow, N., Wolke, D., Bracewell, M. A., and Samara, M. (2005). Neurologic and developmental disability at 6 years of age after extremely preterm birth. *New England Journal of Medicine, 352*, 9-19.

Pietz, J., Peter, J., Graf, R., Rauterberg-Ruland, I., Rupp, A., Sontheimer, D., and Linderkamp, O. (2004). Physical growth and neurodevelopmental outcome of non handicapped low-risk children born preterm. *Early Human Development, 79*, 131-143.

Pritchard, V.E., Clark, C.A., Liberty, K., Champion, P.R., Wilson, K., and Woodward, L.J. (2009). Early school-based learning difficulties in children born very preterm. *Early Human Development, 85*, 215-224.

Rakic, P. (2006). A century of progress in corticoneurogenesis: from silver impregnation to genetic engineering. *Cerebral Cortex, 16,* i13-i17.

Rees, S., and Inder, T. (2005). Fetal and neonatal origins of altered brain development. *Early Human Development, 81*, 753-761.

Reilly, S., Bavin, E.L., Bretherton, L., Conway, L., Eadie, P., Cini, E., Prior, M., Ukoumunne, O., and Wake, M. (2009). The early language in Victoria Study ELVS: a prospective, longitudinal study of communication skills and expressive vocabulary development at 8, 12 and 24 months. *International Journal of Speech-Language Pathology, 11*(5), 344-357.

Reissland, N., and Stephenson, T. (1999). Turn-taking in early vocal interaction: a comparison of premature and term infants' vocal interaction with their mothers. *Child: Care, Health and Development, 25*, 447-456.

Riley, K., Roth, S., Sellwood, M., and Wyatt, J. S. (2008). Survival and neurodevelopmental morbidity at 1 year of age following extremely preterm delivery over a 20-year period: a single centre cohort study. *Acta Paediatrica, 97*, 159-165.

Saigal, S., and Doyle, L. W. (2008). An overview of mortality and sequelae of preterm birth from infancy to adulthood. *The Lancet, 371*, 261-269.

Saigal, S., den Ouden, L., Wolke, D., Hoult, L., Paneth, N., Streiner, D.L., Whitaker, A., and Pinto-Martin, J. (2003). School-age outcomes in children who were extremely low birth weight from four international population-based cohorts school-age outcomes in children who were Extremely Low Birth Weight. *Pediatrics, 112*, 943-950.

Salerni, N., Suttora, C., and D'Odorico, L. (2007). A comparison of characteristics of early communication exchanges in mother-preterm and mother-full-term infant dyads. *First Language, 27,* 329-346.

Sansavini A., Guarini A., Justice L. M., Savini S., Broccoli S., Alessandroni R., and Faldella G. (2010). Does Preterm Birth Increase a Child's Risk for Language Impairment? *Early Human Development, 86,* 765-772.

Sansavini, A., and Guarini, A. (2010). Nascita pretermine e sviluppo cognitivo e linguistico. In S. Vicari and M.C. Caselli (Eds.), *Neuropsicologia dello sviluppo* (pp. 281-292). Bologna: Il Mulino.

Sansavini, A., Bello, A., Guarini, A., Savini, S., Stefanini, S., and Caselli, M.C. (2010). Early development of gestures, object-related-actions, word comprehension and word production and their relationships in Italian infants: a longitudinal study. *Gesture, 10* (1), 52-85.

Sansavini, A., Guarini, A., Alessandroni, R., Faldella, G., Giovanelli, G., and Salvioli, G.P. (2006). Early relations between lexical and grammatical development in very immature Italian preterms. *Journal of Child Language, 33*, 199-216.

Sansavini, A., Guarini, A., Alessandroni, R., Faldella, G., Giovanelli, G., and Salvioli, G.P. (2007). Are early grammatical and phonological working memory abilities affected by preterm birth? *Journal of Communication Disorder, 40*, 239-256.

Sansavini, A., Guarini, A., Savini, S., Alessandroni, R., Faldella, G. (2008). Relations between phonological short-term memory and language at 3½ and 6 years in typically developing and preterm children. In N.B. Johansen (Ed.) *New Research on Short -Term Memory* (241-265). Hauppauge, NY: Nova Science Publishers, Inc.

Sansavini, A., Rizzardi, M., Alessandroni, A., Giovanelli, G. (1996). The development of Italian low- and very-low-birthweight infants from birth to 5 years: The role of biological and social risks. *International Journal of Behavioral Development, 19 (3),* 533-547.

Sansavini, A., Savini, S., Guarini, A., Broccoli, S., Alessandroni, R., and Faldella, G. (2010). The effect of gestational age on developmental outcomes: a longitudinal study in the first two years of life. *Child: Care, Health and Development, 37* (1), 26-36.

Schafer, R.J., Lacadie, C., Vohr, B., Kesler, S.R., Katz, K.H., Schneider, K.C., Pugh, K.R., Makuch, R.W., Reiss, A.L., Constable R.T., and Ment, L.R. (2009). Alterations in functional connectivity for language in prematurely born adolescents. *Brain, 132*, 661-670.

Smith, K.E., Landry, S.H., Swank, P.R., Baldwin, C.D., Denson, S.E., and Wildin, S. (1996). The relation of medical risk and maternal stimulation with preterm infants' development of cognitive, language and daily living skills. *Journal of Child Psychology and Psychiatry and Allied Disciplines, 37* (7), 855-864.

Stolt, S., Haataja, L., Lapinleimu, H., and Lehtonen, L. (2009). The early lexical development and its predictive value to language skills at 2 years in very-low-birth-weight children. *Journal of Communication Disorders, 42,* 107-123.

Taylor, H.G., Minich, N.M., Klein, N., and Hack, M. (2004). Longitudinal outcomes of very low birth weight: neuropsychological findings. *Journal of the International Neuropsychological Society, 10*, 149-163.

The Victorian Infant Collaborative Study Group. (1997). Improved outcome into the 1990s for infants weighing 500-999 g at birth. *Archives of Disease in Childhood Fetal and Neonatal Edition, 77*, F91-F94.

Thomas, M.S.C., Annaz, D., Ansari, D., Scerif, G., Jarrold, C., and Karmiloff-Smith, A. (2009). Using developmental trajectories to understand genetic disorders. *Journal of Speech and Hearing Research, 52*, 336-358.

Van Lierde, K.M., Roeyers, H., Boerjan, S., and De Groote, I. (2009). Expressive and receptive language characteristics in three-year-old preterm children with extremely low birth weight. *Folia Phoniatrica et Logopaedica, 61*, 296-99.

Vohr, B.R., Wright, L.L., Dusick, A.M., Mele, L., Verter, J., Steichen, J. J., Simon, N.P., Wilson, D.E., Broyles, S., Bauer, C.R., Delaney-Black, V., Yolton, K.A., Fleisher, B. E., Papile, L.A., and Kaplan, M.D. (2000). Neurodevelopmental and functional outcomes of extremely low birth weight infants in the National Institute of Child Health and Human Development Neonatal Research Network, 1993-1994. *Pediatrics, 105*, 1216-1226.

Volpe, J.J. (1995). *Neurology of the Newborn, 3rd ed.,* Philadelphia: W.B. Saunders Company.

Volpe, J.J. (2008). Brain injury in premature infants: a complex amalgam of destructive and developmental disturbance. *The Lancet Neurology, 8*, 110-124.

Westermann, G., Mareschal, D., Johnson, M.H., Sirois, S., Spartling, M.W., and Thomas, M.S.C. (2007). Neuroconstructivism. *Developmental Science, 2*, 75-83.

Whitfield, M.F., Grunau, R.V.E., and Holsti, L. (1997). Extremely premature (< 800 g) schoolchildren: multiple areas of hidden disability. *Archives of Disease in Childhood, 77,* F85-F90.

Wolke, D., Meyer, R. (1999). Cognitive status, language attainment, and prereading skills of 6-year-old very preterm children and their peers: The Bavarian Longitudinal Study. *Developmental Medicine and Child Neurology, 41,* 94-109.

Wolke, D., Samara, M., Bracewell, M., and Marlow, N. (2008). Specific language difficulties and school achievement in children born at 25 weeks of gestation or less. *Journal of Pediatrics, 152*, 256-262.

Wood, N.S., Marlow, N., Costeloe, K., Gibson, A.T., Wilkinson, A.R., for The EPICure Study Group. (2000). Neurologic and developmental disability after extremely preterm birth. *New England Journal Medicine, 343*, 378-384.

Woodward, L.J., Moor, S., Hood, K.M., Champion, P.R., Foster-Cohen, S., Inder, T.E., and Austin, N.C. (2009). Very preterm children show impairments across multiple neurodevelopmental domains by age 4 years. *Archives of Disease in Childhood Fetal Neonatal Ed, 94,* 339-344.

In: Preterm Infants
Editors: Diogo Contreiras and Johann Sampaio

ISBN 978-1-62081-819-0

Chapter 8

LANGUAGE AND LITERACY IN PRETERM CHILDREN

Annalisa Guarini** and Alessandra Sansavini
Department of Psychology, University of Bologna, Italy

ABSTRACT

Several studies have highlighted how language and literacy can be affected by preterm birth. This review aims at analyzing the effects of preterm birth on specific language (lexicon, grammar and phonological awareness) and literacy competencies (reading and writing) from the first years of life to adolescence, through the description of studies carried out in the last two decades. The conclusions point out that difficulties found in preterms' language and literacy development do not depend on a slower rhythm of acquisition in all competencies, but on their atypical development. In fact, some competencies are more compromised than others and difficulties in specific competencies emerge at different ages during development. In particular, lexical difficulties become more evident at preschool age, while grammar and phonological awareness are affected by preterm birth since their emergence. With regard to literacy, both reading and writing are affected, but with a greater compromise in the area of writing. This review also highlights that preterm birth does not determine a single developmental trajectory, but several developmental trajectories that relate to the level of neonatal immaturity, the presence of neurological damage, and the biological and environmental risk factors associated to preterm birth. Preterms with a higher immaturity (gestational age <28 weeks and/or birthweight <1000 grams) show diffuse linguistic difficulties from the first years of life to adolescence, while preterms with a moderate neonatal immaturity have more specific difficulties particularly evident from preschool-age.

---

* Corresponding author: Annalisa Guarini, PhD, Department of Psychology, University of Bologna, viale Berti Pichat 5, 40127 Bologna, Italy. Phone: +39 051 2091875. Fax: +39 051 243086. E-mail: annalisa. Guarini @unibo.it.

Funding: This review was supported by research grants from University of Bologna: Basic Oriented Research ex 60% 2004-2009; Strategic Project 2007-2009 "Early communicative-linguistic and cognitive abilities: risks linked to preterm birth" and by a national research grant PRIN 2008 "Gestures and language in children with atypical and at risk developmental profiles: relationships among competences, mother-child interaction modalities and proposals of intervention".

In conclusion, this review provides a useful contribution both for theoretical and clinical aims. At the theoretical level, following a neuroconstructivist approach, it points out how preterm birth is associated with atypical developmental trajectories, since preterms' development occurs in the context of multiple interacting constraints which differ from typical development. At the clinical level, this review highlights the importance to know which specific competencies are particularly affected by preterm birth and need well-timed interventions.

Keywords: Language, literacy, preterm birth

PRETERM BIRTH

Definition and Characteristics

Preterm birth, defined by the World Health Organization as a birth that occurs before 37 weeks (259 days) of gestational age (GA), includes a very heterogeneous group of children. For this reason, in the international literature distinctions related to the degree of neonatal immaturity among mildly preterms (GA<37 weeks), very preterms (GA<32 weeks), and extremely preterms (GA<28 weeks) and among low birthweight -LBW (<2500 grams), very low birth weight -VLBW (<1500 grams), and extremely low birthweight -ELBW (<1000 grams) preterms have been proposed. The majority of preterm infants (approximately 80%) fall into the category mildly preterms (20% between 32 and 33 weeks and 60% between 34 and 36 weeks of GA), 15% in the very preterms' category, and only 5% in the extremely preterms' category (Goldenberg, Culhane, Iams, Romero, 2008). The risk of mortality and morbidity in preterm infants depends not only on the neonatal immaturity, but also on the medical complications often associated with it (e.g., respiratory, cardiovascular, hematologic, gastrointestinal and metabolic-endocrine complications; intra-uterine growth retardation; alteration of the central nervous system –CNS-; sepsis). In severe cases, preterm birth may be associated with neurological damage (e.g., cerebral palsy, periventricular leukomalacia, hydrocephalus, intraventricular hemorrhage of grade III and IV, blindness, deafness) (Behrman, Kliegman, Jenson, 2000).

Atypical Development in Preterms

Several authors have highlighted how development is determined by the continuous interaction between biological and environmental factors (Elman, Bates, Johnson, Karmiloff-Smith, Parisi, Plunkett, 1996). This model was recently expanded and integrated by the neuroconstructivist approach (Karmiloff-Smith, 1998, 2006, 2007; Mareschal, Johnson, Sirois, Spratling, Thomas, Westermann, 2007; Westermann, Mareschal, Johnson, Sirois, Spratling, Thomas 2007), suggesting that to understand development is necessary to investigate the mutual and continuous interaction among genes, brain development, body, and physical and social environment. According to the neuroconstructivist framework, multiple biological and environmental constraints interacting on different levels (from the gene to the external environment) shape the neural structures that support mental representations and behaviors. Cognitive development can thus be understood as originating from the interplay of these constraints. Developmental disorders depend on an adaptation to multiple alterated constraints that result in atypical developmental trajectories, deflecting the normal path of development (Karmiloff-Smith, 1998).

This complex nature-nurture interaction model proposed by neuroconstructivism appears to the authors of this chapter particularly interesting to understand how the complex interaction between biological and socio-environmental factors associated to preterm birth affects the development of these children characterizing it as atypical. Preterm birth, in fact, constitutes a critical event in terms of both biological and socio-environmental atypical constraints over a period of rapid development of the neural system (Giovanelli, Sansavini, Farneti, 1999; Guarini and Sansavini, 2010; Sansavini and Giovanelli 1995; Sansavini and Guarini, 2010; Sansavini, Savini, Guarini, Broccoli, Alessandroni, Faldella, 2010). In particular, especially in very and extremely preterms, the development of the CNS, the process of neuronal migration and growth of dendrites and synapses, the organization of the sleep-wake cycle and the development of motor and sensory systems do not occur in the uterus but in the neonatal intensive care unit (NICU). During the period of hospitalization in the NICU, the preterm newborn is on one side hypo-stimulated because of lack of prenatal rhythmic (maternal heartbeat and voice) and kinesthetic (continuous motion provided by the mother) stimulations, and because of postural limitations related to lying in the incubator and to medical care (e.g., mechanical ventilation limits the spontaneous motor activity and exploration of the environment). On the other side, the preterm newborn is over-stimulated because of light, continuous noise and the often painful and invasive medical procedures which, when combined with the lack of continuous contact with the mother, determine an increased level of stress. Even the first social interactions constitute a situation of risk for the development of preterm infants, especially for very and extremely preterms who appear not very responsive and are characterized by an immature organization of sleep-wake sucking and attention cycles. In addition, preterms' mothers have a strong sense of guilt, fear, and difficulties in recognizing their suffering newborn as their baby, resulting in difficulties in mother-infant relationship and synchronization that are evident not only in the first weeks of life, but also in the medium and long term (Coppolla, Cassibba, Costantini, 2007; Fava Vizziello, Zorzi, Bottos, 1992; Stern, Karraker, Meldrum-Sopko, Norman, 2000; Salerni, Suttora, D'Odorico, 2007). In fact, some studies showed that preterm birth continues to be a stress factor for both parents until school age with a greater extent when child's neurobehavioral outcomes are more severe (Drotar, Hack, Taylor, Schluchter, Andreias, Klein, 2006). Eventually, neuro-imaging studies confirmed that this complex interaction between biological and socio-environmental atypical constraints determines a different brain development (e.g., different volumes of gray matters, altered neural pathways, abnormal white matter connectivity in preterms with respect to full-terms both in the first weeks of life (at 40 weeks of gestation: Ajayi-Obe, Saeed, Cowan, Rutherford, Edwards, 2000; Limperopoulos et al., 2005) and in the long term (e.g., at 8 years, Peterson et al. 2000; at 12 years, Schafer et al., 2009; in adolescence, Myers et al., 2010).

We can affirm thus that a premature transition from intrauterine to extrauterine life appears to be associated with a different cortical organization during development which has an impact on psychological development in the medium and long term, as described in the following paragraph in relation to some main aspects of language (lexicon, grammar and phonological awareness) and literacy (reading and writing).

LANGUAGE DEVELOPMENT

Lexicon

Lexical development (both comprehension and production) has been investigated in preterm children in different developmental periods from infancy to adolescence.

A few studies have been carried out in extremely preterms, showing a diffuse difficulty both in word comprehension and production. In fact, Grunau, Kaerney and Whitfield (1990) revealed specific difficulties in lexical comprehension and production in ELBW preterm infants at 3 years. These difficulties in ELBW preterms free of any major physical, sensorial and neurological impairments at 3 years were confirmed by a recent study (Van Lierde, Roeyers, Boerjan, De Groote, 2009). Diffuse difficulties persisted also at 6 years both in comprehension and production in preterms born at 25 weeks' gestation or less (Wolke, Samara, Bracewell, Marlow, 2008).

Most of the studies on preterm's lexical development have been carried out with very preterms, that is, examining samples with a wider range of gestational ages. These studies have revealed some discordant results with regard to the effect of preterm birth on lexical development. For example, with respect to lexical comprehension in the first year of life Casiro, Moddemann, Stanwick, Panikkar-Thiessen, Cowan and Cheang (1990) showed greater difficulty in understanding simple questions (e.g. "where is the ball?) or in recognizing objects or body parts in very preterms without severe medical complications with respect to full-term infants. By contrast, Smith, Landry, Swank, Baldwin, Denson and Wildin (1996) revealed an absence of difficulties in language comprehension in very preterms without severe medical complications at 1 year. Very recent longitudinal studies have examined early lexical comprehension at several age points between the first and the second year of life. Results are not concordant, since some studies revealed that lexical comprehension is affected by preterm birth during the second year of life taking into account corrected age (Stolt, Haataja, Lapinleimu, Lehtonen, 2009; Sansavini et al., submitted), while another study observed this disadvantage only when considering chronological age (Cattani, Bonifacio, Fertz, Iverson, Zocconi, Caselli, 2010). With respect to later lexical comprehension, a longitudinal study suggested that from 3 to 12 years very preterms (birtweight <1250 grams) catch-up their difficulty in lexical comprehension, since they started with an average standardized score of 84.1 at 3 years and gained 1.2 points per year across the age period studied (test PPVT-R). This study pointed out also that preterm children with severe brain injury demonstrated slower gains in skills over time, compared with those who did not suffer severe brain injury (Luu et al., 2009).

Concerning lexical production, some precocious difficulties were found in very preterms at 12 months (corrected age) in the production of the first words (Casiro et al., 1990). Lexical production (vocabulary size), as well as lexical comprehension, in the first three years of life has been observed and analyzed in preterms growing up in different countries mainly using the MacArthur-Bates Communicative Developmental Inventory (MB-CDI) in its various translations. These studies revealed three different scenarios. A first scenario emerged from some Finnish studies that showed how vocabulary size of very preterm infants without severe medical complications did not differ significantly from that of full-terms at 2 years of chronological age (Jansson-Verkasalo, Valkama, Vainionpää, Pääkkö, Ilkko, Lehtihalmes,

2004) or of corrected age (Stolt et al., 2007). This result was partially confirmed by a more recent Finnish study which evaluated a sample of preterms including some children with neurological damage (Stolt et al., 2009). This study revealed that at 2 years the entire sample of preterms, including those with neurological damage, had lower linguistic scores with respect to full-terms both for a parental report (MB-CDI) and at a direct evaluation (Reynell Test). However, when only preterms without neurological damage were considered, lower scores than full-terms were found only at the direct evaluation (the Reynell test; Stolt et al., 2009).

A second scenario was depicted by two studies which revealed that very preterms had a smaller vocabulary size than full-terms and this difference became more evident in function of gestational age. In fact, the two studies (one carried out in France, the other in New Zealand) revealed that lexical production at 2 years (corrected age for preterms) of extremely preterms (GA <28 weeks) was significantly lower than that of very preterms (GA 28-32 weeks) and of full-terms and highlighted also differences between very preterms and full-terms (Gayraud and Kern, 2007; Foster-Cohen, Edgin, Champion, Woodward, 2007). However, in the Kern and Gayraud study, the presence of medical complications in the preterm sample was not specified and in the Foster-Cohen and colleagues' study some children with brain damage were included in the preterm sample, which adds complexity to the interpretation of their results.

The third scenario was described by some Italian studies which revealed that very preterms (GA <33 weeks) without cerebral damage did not differ globally from full-terms on their vocabulary size at 2 ½ years (corrected age). However, two specific considerations emerged from these studies. First, preterms characterized by an extremely low birthweight (<1000 grams) and male gender revealed slight delays in lexicon, confirming the effect of a high neonatal immaturity on this ability (Sansavini, Guarini, Ruffilli, Alessandroni, Giovanelli, Salvioli, 2004; Sansavini, Guarini, Alessandroni, Giovanelli, Salvioli, 2006). Second, as confirmed by a more recent study, the percentage of preterms at lexical risk at 2 ½ years (corrected age), that is, with a lexical production $<10^{th}$ percentile of the MB-CDI, is double than that of a full-term comparison sample (Sansavini, Guarini et al., 2010).

Although the three scenarios seem apparently different, they can be integrated. In fact, they suggest how the population of very preterms cannot be considered globally and severely delayed in lexical production in the first three years of life (Jansson-Verkasalo et al., 2004; Sansavini et al., 2006), but linguistic difficulties arise in case of high neonatal immaturity, that is, an extremely low gestational age (Gayraud and Kern, 2007; Foster-Cohen et al., 2007) and/or birthweight (Sansavini et al., 2006), and/or presence of brain damage (Foster-Cohen et al., 2007). Recent Italian longitudinal studies allow us to deeper understand the differences between preterms' and full-terms' development by examining their developmental trajectories at several ages of assessment during the first three years of life. In particular, divergence between preterms and full-terms in lexical production starts to be evidentiated and increases during the second year (Sansavini et al., submitted) and becomes more evident between 2 and 3 years (Fasolo, D'Odorico, Costantini, Cassibba, 2010).

Lexical development in very preterms was also investigated at preschool and school age. Several studies are consistent in indicating more difficulties in lexical development in these children in comparison to full-terms either when preterms with neurological damage are included or not. For example, a study including preterms with neurological damages, found that about 30% of extremely and very preterms presented receptive and expressive language delays at 4 years of corrected age (Woodward et al., 2009). Among studies examining preterms without neurological damages, several specifical lexical competencies have been investigated. Object naming and sensory discrimination of auditory stimuli were found to be less developed at 4 years in healthy very preterm infants compared to full-terms. Since the two abilities were strongly correlated, the authors hypothesized that the difficulty of auditory discrimination in preterm infants may determine difficulties in language development (Jansson-Verkasalo et al., 2003). A poor use of verbs was also highlighted through a qualitative analysis in preterm infants without severe medical complications at the age of 3 ½ and 5 years compared with full-term infants, in contexts of structured play with the examiner (Le-Normand and Cohen, 1999). This study points out the importance of integrating quantitative studies with qualitative observations for understanding the evolutionary trajectory of children born preterm. In addition, in this study a lower rate of acquisition of verb production was found not only in extremely preterms (<1200 grams) and very preterms (1200-1500 grams), but also in mildly preterms (1501- 2210 g), pointing out how the effect of preterm birth on language development was particularly evident and strong at preschool age. Lower scores in lexicon development (both comprehension and production) were found in very preterm infants (GA ≤32 weeks) with respect to those of full-terms at 5 years. Even when children with major neurological deficits were excluded from the preterm group, differences between preterms and full-terms persisted in vocabulary skills, especially in understanding and naming colors and objects (Luoma, Herrgård, Martikainen, 1998). Semantic verbal fluency, but not vocabulary, has instead been found to be lower in healthy preterms (GA <33 weeks) with respect to full-terms at 4 years (Dall'Oglio et al., 2010).

Some difficulties in lexical production in preterm infants have also been detected at later ages. In fact, some Italian studies revealed that very preterms without cerebral damage made more errors in naming than full-terms both at 5-6 years, before starting primary school, and at 8 years (Guarini, Sansavini, Fabbri, Alessandroni, Faldella, Karmiloff-Smith, 2009; Sansavini, Guarini, Savini, Alessandroni, Faldella, 2008; Guarini et al., 2010). In addition, Guarini and colleagues (2009) revealed that a different strategy was employed by preterms for vocabulary production at 6 years compared to full-terms. Thus, when preterm children were unable to access a correct label, they produced a semantically related but incorrect label (e.g., "guitar" instead of "violin") or used words not directly linked to the picture. By contrast, full-term children seemed more aware of their difficulty to access a label, as shown by their significantly higher number of circumlocutions (e.g., "It is not a guitar…It is an instrument that you can play"). Such differences in strategy are important indicators of the specific processes by which preterms and full-terms process language. Lexical production was also investigated from school age to adolescence. Children born preterm (GA <32 weeks) at 9 years were slower in naming colors and objects, but these differences were no longer present at age 16 (Saavalainen et al., 2006). Thus, the authors suggest that a reduction in difficulties during adolescence occurs.

In the end, lexical production was investigated in mildly preterm children. A recent study revealed that preterms with a gestational age between 34-36 weeks of gestation did not differ from full-terms on naming at 4 years (Baron, Erickson, Ahronovich, Coulehan, Baker, Litman, 2009).

In sum, lexical development appears to be affected by preterm birth in function of neonatal immaturity. In fact, when neonatal immaturity is particularly high, both lexical comprehension and production are typically delayed from the first years of life. By contrast, the findings on preterms with a moderate neonatal immaturity are discordant, showing how lexical development (both comprehension and production) is not globally compromised in the first three years of life in the whole sample, but in subgroups with higher biological immaturity and/or brain damage, while becomes gradually characterized by diffuse difficulties which are apparent at preschool and school age but seem to decrease in adolescence. New longitudinal studies in this direction are needed from preschool to school age and adolescence to deeper understand the lexical developmental trajectory in preterms.

Grammar Development

The studies on the acquisition and consolidation of grammatical competencies in preterm children have showed a different developmental trajectory from that described with regard to lexicon, highlighting more widespread difficulties from the first years of life to school age.

Grammar development in extremely preterms has been scarcely investigated. Van Lierde and colleagues' study (2009) found that ELBW preterms free of any major physical, sensorial and neurological impairments have difficulties in morphosyntactic abilities at 3 years with respect to full-terms.

Several studies on preterms' grammar development have been carried out with more heterogeneous samples of very preterms. In the first years of life, healthy VLBW preterms showed a lower mean length of utterance –MLU- at 2 years (corrected age) in comparison to full-terms (Jansson-Verkasalo et al., 2004). Similar results emerged in another study that revealed how maximum length of utterance (henceforth MaxLU) reported by parents (MB-CDI) of extremely preterms (GA <28 weeks) and very preterms (GA 28-32 weeks) was significantly shorter than that of mildly preterm (GA 33-36 weeks) and full-term infants (Gayraud and Kern, 2007). In relation to the Italian language, children born preterms (GA≤ 33 weeks) without brain damage did not differ significantly from the full-term sample in the MLU score at 2 ½ years (corrected age), while difficulties were found in a subsample characterized by a high neonatal immaturity (GA<31 weeks) and male gender (Sansavini et al., 2006). By contrast, at 3 ½ years of age preterms showed a lower MLU score compared with full-term infants and the degree of neonatal immaturity was no longer a specific effect as in 2 ½ years, since the difference in MLU score concerned the whole group of preterm infants (Sansavini, Guarini, Alessandroni, Faldella, Giovanelli, Salvioli, 2007). The authors also found more difficulties in preterm infants in phonological short-term memory (non-word repetition) and strict relationships between MLU scores and phonological short-term memory indicating mutual influence in their development (Sansavini et al., 2007). A recent Italian longitudinal study found also that the percentage of preterms at risk for language impairment, characterized by MLU scores and compared both with normative data and a full-term sample, increased significantly from one in four at 2 ½ to one in three preterms at 3 ½ years (Sansavini, Guarini et al., 2010). Another recent Italian longitudinal study on a small sample of preterms found that their increase in MLU from 2 to 3 years was less than that of full-terms, with heterogeneous profiles, since some preterms had a typical development, some a general linguistic delay, and some a grammar but not lexical impairment (Fasolo et al., 2010).

Grammar development was affected by preterm birth even after the third year of life, as indicated by a longitudinal study that has found a lower MLU and differences in the use of verbs in preterms without brain damage compared with full-terms at 2, 3 ½ and 5 years

(Crunelle, Le Normand, Delfosse, 2003). Other studies have revealed that preterm children without neurological damage scored significantly lower than their peers on a test of morphosyntactic comprehension at 4 years (Dall'Oglio et al., 2010), had less developed grammatical skills at 5 years (Largo, Molinari, Comenale-Pinto, Weber, Duc, 1986), showing a greater number of difficulties in the use of grammatical roles, in verb conjugation, and noun-adjective declination (Wolke and Meyer, 1999).

Grammar difficulties in preterm children persisted also at school age. In fact, difficulties in grammar skills (comprehension of logical grammatical constructions) were found even at the age of 6 ½ years in very preterms (GA<32 weeks, Jennische and Sedin, 2001). Difficulties in grammar comprehension were also confirmed by two Italian studies on preterm infants (GA≤33 weeks) without cerebral damage. Preterms made more errors than full-terms in grammar comprehension both before entering primary school (Guarini et al., 2009; Sansavini et al., 2008) and at 8 years (Guarini et al., 2010).

Difficulties in grammar production at school age emerged also in a study on mildly preterms, which found that preterms made more errors than full-terms in the use of proper grammatical forms to complete statements at age 7 (Pietz et al., 2004).

To summarize, the findings described in this paragraph show the presence of diffuse difficulties (both in comprehension and in production) in grammatical skills from the first years of life until school age, highlighting how this language ability is particularly vulnerable and affected by preterm birth. Moreover, these diffuse difficulties in grammar development do not concern only preterms with a high or moderate neonatal immaturity, but also preterms with a mild immaturity, even if more studies on these children are needed to deeper understand different individual profiles in the preterm population.

Phonological Awareness

A very few studies have described phonological awareness in preterm infants, even if this linguistic ability has strong relationships with children's acquisition of literacy, as revealed by studies on typical development (Bradley and Bryant, 1983).

One study examined phonological awareness in extremely preterm children with a high neonatal immaturity (GA<25 weeks). These children were more likely to have difficulties at 6 years on rhyme detection, phoneme deletion beginning sounds, phoneme deletion end sounds and letter knowledge in comparison to full-terms (Wolke et al., 2008).

Phonological awareness has also been studied in very preterms. Wolke and Meyer's study (1999) showed that preterm children, without cerebral damage, had lower phonological awareness skills, making more errors in rhymes, phoneme recognition, letter knowledge. The presence of difficulties in phonological awareness was confirmed by some Italian studies conducted with preterm children (GA≤ 33 weeks) without cerebral damage (Guarini et al., 2009; Guarini et al., 2010; Sansavini et al., 2008). These studies revealed that at 6 years, before entering primary school, preterms showed more difficulties than full-terms in phonological awareness tasks and in particular in recognition of the first syllable, recognition of rhyme and syllabic segmentation (Guarini et al., 2009; Sansavini et al., 2008). Some difficulties in phonological awareness persisted even at 8 years, as shown by more errors in phonemic synthesis and deletion of the first syllable (Guarini et al., 2010).

All the described studies seem to indicate that the difficulties in phonological awareness in preterm children without brain damage brain are diffuse in the acquisition phase of these abilities (5-6 years) and in their consolidation (8 years) both in extremely and very preterms. However, few authors have investigated phonological awareness in preterms and more studies are needed to better understand preterms' trajectory on this ability.

LITERACY: READING AND WRITING

Several studies have investigated preterm's academic skills, showing that the incidence of difficulties and impairments becomes particularly evident at school age, with greater need for educational support (Marlow, 2004; Marlow, Roberts, Cooke, 1993; Walther, den Ouden, Verloove-Vanhorick, 2000). However, different results emerged in function of neonatal immaturity, medical complications and neurological damages.

Diffuse difficulties in extremely preterms were found at school age both in reading and writing abilities, as revealed by some studies which mainly concern the English language. In particular, healthy ELBW preterms (birthweight ≤800 grams) assessed at school age (6 to 14 years) and compared with full-terms had less advanced skills in reading and writing, and these differences persisted even when children with cognitive difficulties were excluded (Whitfield, Grunau, Holsti, 1997). Similar results emerged from the epidemiological study conducted by Anderson, Doyle and the Victorian Infant Collaborative Study Group (2003), examining a large cohort of ELBW preterm infants. In this study preterms showed at 8 years lower scores than the control group both in reading and writing. These differences persisted, even when preterms with brain and sensorial damage were excluded. Other studies revealed that preterms with a birthweight <750 g and without neurosensory disorders had higher rates of learning disabilities in reading and math than controls at 11 years children, showing that learning problems emerge early in schooling and persist over time (Litt, Taylor, Klein, Hack, 2005; Taylor, Klein, Minich, Hack, 2000). These authors highlighted that changes in outcomes from 7 to 11 years were less positive in preterms with respect to full-terms. This increasing gap between extreme preterms and full-terms can be due to preterms' difficulties in taking advantage of learning opportunities, to sequelae emerging when more complex competencies are required from the environment, and to motivational problems. It is relevant to highlight that the difficulties found in preterms with a high neonatal immaturity were not specific for reading and writing skills, but referred to a lower general competence, as evidenced by lower scores in IQ and math skills. These studies therefore reveal that learning disabilities in preterm infants are not isolated and independent, but closely related and concurrent (Grunau, Whitfield, Davis, 2002). Difficulties in literacy in ELBW preterms were also confirmed by a cross-cultural study carried out with children from 8 to 11 years in the U.S., Canada, Germany and Holland (Saigal et al., 2003).

Besides these studies, which have identified pervasive impairments in preterm infants with high neonatal immaturity, other studies have revealed specific difficulties in writing skills in very preterms. These difficulties emerged already in the first year of primary school. Healthy preterm infants (birth weight <1250g) showed less competence than full-term infants in handwriting legibility and speed of writing (Feder, Majnemer, Bourbonnais, Platt, Blayney, Synnes, 2005). The authors attribute these results to difficulties encountered by preterms in visual-motor skills, such as coordination and manipulative skills and visual-motor integration. Difficulties in academic skills in preterm children (GA≤33 weeks) at 6 years were also confirmed by a recent study which used standardized measures, teacher reports and school administered curriculum-based tests (Pritchard, Clark, Liberty, Champion, Wilson, Woodward, 2009). This study revealed that, when children with severe neurodevelopmental impairments were included in the sample, pervasive educational delays (math, reading and writing) were found. By contrast, when these infants were excluded the difficulties persisted in math and writing, but not in reading since the difference found in this skill was largely explained by group differences in neurodevelopmental impairment and SES. They pointed out that the area of academic achievement in which the poorest performance was observed was math. Specific difficulties in preterms (GA≤33 weeks) without major cerebral damage were also present at 8 years, as revealed by a recent Italian study (Guarini et al., 2010). Preterms had lower scores than full-terms in reading speed and writing accuracy, while no differences emerged in other academic abilities (comprehension of written text and reading accuracy) and on IQ. The authors pointed out how writing skills seemed particularly affected by preterm birth. Difficulties in writing persisted also in adolescence. In fact, healthy very preterms (birth weight <1500g) at 12 years showed difficulties in writing and mathematical skills but not in reading (Chaudhari, Otiv, Chitale, Pandit, Hoge, 2004). All the results obtained in preterms with moderate immaturity pointed out the importance of investigating reading and writing not merely as a whole, but with particular attention to each competence and their relationships. In fact, preterm birth seems to have partially differentiated effects on reading and writing and to affect other academic skills such as math.

With regard to mildly preterms, a study revealed that the preterm group scores at 8 years were significantly worse than the full-term group scores in math, but not in literacy (reading and spelling achievement), even if literacy scores for the preterm groups were on average 10 points lower than the full-term group (Sullivan and McGrath, 2003). This study showed that in preterms with a mild immaturity, as already described for very preterms (Chaudhari et al., 2004; Pritchard et al., 2009), math was the area of academic achievement in which the poorest performance was observed. Some difficulties in reading and writing abilities where found also in adolescents born preterm (GA<35 weeks) at 16 years in comparison to a full-term sample. However, these differences disappeared at 19 years, indicating a possible recovering of difficulties in preterm children with mild neonatal immaturity at the end of schooling (Tideman, 2000). The results of these studies demonstrate the importance of investigating preterms' skills at different ages and highlight the existence of different developmental trajectories.

Difficulties in literacy become more evident when preterm birth is associated with medical complications and/or neurological damages. For example, children with broncho-pulmonary dysplasia had lower scores in reading compared to preterm infants without this complication (Gray, O'Callaghan, Rogers, 2004). The results of this study show that within the population of preterm infants, different trajectories with specific drops can emerge in function of specific neonatal pathologies. Another study revealed that VLBW (birth weight <1500g) preterms including children with brain and sensorial damage, showed greater difficulties in reading tests at 8 years compared to the control group (Hall, McLeod, Counsell, Thomson, Mutch, 1995). These findings confirm the need to take into account the type of sample selection criteria of each study for the generalization of its results.

In sum, as already indicated for language development, literacy appears to be affected by preterm birth as a function of neonatal immaturity. In fact, when neonatal immaturity is particularly high, both reading and writing are delayed from the first acquisitions. By contrast, difficulties in preterms with a moderate neonatal immaturity are less diffuse, with a wider compromising of writing than reading. Finally, preterms with a mildly neonatal immaturity show specific difficulties in literacy which apparently decrease in adolescence.

CONCLUSION

This review pointed out how preterm birth causes not only difficulties in the first years of life that can be compensated for during development, but gives rise to an atypical developmental trajectory, which is characterized by different rates of development in specific linguistic abilities. In fact, some competencies are more compromised than others and difficulties in specific competencies emerge at different ages during development. If, for example, the lexicon shows more diffuse difficulties in very preterms mainly from preschool age with a catch up in adolescence, grammatical skills and phonological awareness are delayed in these children already in the first acquisitions. These studies show the importance of comparing developmental trajectories of preterms with those of typically developing children revealing how difficulties of preterm infants are not constituted by a slower rate of acquisition in all linguistic skills. Most of the studies in the literature are cross-sectional, while few are longitudinal with several age points of assessment which have studied preterms' developmental trajectories compared to those of full-terms over time. More longitudinal studies are thus needed with special attention to the periods of transition in order to understand how specific difficulties in basic skills may affect complex abilities in later stages of development.

The present review has also highlighted how preterm birth does not determine a single developmental trajectory, but different atypical paths depending primarily on the degree of neonatal immaturity. For example, with respect to literacy, extremely preterms show diffuse difficulties both in reading and writing, while very preterms were more compromised in writing than in reading. Furthermore, mildly preterms recover their difficulties in adolescence. The level of neonatal immaturity at birth is therefore important in determining the developmental trajectories of preterm infants not only in the short, but also in the medium and long term.

We presume that since extremely preterm birth is characterized by extremely atypical constraints (high risk for brain insults, association with other neonatal complications, hypo- and hyper-stimulation, diffuse difficulties in mother-infant interaction and synchronization, etc.) a more compromised development can occur. At the same time, we stress the relevance of carrying out new studies on the important interplay among atypical constraints in preterm children in order to better understand their developmental trajectories and which are the critical transition needing well-time interventions.

REFERENCES

Ajayi-Obe, M., Saeed, N., Cowan, F.M., Rutherford, M.A., Edwards, A.D. (2000). Reduced development of cerebral cortex in extremely preterm infants. *The Lancet,* 356, 1162-1163.

Anderson, P., Doyle, L.W., Victorian Infant Collaborative Study Group (2003). Neurobehavioral outcomes of school-age children born extremely low birth weight of very preterm in the 1990s. *The Journal of the American Medical Association,* 289, 3264 - 3272.

Baron, I.S., Erickson, K., Ahronovich, M.D., Coulehan, K., Baker, R., Litman, F.R. (2009). Visuospatial and verbal fluency relative deficits in 'complicated' late-preterm preschool children. *Early Human Development,* 85(12), 751-754.

Behrman R.E., Kliegman R.M., Jenson H.B. (2000). *Nelson Textbook of pediatrics* (16th edition). Philadelphia: Harcourt Brace.

Bradley, L. Bryant, P.E. (1983). Categorizing sounds and learning to read – a causal connection. *Nature,* 301, 419–21.

Casiro, O.G., Moddemann, D.M., Stanwick, R.S., Panikkar-Thiessen, V.K., Cowan, H., Cheang, M.S. (1990). Language development of very low birth weight infants and fullterm controls at 12 months of age. *Early Human Development,* 24, 65-77.

Cattani, A., Bonifacio, S., Fertz, M., Iverson, J.M., Zocconi, E., Caselli, M.C. (2010). Communicative and linguistic development in preterm children: A longitudinal study from 12 to 24 months. *International Journal of Language and Communication Disorders,* 45(2), 162-173.

Chaudhari, S., Otiv, M., Chitale, A., Pandit, A., Hoge, M. (2004). Pune low birth weight study – Cognitive abilities and educational performance at twelve years. *Indian Pediatrics,* 41, 121-128.

Coppola, G., Cassibba, R., Costantini, A. (2007). What can make the difference? Premature birth and maternal sensitivity at 3 months of age: the role of attachment organization, traumatic reaction and baby's medical risk. *Infant Behaviour and Development,* 30, 679-684.

Crunelle, D., Le Normand, M.T., Delfosse, M.J. (2003). Langage orale et écrit chez des enfants prématurés: résultats à 7½ ans. *Folia Phoniatrica et Logopaedica,* 55, 115-127.

Dall'Oglio, A. M., Rossiello, B., Coletti, M. F., Bultrini, M., De Marchis, C., Ravà, L., Caselli, M.C., Paris, S., Cuttini, M.. (2010). Do healthy preterm children need neuropsychological follow-up? Preschool outcomes compared with term peers. *Developmental Medicine and Child Neurology,* 52(10), 955-961.

Drotar, D., Hack, M., Taylor, G., Schluchter, M., Andreias, L., Klein, N. (2006). The impact of extremely low birthweight on the families of school-aged children. *Pediatrics,* 117, 2006-2013.

Elman, J.L., Bates, E.A., Johnson, M.H., Karmiloff-Smith, A., Parisi, D., Plunkett, K. (1996). *Rethinking innateness.* Cambridge: The MIT Press.

Fasolo, M., D'Odorico, L., Costantini, A., Cassibba, L (2010). The influence of biological, social, and developmental factors on language acquisition in pre-term born children. *International Journal of Speech-Language Pathology,* 13(3), 1-11.

Fava Vizziello, G., Zorzi, C., Bottos, M. (1992). *Figli delle macchine.* Milano: Masson.

Feder, K.P., Majnemer, A., Bourbonnais, D., Platt, R., Blayney, M., Synnes, A. (2005). Handwriting performance in preterm children compared with term peers at age 6 to 7 years. *Developmental Medicine and Child Neurology,* 47, 163-170.

Foster-Cohen, S., Edgin, J.O., Champion, P.R., Woodward, L.J. (2007). Early delayed language development in very preterm infants: evidence from the MacArthur-Bates CDI. *Journal of Child Language,* 34, 655-675.

Gayraud, F., Kern, S. (2007). Influence of preterm birth on early lexical and grammatical acquisition. *First Language,* 27, 159-173.

Giovanelli, G., Sansavini, A., Farneti, A. (1999). Perception of sound, rhythm and speech from pre-natal to post-natal life. In A.F. Kalverboer, M.L. Genta, J.B. Hopkins (eds), Current issues in developmental psychology. *Biopsychological perspectives* (pp. 137-159). Dordrecht, The Netherlands: Kluwer Academic Publisher.

Goldenberg, R.L., Culhane, J.F., Iams, J.D., Romero, R. (2008). Epidemiology and causes of preterm birth, *Lancet,* 371, 75-84.

Gray, P.H., O'Callaghan, M.J., Rogers, Y.M. (2004). Psychoeducational outcome at school age of preterm infants with bronchopulmonary dysplasia. *Journal of Paediatrics and Child Health,* 40, 114-120.

Grunau, R.V., Kearney, S.M., Whitfield, M.F. (1990). Language development at 3 years in pre-term children of birth weight below 1000g. British *Journal of Disorders of Communication,* 25, 173-182.

Grunau, R.V., Whitfield, M.F., Davis, C.D. (2002). Pattern of learning disabilities in children with extremely low birth weight and broadly average intelligence. *Archives of Pediatrics and Adolescent Medicine,* 156, 615-620.

Guarini, A., Sansavini, A. (2010). Sviluppo cognitivo e competenze linguistiche orali e scritte nei nati pretermine: traiettorie evolutive a rischio o atipiche? *Psicologia Clinica dello Sviluppo,* 14, 3-32.

Guarini A., Sansavini A., Fabbri C., Alessandroni R., Faldella G., Karmiloff-Smith A. (2009). Reconsiderig the impact of preterm birth on language outcome. *Early Human Development,* 85, 639 – 645.

Guarini A., Sansavini A., Fabbri C., Savini S., Alessandroni R., Faldella G., Karmiloff-Smith A. (2010). Long-term effects of preterm birth on language and literacy at eight years. *Journal of Child Language,* 37, 865 – 885.

Hall, A., McLeod, A., Counsell, C., Thomson, L., Mutch, L. (1995). School attainment, cognitive ability and motor function in a total Scottish very-low-birth-weight population at eight years: a controlled study. *Developmental Medicine and Child Neurology,* 37, 1037-1050.

Jansson-Verkasalo, E., Čeponiene, R., Valkama, M., Vainionpää, L., Laitakari, K., Alku, P., Suominen, K., Näätäneng, R. (2003). Deficient speech-sound processing, as shown by the electrophysiologic brain mismatch negativity response, and naming ability in prematurely born children. *Neuroscience Letters,* 348, 5–8.

Jansson-Verkasalo, E., Valkama, M., Vainionpää, L., Pääkkö, E., llkko, E., Lehtihalmes, M. (2004). Language development in very low birth weight preterm children: A follow-up study. *Folia Phoniatrica et Logopaedica,* 56, 108-119.

Jennische, M., Sedin, G. (2001). Linguistic skills at 6 ½ years of age in children who required neonatal intensive care in 1986-1989. *Acta Paediatrica,* 90, 199-212.

Karmiloff-Smith, A. (1998). Development itself is the key to understanding developmental disorders. *Trends in Cognitive Sciences,* 10, 389-398.

Karmiloff-Smith, A. (2006). The tortuous route from genes to behavior: a neuroconstructivist approach. *Cognitive Affective and Behavioral Neuroscience,* 6, 9-17.

Karmiloff-Smith, A. (2007). Atypical epigenesis. *Developmental Science*, 10, 84-88.

Largo, R.H., Molinari, L., Comenale-Pinto, L., Weber, M., Duc, G. (1986). Language development of term and preterm children during the first five years of life. *Developmental Medicine and Child Neurology,* 28, 333-350.

Le-Normand, M.T., Cohen, H. (1999). The delayed emergence of lexical morphology in preterm children: the case of verbs. *Journal of Neurolinguistics,* 12, 235-246.

Limperopoulos, C., Soul, J.S., Gauvreau, K., Huppi, P.S., Warfield, S.K., Bassan, H., Robertson, R.L., Volpe, J.J., du Plessis, A.J. (2005). Late gestation cerebellar growth is rapid and impeded by premature birth. *Pediatrics,* 115, 688-695.

Litt, J., Taylor, G., Klein, N., Hack, M. (2005). Learning disabilities in children with very low birthweight: Prevalence, neuropsychological correlates and educational interventions. *Journal of Learning Disabilities,* 38, 130-141.

Luoma, L., Herrgård, E., Martikainen, A. (1998). Neuropsychological analysis of the visuomotor problems in children born preterm at 32 weeks of gestation: a 5 year prospective follow-up. *Developmental Medicine and Child Neurology*, 40, 21-30.

Luu, T.M., Vohr, B.R., Schneider, K.C., Katz, K.H., Tucker, R., Allan, W.C., Ment, L.R. (2009). Trajectories of receptive language development from 3 to 12 years of age for very preterm children. *Pediatrics,* 124(1), 333-341.

Mareschal, D., Johnson, M.H., Sirois, S., Spratling M.W., Thomas, M.S.C., Westermann, G. (2007). Neoroconstructivism. *How the brain constructs cognition (Vol. 1).* Oxford: Oxford University Press.

Marlow, N., Roberts, L. Cooke, R. (1993). Outcome at 8 years for children with birth weights of 1250 g or less. *Archives of Disease in Childhood,* 68, 286–90.

Marlow, N. (2004). Neurocognitive outcome after very preterm birth. *Archives of Disease Childhood- Fetal and Neonatal Edition,* 89, F224–F228.

Myers, E.H., Hampson, M., Vohr, B., Lacadie, C., Frost, S.J., Pugh, K.R., Katz, K.H., Schneider, K.C., Makuch, R.W., Constable, R.T., Ment, L.R. (2010). Functional connectivity to a right hemisphere language center in prematurely born adolescents. *NeuroImage,* 51(4), 1445-1452.

Peterson, B.S., Vohr, B., Staib, L.H., Cannistraci, C.J., Dolberg, A., Schneider, K.C., Katz, K.H., Westerveld, M., Sparrow, S., Anderson, A.W., Duncan, C.C., Makuch, R.W., Gore, J.C., Ment, L.R. (2000). Regional brain volume abnormalities and long-term cognitive outcome in preterm infants. *The Journal of the American Medical Association,* 284, 1939-1947.

Pietz, J., Peter, J., Graf, R., Rauterberg-Ruland, I., Rupp, A., Sontheimer, D., Linderkamp, O. (2004). Physical growth and neurodevelopmental outcome of nonhandicapped low-risk children born preterm. *Early Human Development,* 79, 131–143.

Pritchard, V.E., Clark, C.A.C., Liberty, K., Champion, P.R., Wilson, K., Woodward, L.J. (2009). Early school-based learning difficulties in children born very preterm. *Early Human Development,* 85(4), 215-224.

Saavalainen, P., Luoma, L., Bowler, D., Timonen, T., Määttä, S., Laukkanen, E., Herrgård, E. (2006). Naming skills of children born preterm in comparison with their term peers at the ages of 9 and 16 years. *Developmental Medicine and Child Neurology,* 48, 28–32.

Saigal, S., den Ouden, L., Wolke, D., Hoult, L., Paneth, N., Streiner, D.L., Whitaker, A., Pinto-Martin, J. (2003). From four international population-based cohorts school-age outcomes in children who were Extremely Low Birth Weight. *Pediatrics,* 112, 943-950.

Salerni, N., Suttora, C., D'Odorico, L. (2007). A comparison of characteristics of early communication exchanges in mother-preterm and mother-full-term infant dyads. *First Language,* 27, 329-346.

Sansavini, A., Giovanelli, G. (1995). La nascita pretermine e il peso alla nascita basso o inadeguato per l'età gestazionale come possibili fattori di rischio per lo sviluppo. In M. D'Alessio, P. E. Ricci Bitti, G. Villone Betocchi (eds), *Gli indicatori psicologici e sociali del rischio. Modelli teorici e ricerca empirica* (pp. 91-116). Napoli: Gnocchi.

Sansavini, A., Guarini, A. (2010). Nascita pretermine e sviluppo cognitivo e linguistico. In S. Vicari and M.C. Caselli (eds.) *Neuropsicologia dello sviluppo* (pp. 281-292). Bologna: Il Mulino.

Sansavini, A., Guarini, A., Alessandroni, R., Faldella, G., Giovanelli, G., Salvioli, G. (2006). Early relations between lexical and grammatical development in very immature Italian preterms. *Journal of Child Language,* 33, 199-216.

Sansavini, A., Guarini, A., Alessandroni, R., Faldella, G., Giovanelli, G., Salvioli, G. (2007). Are early grammatical and phonological working memory abilities affected by preterm birth? *Journal of Communication Disorders,* 40, 239-256.

Sansavini A., Guarini A., Justice L. M., Savini S., Broccoli S., Alessandroni R., Faldella G. (2010). Does preterm birth increase a child's risk for language impairment? *Early Human Development,* 86, 765-772.

Sansavini, A., Guarini, A., Ruffilli, F., Alessandroni., R., Giovanelli, G., Salvioli, G.P. (2004). Fattori di rischio associati alla nascita pretermine e prime competenze linguistiche rilevate con il MacArthur. *Psicologia Clinica dello Sviluppo*, 8, 47-67.

Sansavini, A., Guarini, A., Savini, S., Alessandroni, R., Faldella, G. (2008). Relations between phonological short-term memory and language at 3½ and 6 years in typically developing and preterm children. In N.B. Johansen (ed), *New Research on Short -Term Memory* (pp. 241-265). Hauppauge, NY: Nova Science Publishers, Inc.

Sansavini, A., Savini, S., Guarini, A., Broccoli, S., Alessandroni, R. Faldella, G. (2010). The effect of gestational age on developmental outcomes: a longitudinal study in the first two years of life. *Child: Care, Health and Development,* 37, 26-36.

Schafer, R.J., Lacadie, C., Vohr, B., Kesler, S.R., Katz, K.H., Schneider, K.C., Pugh, K.R., Makuch, R.W., Reiss, A.L., Constable, R.T., Ment, L.R. (2009). Alterations in functional connectivity for language in prematurely born adolescents. *Brain,* 132(3), 661-670.

Smith, K.E., Landry, S.H., Swank, P.R., Baldwin, C.D., Denson, S.E., Wildin, S. (1996). The relation of medical risk and maternal stimulation with preterm infant's developmental of cognitive, language and daily living skills. *Journal of Child Psychology and Psychiatry,* 37, 855-864.

Stern, M., Karraker, K., Meldrum-Sopko, A., Norman, S. (2000). The prematurity stereotype revisited: impact on mother's interactions with premature and full-term infants. *Infant Mental Health Journal,* 21, 495-509.

Stolt, S., Haataja, L., Lapinleimu, H., Lehtonen, L. (2009). Associations between lexicon and grammar at the end of the second year in finnish children. *Journal of Child Language,* 36(4), 779-806.

Stolt, S., Klippi, A., Launonen, K., Munck, P., Lehtonen, L, Lapinleimu, H., Haataja, L., the Pipari study group (2007). Size and composition of the lexicon in prematurely born very-low-birth-weight and full-term Finnish children at two years of age. *Journal of Child Language,* 34, 283–310.

Sullivan, M.C., McGrath, M.M. (2003). Perinatal morbidity, mild motor delay, and later school outcomes. *Developmental Medicine and Child Neurology,* 45, 104–112.

Taylor, H.G., Klein, N., Minich, N.M., Hack, M. (2000). Middle school age outcomes in children with very low birthweight. *Child Development,* 71, 1495-1511.

Tideman, E. (2000). Longitudinal follow-up of children born preterm: cognitive development at age 19. *Early Human Development,* 58, 81–90.

Van Lierde, K.M., Roeyers, H., Boerjan, S., De Groote, I. (2009). Expressive and receptive language characteristics in three-year-old preterm children with extremely low birth weight. *Folia Phoniatrica et Logopaedica*, 61(5), 296-299.

Walther, F.J., den Ouden, A.L., Verloove-Vanhorick, S.P. (2000). Looking back in time: outcome of a national cohort of very preterm infants born in the Netherlands in 1983. *Early Human Development,* 59, 175-191.

Westermann, G., Mareschal, D., Johnson, M.H., Sirois, S., Spratling, M.W., Thomas, M.S.C. (2007). Neuroconstructivism. *Developmental Science,* 10, 75-83.

Whitfield, M.F., Grunau, R.V.E., Holsti, L. (1997). Extremely premature (< 800 g) schoolchildren: multiple areas of hidden disability. *Archives of Disease in Childhood, 77,* F85–F90.

Wolke, D., Meyer, R. (1999). Cognitive status, language attainment, and prereading skills of 6-year-old very preterm children and their peers: The Bavarian Longitudinal Study. *Developmental Medicine and Child Neurology,* 41, 94-109.

Wolke, D., Samara, M., Bracewell, M., Marlow, N. (2008). Specific language difficulties and school achievement in children born at 25 weeks of gestation or less. *Journal of Pediatrics,* 152(2), 256-262.

Woodward, L.J., Moor, S., Hood, K.M., Champion, P.R., Foster-Cohen, S., Inder, T.E., Austin, N.C. (2009). Very preterm children show impairments across multiple neurodevelopmental domains by age 4 years. *Archives of Disease in Childhood: Fetal and Neonatal Edition*, 94(5), F339-F344.

Reviewed by Laura M. Justice, School of Teaching and Learning, The Ohio State University, United States.

In: Preterm Infants
Editors: Diogo Contreiras and Johann Sampaio

ISBN 978-1-62081-819-0

Chapter 9

DEVELOPMENTAL OUTCOMES OF PRETERM BIRTH: COGNITIVE AND BEHAVIOURAL PROBLEMS IN MODERATELY PRETERM CHILDREN AT PRESCHOOL AGE

Giovanna Perricone*, M. Regina Morales, and Concetta Polizzi
Department of Psychology, University of Palermo, Italy

ABSTRACT

The chapter proposes a research study on the likely developmental outcomes of preterm birth and, in particular, on cognitive and behavioural problems in moderately preterm children at preschool age.

The objective of the study is to investigate the likely occurrence of precursors of ADHD, meant as a complex disorder, in moderately preterm children at preschool age, characterised by distraction, impulsiveness and hyperactivity, at school and home. Therefore, the study is aimed at broadening the knowledge on some specific features of the evolutional paths of moderately preterm children, in order to provide directions for the activation of the training, useful for improving their life quality.

The research has involved 55 moderately preterm children (M: 34,6-week gestational age, SD: 2) without any medical and/or neurological neonatal complications, and low birth weight (M:2100 g, SD: 350 g); a control group of 55 full term children without any pre- and perinatal complications (M: 40-week gestational age, SD: 2). Parents and reference teachers of children were administered specific questionnaires and Italian scales (IPDDAI - *Attention Deficit Hyperactivity Disorder Early Detection for Teachers;* IPDAG - *Attention Deficit Hyperactivity Disorder Early Detection for Parents*; IPDA- *Early Learning Deficit Detection Questionnaire*) to detect attention deficit and hyperactivity in the child's everyday and school life.

The results show a profile of moderately preterm children at risk of attention deficit and hyperactivity, and highlight statistically significant differences related to gender (IPDDAI [$F_{(2,\ 110)}$ = 2.9, p=.04]), birth (IPDAG [$F_{(2,\ 110)}$ = 3, p =.04]) and interaction

* Corresponding author: Giovanna Perricone, Email addresses: giovanna.perricone@unipa.it, Telephone number: +3909123897740

(IPDDAI [$F_{(2, 110)} = 2$, p=.01]). The moderately preterm children show a deficit in self-regulation and self-control (IPDAG [$F_{(1)} = 3.6$, p=.04], and attention deficit in both everyday family (IPDAG [$F_{(1)} = 5.7$, p=.02]) and school life (IPDDAI [$F_{(1)} = 2.9$, p=.04]. In particular, preterm young girls show a higher risk of disattention, compared to young boys.

The outcomes would suggest assessment paths, aimed at monitoring the aspects of cognitive, motor and behavioural development of moderately preterm children, recognised as signs of problematic functioning profiles.

Therefore, the chapter suggests the activation of training for children showing precursors of ADHD at preschool age. The training would involve children in experiential activities, which are aimed at improving the management of their attention and self-regulation processes, in order to prevent ADHD syndrome from occurring.

INTRODUCTION

The chapter proposes a research study on the likely developmental outcomes of preterm birth and, in particular, on cognitive and behavioural problems in moderately preterm children at preschool age.

In fact, preterm birth (gestational age between 32 and 34/5 weeks), especially when occurs together with low birth weight (1500 - 2500g), would seem to be an evolutional risk condition at cognitive, behavioural and socio-relational levels (Aylward, 2005; Huddy, Johnson and Hope, 2001; Bhutta, Cleves, Casey, Cradock and Anand, 2002). Some studies, in fact, have highlighted that the interruption of the foetal maturation, which occurs at 32nd and 36th gestational week, includes a cerebral immaturity at birth (Inder, Warfield, Wang, Huppi and Volpe, 2005; van Baar, Vermaas, Knots, de Oleine and Soons, 2009; Heinonen, Räikkönen, Pesonen, Andersson, Kajantie, Eriksson, Wolke and Lano, 2010) and, then, likely risks for the cognitive development of preterm children (Kinney, 2006; Espy, Senn, Charack, Tayler and Wieber, 2007; Peterson, Anderson, Ehrenkranz, Staib, Tageldin, Colon, Gore, Duncan, Makuch and Ment, 2003). That means attentive, metacognitive, self-regulation impairments, which would lead to symptomatic configurations of attention and hyperactivity deficit (ADHD) (Krain & Castellanos, 2006), and/or learning disorders and lower scholar marks (McGrath & Sullivan, 2002; O'Keeffe, O'Callaghan, Williams, Najmanm and Bor, 2003). Such studies would seem to stress that moderately preterm children (gestational age < 32 weeks), besides severely preterm cases, also show general self-control and attention disorders since (pre-)school age, though at a less severe level (Chyi, Lee, Hintz, Gould and Sutcliffe, 2008; Huddy et al., 2001; Van Baar et al., 2009; Heinonen et al., 2010). These disorders are usually detected at school age, when a problematic configuration of them becomes easy to be diagnosed (ibid.). They may clearly be revealed by symptomatic disadaptive behaviour in the child's reference educational contexts such as family, group of peers, etc. (ibid.) and, especially at school, since it is characterized by a specific time and spaces, organized by a discipline referring to metacognitive process, and the use of diversified languages and multiple modalities of elaboration of information.

In the light of such considerations, this study focuses its attention on the likely presence of precursors of ADHD, meant as a neurobiological complex disorder (American Psychological Association [APA], 1994; Byrne, Bawden, Beattie and De Wolfe, 2000; Curatolo, D'Agati and Moavero, 2010; Daley, 2006), in moderately preterm birth children at (pre-)school age, characterised by distraction, impulsiveness and hyperactivity. Hence, the study is aimed at broadening knowledge on some specific features of the evolutional paths, in order to provide directions for the activation of the training (Tenuta, 2007), useful for improving the moderately preterm children life quality (Theunissen, Veen, Fekkes, Koopman, Zwinderman, Brugman and Wit, 2001).

The study deals, in particular, with some cognitive and behavioural functioning of moderately preterm children at (pre-)school age, detected as likely precursors of ADHD which, at school age, may lead not only to the real syndrome, but also to learning disorders which impair children school functioning (Als, Gilkerson, Duffy, Mcanulty, Buehler, Vendenberg, Sweet, Sell, Parad, Ringer, Butler, Blickman and Jones, 2003; Cherkes-Julkowski, 1998). It is a model for reading specific indicators of the precursors of ADHD, such as *disattention/inattention*, meant as a distraction during school and recreational activities and to fulfil an activity in later instructions. A wide literature has highlighted that preterm children are easily distracted and less capable to sustain their attention to an object, or what they are doing at that moment (Gillberg, 2003; Espy, et al., 2007), impairing the activation of cognitive processes (gathering and selecting information, concentration…) useful for a more rational adjustment to situations (ibid.), especially for the cases of severe prematurity (Shum, Neulinger, O'Callaghan and Mohay, 2008; Lawson & Ruff, 2004).

Hyperactivity, which includes restlessness, difficulties in performing "calm" ludic activities and motor activity modulation disorder, leading to perform clumsy and uncoordinated not-oriented movements with a reckless motor behaviour (Byrne, et al., 2000; Curatolo et al., 2010; Daley, 2006). It would seem that when such processes lack in preterm children, especially in extremely preterm children, as verified by specific studies (Foulder-Hughes & Cooke, 2003; Hemgren & Persson, 2006), some motor developmental impairments occur particularly with regard to the capacity of modulation of fine motor skills and visuo-spatial coordination (ibid.). One more indicator, linked to the previous one, is *impulsivity*, meant as behavioural self-regulation, motor skills and self-control impairments. Children find it hard to respect roles, modulate his/her relationship with the other, join to and "invade" the others' activities (plays, conversations, etc.), wait before speaking and (Clark, Woodward, Horwood and Moor, 2008), due to their impulsivity.

The reading model of the precursors of ADHD, according to the literature of the field, recognizes that males are likely to be more affected by the precursors of ADHD than females (McGrath, Sullivan, Devin, Fontes-Murphy, Barcelos, DePalma and Faraone 2005; Befera & Barkley, 1985), especially with respect to hyperactivity. It also detects, in preterm children, the probable concomitance, related to hyperactivity and attention disorders, of deficit of specific skills useful for (pre-)school learning such as linguistic comprehension, oral expression, metacognition, memory, orientation, pre-mathematics and pre-literacy (pre-reading and pre-writing) (Sansavini, Guarini, Ruffilli, Alessandrini, Giovanelli and Salvioli, 2004; Chyi et al., 2008; Cherkes-Julkowski, 1998; Delobel-Ayoub, Arnaud, White-Koning, Casper, Pierrat, Garel, Burguet, Roze, Matis, Picaud, Kaminski and Larroque 2009; Egeland, Kalkoske, Gottesman and Erickson, 1990; Saigal, den Ouden e Wolke, 2003; Taylor, Klein, Munich and Hack, 2000).

METHODS

Study Objects and Hypothesis

In the light of the previous considerations, and according to the above-mentioned model, the study is aimed to investigate behavioural and cognitive precursors of ADHD in moderately preterm children at school age. It has been verified:

- the presence of statistically significant differences between moderately preterm young boys/girls, and full term young boys/girls at school age, with relation to the indicators of precursors of ADHD (distraction, hyperactivity/impulsivity);
- the presence of statistically significant differences between moderately preterm young boys/girls, and full term young boys/girls at school age, with relation to various general and specific skills, useful for (pre-)school learning (cognitive skills such as memory, orientation, linguistic comprehension, oral expression, metacognition, prerequisites of reading/writing and mathematics).

Participants

The research has involved an experimental group, so defined according to the "preterm birth" variable, consisted of 55 moderately preterm children (M: 34,6-week gestational age, SD: 2) without any medical neonatal and/or complications and low birth weight (M: 2100g, SD: 350 g), selected according to the following criteria: gestational age <35 weeks, birth weight 1500 to 2500 g. without any neurological pathology, sensorial and genetic pathology deficit nor malformative syndrome.

A control group made up of 55 healthy full term children (M: 40-week gestational age, without any pre and perinatal complications), has also been involved and can be superimposed to the previous one for their anamnestic and sociocultural features (see table 1). The selection criteria of the control group were: birth at about 40th post conceptional week (range= 39 to 41 weeks of gestation); birth weight > 2500 g; absence of pre and perinatal complications, neurologic pathology, sensorial and genetic pathology deficit and malformative syndrome.

All the involved children, of whom the ADHD precursors have been studied, were at the average age of 5 years and two months; the 90% of them had siblings (two on average), belonged to social middle class one-income families with secondary school education on the average. The children attended the last year of Italian pre-school (namely the English equivalent for the first year of primary school) at school institutes of Palermo and its province.

The research group children were involved after their parents had signed the declaration of informed consent, according to the D.LGS. 196/2003 art.13 related to the personal data protection.

Table 1. Characteristics of the sample by term and preterm birth

Prenatal and family characteristics						
Characteristics of moderately preterm children* (=55)				Characteristics of full term children (=55)		
Variable	*mean*	*sd*	*range*	*mean*	*sd*	*range*
Child age (months)	62	4	57-67	64	2.5	61-66
Birth gestational age	34,6	2	31–35	40	2.5	38–41
Birth weight (g)	2100	350	1450-2400	3100	350	2750-3450
Days of hospitalization	15	8	8–23	2	1.5	2–3
Female %	54%			51%		
Male %	46%			49%		
Family background of preterm children				Family background of full term children		
Variable	*mean*	*sd*	*range*	*mean*	*sd*	*range*
Mother's age (years)	30,6	6	24-37	32,6	5	28-38
Parental educational attainment (years)	13	8	8-23	12	8	8-22
Number of children	2	1.5	1-3	2	1.5	1-4

* Healthy Preterm (HPT): No medical/neurological complications

Procedures and Instruments

The following instruments have been utilised in order to investigate the research field

- IPPDDAI Italian scale (*Attention Deficit Hyperactivity Disorder Early Detection for Teachers*) (Marcotto, Paltenghi and Cornoldi, 2002), a specific questionnaire, articulated in 18 items, which allows to investigate distraction and hyperactivity symptoms in children, 5 to 6 years old, attending the equivalent English first year of primary school. Such development stage is the best moment for evaluating the self-control grade, gained by the subject. It is due to the mild behavioural variability among children and their coming up to the important phase of primary school (ibid.). The children's reference teachers filled in the questionnaire. They were asked to evaluate how frequently they detected certain skills and behaviours showed by children in the classroom, by means of Likert-type Scale 4 response levels (0= not at all/never; 1=rarely/sometimes; 2=quite frequently/most of the times; very frequently/always). The 14 items of questionnaire refer to the dimensions of *disattention*, meant as the difficulty the child has in focusing on details and prolong his/her attention during an activity and of *hyperactivity/impulsivity*, meant as motor skills restlessness and self-control and self-regulation disorders. The last four items are related to the likely risk factors that may affect the persistency, grade and development of ADHD symptoms such as a socio-cultural disadvantage, poor cognitive potentialities, presence of emotional and/or relational impairments and likely family troubles. The analysis of data allows to distinguish scores related to each subscale (*disattention* and *hyperactivity/impulsivity*). To be more precise, the score equal to or lower than 10 percentile (raw score equal to or higher than 14 points per dimension), shows a case at risk; the score between 11 and 24 percentile (score equal to or higher than 9), is an edge case; the score equal to or higher than 25 percentile is a non problematic case.

The instrument has been designed according to the Italian normative sample. It has been performed a factorial analysis on the items that, as a general rule, refer to diagnostic criteria of DSM-IV and Kendall & Wilcox's Scale (1979). Such analysis allowed to assess appreciable levels of saturation of each item, with respect to the two dimensions that the instrument need to evaluate. The predictive quality of the instrument has also been assessed through the administration of other instruments, useful for the detection of children with attention and hyperactivity deficit, at school age, and it proved to be quite trustworthy.

- IPDDAG Italian Scale (*Attention Deficit Hyperactivity Disorder Early Detection for Parents*) (Riello, Re and Cornoldi, 2005), a specific questionnaire, aimed to the detection of subjects defined "at risk" of ADHD, during the (pre-)school age, performed through the assessment of parents. To be more precise, the questionnaire has been administered to parents of children attending the last year of Italian pre-school, namely the English equivalent for the first year of primary school. Parents were asked to evaluate, through the Likert-type scale 4 response levels (0= not at all/never; 1= rarely/sometimes; 2=quite frequently/most of the time; very frequently/always), how frequently they had observed the behaviour that their children display at home. The questionnaire is made up of 14 items expressed in a negative form, whose odd items refer to disattention, related to the difficulty the child has in prolonging his/her attention on an activity and plays at home, while the evens refer to *impulsivity/hyperactivity* meant as motor restlessness and self-control and self-regulation disorders. Five more final items are also to be considered related to risk factors (forms of socio-cultural disadvantage, poor cognitive potentialities, presence of emotional and/or relational impairments and likely family troubles). The content of items refers to other previous questionnaires, namely IPDDAI scale and SDAG scale (addressed to parents in order to assess disattention and hyperactivity behaviour of children at school age) and DSM-IV criteria. The validity of the scale has been verified through a factorial analysis whose results show that the division of items in components (disattention and hyperactivity), hypothesized during the design of the instrument, have been realized. Moreover, the values of Pearson's coefficients of correlation and Cronbach's alpha value showed appreciable internal coherence of the instrument.

  It has to be specified that the higher the score is, the larger the presence of pathognomonic tracts of the disorder occurs. Therefore, the case of a child who gets a score equal to, or higher than 14 marks in each scale (Hyperactivity/impulsivity average score= 13,7 ds=4,30; Disattention Scale average score=11,7 ds=3,78), is at risk.
- IPDA Italian Questionnaire (*Early Learning Deficit Detection Questionnaire*) (Terreni, Tretti, Corcella, Cornoldi and Tressoldi, 2002), an instrument aimed to assess behavioural disorders at (pre-)school age, detecting some aspects related to ADHD precursors, particularly those linked to *hyperactivity/impulsivity* (*motor skills* and *behavioural aspects* scales) and *Disattention* (*Metacognition Scale, Other cognitive skills, Oral expression* and *Linguistic comprehension*). It also detects

further deficiencies of children's learning skills (pre-mathematics and pre-literacy). The questionnaire has been filled in, by the children's reference teachers who were asked to evaluate, by means of the Likert-type Scale 4 response levels (0= not at all/never; 1= rarely/sometimes; 2=quite frequently/most of times; very frequently/always), how frequently they detected certain skills and behaviours, displayed by the children in the classroom. The questionnaire is made up of 43 items, divided into two sections, where the first section deals with general skills related to learning "aptitude" (ibid.), and the second one focuses on specific skills, namely reading-writing and mathematics prerequisites. The first section includes the *behavioural aspects scale*, related to the capability of children to adjust themselves to rules, to self-control, to collaborate and work autonomously, and the skill of concentration and interest related to the field of *impulsivity*; the *Motors skills* scale, which assesses the quality of the general movement coordination, the fine motor skills and, therefore, the impaired capabilities in case of hyperactivity; the *Linguistic comprehension* and *Oral expression* are centred on the capability of being concentrated on the other's discourse, following and listening to teacher's directions, and the capabilities of expository and descriptive clarity, which would lack in case of disattention and hyperactivity. Finally, the *Metacognition* scale, which investigates the child's ability to use strategies better to understand the persistence in exercises, the capability of realizing that particular noise, or other activities may distract him/her, is usually related to appreciable levels of attention; the scale of *Other cognitive abilities* that investigates memory, space orientation and visual-motor coordination. *Pre-literacy* scale about metalinguistic skills and *Pre-mathematics* scale about reasoning, use of quantities and mathematical operations skills, are included in the section related to the requested skills successfully to face learning.
As for reading and interpreting the result, it has to be specified that a score, equal to or lower than 113, shows the presence of a likely risk of learning disorders, potentially linked to attention and cognitive skills deficiency, and self-regulation difficulties; furthermore, the procedure includes the comparison with reference normative scores for each scale, collected through the process of validation of the instrument on Italian sample, which proved to have appreciable levels of validity and trustworthiness.

RESULTS

Data Treatment and Analysis

The statistic programme for Social Sciences – SPSS 16 has analysed the data codified.

The survey about the likely differences between moderately preterm and full term young boys/girls, detected in the different fields precursors of ADHD (*disattention, hyperactivity/impulsivity*), besides of general skills useful to school learning (*Behaviour, motor skills, cognitive skills, linguistic comprehension, oral expression, metacognition, prerequisites of the reading-writing* and *mathematics*), has been performed through the analysis of the multivariate variance (MANOVA), with continuous variables (scores related to the different scales) 2 (birth) X 2 (gender) and the one-varied variance (ANOVA). To be more precise, the likely differences between the scores of the various scales (dependent variables) have been analyzed considering as independent variables, birth (Term/Preterm) and gender (F/M), both jointly (interaction effect through MANOVA) and independently (single effect through ANOVA). So, the effect of each separately independent variable (birth/gender) and the likely effect of interaction between the two (birth X gender) have been verified. A value of p=0,05 has been used for the text of significativity.

Concerning the presence of precursors of attention deficit and hyperactivity, and the likely differences between the two groups in scores, collected through the assessments by the teachers (IPDDAI) and the parents (IPDAG), the results of MANOVA (table 2) highlight both the presence of single effects, statistically significant linked to gender (IPDDAI, [lambda $_{(2,\ 110)}$ = 2.9, p=.04]) and birth (IPDDAG, [lambda $_{(2,\ 110)}$ = 3, p =.04]), and the relative effects (IPDDAI, [lambda $_{(2,\ 110)}$ = 2.03, p=.01]). Therefore, in parents' evaluation, moderately preterm and full term children differ with relation to the presence of ADHD precursors while, in teachers' assessment, such difference seems to occur both with relation to the "gender" variable and jointly to "birth" variable, namely, moderately preterm young boys/girls, when compared to full term children, have different attention deficits and behavioural self-regulation disorders.

Concerning the differences related to general abilities at the (pre-)school age useful for school learning, as evaluated by teachers (IPDA), there are statistically significant differences with regard to "gender" variable [lambda $_{(8,\ 110)}$ = 2.3, p=.02] and the two jointly [lambda $_{(8,\ 110)}$ = 2.1, p=.03]. Therefore, moderately preterm young boys/girls gained different scores in comparison with full term young boys/girls.

Table 2. ADHD precursors in moderately preterm and full term children

Instruments	Effect*		
	Birth (MPT/T)	Gender (M/F)	Gender * Birth
IPDAG	$F_{(df2,\ 110)}$ 3 Sign .04	$F_{(df2,110)}$ 1.8 Sign.17	$F_{(df2,\ 110)}$ 1.3 Sign .8
IPDDAI	$F_{(df2,\ 110)}$ .5 Sign .6	$F_{(df2,110)}$ 2.9 Sign .04	$F_{(df2,\ 110)}$ 2.03 Sig .01
IPDA	$F_{(df8,\ 110)}$ 1.4 Sig .06	$F_{(df8,110)}$ 2.3 Sig .02	$F_{(df8,110)}$ 2.1 Sig .03

* Multivariate Test: Wilks' Lambda.

Legend: IPDDAI - Attention Deficit Hyperactivity Disorder Early Detection for Teachers; IPDAG: Attention Deficit Hyperactivity Disorder Early Detection for Parents; IPDA: Early Learning Deficit Detection Questionnarie.

Particularly, the univariate analysis of the variance highlight, in teachers' assessment performed through the IPDDAI, statistically significant differences, related to the interaction between gender and birth, in disattention [$F_{(1)}$ = 2.9, p=.04]. Preterm young girls, as highlighted by mean scores of the research group (table 3), have higher scores in comparison with preterm and full term young boys and girls. It seems that preterm young girls mostly show difficulty in sustaining their attention to homework and (pre-)school activities, so they are often distracted; they try to avoid those activities which require a mental effort or attention to details or organize activities.

Table 3. Mothers and teacher'sRating on Attention Deficit and Hyperactivity/ Impulsivity in Moderately Preterm and full Term children

Mothers - IPDDAG Questionnarie									
	MPT			*T*			*Tests of Between-Subjects Effects*		
Scales	*Mean (SD)*	*Mean Female (SD)*	*Mean Male (SD)*	*Mean (SD)*	*Mean Female (SD)*	*Mean Male (SD)*	*Birth (MPT/T)*	*Sex (M/F)*	*Sex * Birth*
Inattention	10.01 (.54)	10.7 (5.9)	9.8 (5.9)	8 (5.3)	7 (4.7)	9 (5.9)	$F_{(dfl)}$ 5.7 sign. .02	$F_{(dfl)}$ .34 sign. .5	$F_{(dfl)}$2.5 sign. .12
Hyperactivity/ Impulsivity	15.67 (.51)	15.7 (6.6)	15.2 (6.7)	13.5 (6.5)	13 (6.3)	14.4 (6.6)	$F_{(dfl)}$3.6 sign. .04	$F_{(dfl)}$. 07 sign. .8	$F_{(dfl)}$4 sign. .52
Teachers - IPDDAI Questionnarie									
	MPT			*T*			*Tests of Between-Subjects Effects*		
Scales	*Mean (SD)*	*Mean Female (SD)*	*Mean Male (SD)*	*Mean (SD)*	*Mean Female (SD)*	*Mean Male (SD)*	*Birth (MPT/T)*	*Sex (M/F)*	*Sex * Birth*
Inattention	9 (5.2)	7 (5.3)	5.3 (4.8)	5.6 (4.9)	5.1 (4.8)	6.1 (5)	$F_{(dfl)}$ .45 sign. .5	$F_{(dfl)}$ .16 sign. .69	$F_{(dfl)}$ 2.9 sign. .04
Hyperactivity/ Impulsivity	13.04 (5.3)	6.3 (5.4)	6.3 (5.4)	5.3 (5.2)	4.6 (5.1)	6.1 (5.2)	$F_{(dfl)}$ .86 sign. .35	$F_{(dfl)}$. 52 sign. .47	$F_{(dfl)}$ 1.02 sign. .31

Legend: MPT: Moderately Preterm; T: Term children; SD: Std. Deviation.

Such datum is also confirmed by information given by parents (IPDAG) that highlight statistically significant differences related to preterm birth in both *hyperactivity/impulsivity* [$F_{(1)}$ = 3.6, p=.04] and *disattention* [$F_{(1)}$ = 5.7, p=.02], where preterm children get higher scores in these two dimensions compared to full term children (table 3). The parents gave a description of moderately preterm children' behaviour as children who, besides their gender, not only show attention deficit at home concurring the valuation of behaviour in the classroom provided by the teachers, but they also show fidgets, excessive and restless movements, difficulties in modulating motor skills activities with clumsy uncoordinated reckless not aimed movements.

In the light of such data, it has to be considered the relevance of scores of preterm children with regard to hyperactivity and disattention precursors, since they are higher than the cut off score fixed in the questionnaire. In detail, considering the cases when parents and teacher agree (Cohen's agreement inter rater reliability k index has been calculated, and it has highlighted acceptable levels of agreement – IPDAG and IPDA=.90; IPDDAI and IPDAG= .73), the 30% of moderately preterm children exceed the cut off score, being at risk of attention deficit, while 15% is on the edge, whereas only the 15% of full term children seem to be at risk and the 7% on the edge. With regards to hyperactivity, the 55% of preterm seem to be at risk, and 15% on the edge differing from the 20% of full term children and 6% on the edge.

As for the data related to the risk of precursors of likely disorders of learning (IPDA) (table 4), ANOVA instrument only highlights, according to some scales, statistically significant differences in relation to the "gender" variable. To be more precise, males, unlikely females, have lower scores in *Metacognition*[$F_{(1)}$ = 3.7, p=.05], in *Other cognitive skills* [$F_{(1)}$ = 5, p=.02], and in *Pre-mathematics* [$F_{(1)}$ = 1.8, p=.001]. With regard to learning skill, young boys in comparison with young girls, are described by teachers as being less able to interpret their own activated cognitive processes, having poorer skills of persistence in exercises, fewer mnemonic, space orientation and visual-motor skills besides poorer skills of mathematic reasoning.

Table4. Learning performance of the children Moderately Preterm and Term at (pre-)school age

Scales IPDA Questionnaire	MPT			T			Tests of Between-Subjects Effects		
	Mean MPT (SD)	Mean Female (SD)	Mean Male (SD)	Mean (SD)	Mean Female (SD)	Mean Male (SD)	Birth (MPT/T)	Sex (M/F)	Sex * Birth
Behaviour	3 (.73)	3.1 (.78)	2.9 (.65)	3.1 (.63)	3.2 (.52)	2.3 (.72)	F (dfl) .45 sign. .5	F (dfl) 2.4 sign. .12	F (dfl) .09 sign. .75
Motor skills	3.3 (.77)	3.3 (.67)	3.1 (.89)	3.4 (.57)	3.4 (.59)	3.4 (.56)	F (dfl)2.9 sign. .09	F (dfl) .6 sign. .44	F (dfl) 1 sign. .3
Linguistic comprehension	3.3 (.6)	3.4 (.59)	3.29 (.62)	3.41 (.59)	3.46 (.53)	3.36 (.66)	F (dfl) .17 sign. .67	F (dfl) 1.4 sign. .24	F (dfl) .04 sign. .83
Metacognition	2.9 (.85)	3.07 (.78)	2.7 (.91)	2.9 (.74)	3.01 (.71)	2.8 (.77)	F (dfl) .06 sign. .8	F (dfl) 3.7 sign. .05	F (dfl) .42 sign. .5
Other cognitive abilities	3.3 (.67)	3.4 (.49)	3.08 (.82)	3.42 (.51)	3.4 (.49)	3.4 (.54)	F (dfl) 2.7 sign. .1	F (dfl) 5 sign. .02	F (dfl) 2.7 sign. .1
Pre-literacy	3.25 (.82)	3.30 (.53)	3.19 (1.1)	3.3 (.7)	3.4 (.61)	3.2 (.75)	F (dfl) .26 sign. .6	F (dfl) 1.8 sign. .18	F (dfl) 2.3 sign. .62
Pre-mathemat.	3.4 (.80)	3.6 (.43)	3.1 (1,04)	3.5 (,63)	3.6 (.51)	3.4 (.71)	F (dfl) 2.5 sign. .12	F (dfl)12 sign. .001	F (dfl)1.2 sign. .26
Total score	133.8 (27,1)	136.9 (22,6)	129.7 (32,3)	139.8 (22,4)	143.1 (19,9)	136.1 (24.4)	F (dfl) 2.4 sign. .12	F (dfl) 3.1 sign. .08	F (dfl) 0 sign. .9

Legend: MPT: Moderately Preterm; T: Term children; SD: Std. Deviation

From a descriptive point of view, it seems interesting that both scores related to such scales and those collected from all other scales of the questionnaire, are lower in moderately preterm young boys (=129) when compared to full term children (males and females) and preterm young girls. Finally, considering the total score of IPDA (table 4), the two groups on average do not reach the cut off score (equal to 113), so it is not enough to detect the presence of precursors of learning disorders. Hence, moderately preterm young boys are not mostly at risk in comparison with full term children (tot > 113). In fact, in the two groups there is the same percentage of subject at risk (about 20%).

DISCUSSION

The data gained by the research highlight the presence of a profile of moderately preterm children who, even at (pre-)school age are "at risk" of attention deficit and hyperactivity disorder. Preterm children of the research group are described, especially at home, as hyperactive and restless, children, showing a certain difficulty in self-regulating and self-controlling during calm play activities.

A further remarkable element underlined by data and related to disattention, is that parents and teachers agree in reporting that moderately preterm children show, both at school and home, attention difficulties that are at risk of attention deficit at (pre-)school age. Therefore, the children do not succeed in prolonging their attention on homework to be done at school, and plays at home; they seem almost to divert their mind while performing school and game activities, showing difficulties in listening to direct speech, following the directions given to fulfil a game or homework. Such datum seem to be connected to the literature of the field, which highlights how preterm children are more distractible, and less able to monitor what happens, what they do, or sustain their attention on an object, than full term children are (Gillberg, 2003; Espy et al., 2007; Shum et al., 2008; Lawson & Ruff, 2004).

This aspect seems to be strongly characterized in terms of gender typization. With regard to *hyperactivity,* in fact, teachers, unlike parents, do not diversify children because of birth but rather of gender, attributing to males a higher risk of hyperactivity, while, in respect of *disattention,* both parents and teachers recognize such difficulty in moderately preterm children, even if teachers detect a higher impairment in females (see Tabb. 2 and 3).

Such data trace a similarity between the maturity and developmental path of severely preterm children (< 32 weeks) and that of moderately preterm ones (van Baar et al., 2009) highlighting, even in the latter case, potential risks linked to moderately preterm birth. Such data are linked to those studies that have highlighted that severe prematurity and low birth weight, occurring together or separately, are factors that may affect (ibid.; Strang-Karlsson, Raikkonen, Pesonen, Kajantie, Paavonen, Lahti, Hovi, Heinonen, Jarvenpaa, Eriksson and Andersson, 2008) the development of impulsivity regulation, self-regulation and behaviour and motor self-control processes (as well as concentration and attention skills). Prematurity and low birth weight (aside from gestational age of foetus), are important factors which lead to underline that children of the research group are characterized by a moderately prematurity (32-34 weeks), without any neurologic sequence, cognitive impairments, prolonged hospitalizations in UTIN (on the average 15 days), nor surgical interventions, but a low birth weight (mean =2100 g). The levels of maturity of physiological brain processes of foetus, reached before the interruption caused by birth at 34 weeks (Allin, Henderson and Suckling, 2004) are noteworthy too, because, together with genetic and environmental factors (early interaction with hospital environment, medical treatments, relationships with parents, external stimuli…), contribute to trace problems and slight disorders only occurring in terms of "slowness" and/or difficulty at (pre-)school and school age.

It has to be noticed that the evolutional level of the moderately preterm children, involved in the research group, seems to be less problematic than that of severely preterm children, aside from likely risks related to attention deficit and hyperactivity at (pre-)school age, when specific resources are highlighted. The data, in fact, show the lack of disorders and learning retardation, showing levels of (pre-)school performance that, even if poorer than that of full term children, is not a risk of future school failure as it could be in case of severe prematurity.

ADHD Risk Training in Moderately Preterm Children at Preschool Age

The research seems to suggest some implications related to the intervention of prevention of ADHD risk in moderately preterm children. This study, in fact, reports a specific early training course, addressed to preschoolers to develop self-regulation skills (emotional, cognitive, relational, behavioural skills); to parents, to develop their parental competencies, useful for facing their child behavioural problems related to everyday life; finally, specific preschool and school educational paths, addressed to the teachers to manage didactical strategies, oriented to the development of cognitive and meta-cognitive competencies in children.

Table 5. Training path for the ADHD risk at preschool age

Subjects involved	1st month	2nd month	3rd month	4th month	5th month	6th month
Children	First meeting Attention focus group Self-regulation focus group Metacognition focus group	Laboratories focusing on the task "knowing the world"	Laboratories focusing on the task "the self and the other"	Laboratories focusing on the task "body and movement"	Laboratories focusing on the task "talks and words"	Laboratories focusing on "languages, creativity and expression"
Parent	Forum "attention and self-regulation difficulties" child's behaviour observation through the catalogue technique Laboratories focusing on child's behavioural repertoire	Administration of the Q-sort on parental competence Task-based laboratories on the connection between educational practices and dysfunctional behaviours of children Task-based laboratories on the transformation of parental behaviour	Homework Parole with group of parents	Counselling setting for each parental couple	Home-work	Supervision through phone counselling Administration of narrative interview and the assessment questionnaire (IPDAG)
Teacher	Forum on "attention and self-regulation difficulties" Task-based Laboratory on the guidelines for the prevention of ADHD	Task-based Laboratory on planning interventions to be activated in the classrooms	Homework	Super-vision with counselling setting	Home-work	Supervision Administration of a questionnaire and of the assessment questionnaires (IPDA e IPDDAI)
Pediatrician	Administration of a narrative interview		Administration of a narrative interview			Administration of a narrative interview

The main guidelines for the treatment of ADHD (Kirby & Grimley, 2007; Consensus Conference, 2003;Chiarenza, Bianchi and Marzocchi, 2006), and other several scientific contribution of the field (Barkley, 1990; 1997; Conners, Epstein, March, Angold, et al., 2001) suggest, in fact, the importance of elaborate training interventions concurrently addressed to child, parents, teachers and family pediatricians. Therefore, it has been created a "combined" intervention programme (table 5), since every subject (child, parents, teachers and family pediatricians) will be involved at the same time, and each of them will be the author of a path monitoring the likely change in the child's behaviour. The programme will be performed after disclosing to parents and teachers, the outcomes of the above-mentioned assessment activated with children at school. The disclosure of the outcomes, will allow parents to take part, consciously and proactively, in their own training, and to involve their children, identified as at risk of ADHD.

Parent Training

With respect to work with parents, the programme implies a parent training aimed to the redefinition of parental competence, useful for the management of the problem behaviour of children at preschool age, which may lead to ADHD at school age. It is a parental training, whose purpose is fostering the proper management of some relevant parental functions such as

- The *assessment* function, which is related to the recognition of child's skills and behaviours characterising his/her everyday life. This function is aimed clearly to distinguish what is a developmental resource of the child, from what may be a likely "signal" (problem behaviour) as a precursor of the syndrome.
- The *cognitive* and *emotional coping,* which is related to parents' skill of properly managing their own emotions, while facing their child's difficult behaviours and, at the same time, of detecting the possibilities of change and future planning.
- The *scaffolding* function, which is meant as a cognitive orientation and emotional support addressed to the child. It is aimed to stimulate the child to convert his/her problem behaviours, which are potential precursors of ADHD.
- The *caregiving* function, which is meant as the parents' skill of meeting the "special" developmental needs of their child.

This parent training implies, in respect of procedure and method, a path that comprises interventions to be performed over the course of six months, together with each participant parental couple, and a group consisting of up to a maximum of eight couples selected from them.

To be more precise, the training implies an *earlier phase* performed through the activation of one *Forum* on "attention deficit and self-regulation difficulties in children at preschool-age", as a group method aimed to valorise the different perspectives, ideas and representations (Perricone Briulotta, 2005; 2011) that every participant parent has about the issue to be tackled. The forum implies the activation of a debate on a narrative text concerning the "case" of a child displaying certain behaviours, at both home and school, that may be a sign of hyperactivity and impulsivity disorder and attention deficit. Such an intervention would allow the trainer, together with parents, to "draw" a spectrum not only of every likely implications and problems connected to such difficulties, but also of the likely resources.

The *treatment phase* implies the activation, with each parental couple, of an assessment path focused on their child's competences and developmental impairments, by means of descriptive techniques of observation and, in particular, behavioural catalogue technique and the Q-Sort technique (Perricone Briulotta, 2003), besides some laboratory methods. In detail:

- the administration to parents of a *catalogue* made up of a list of thirty behaviours displayed by children during their everyday life at home. These behaviours are related to the attention processes (10 items), self-regulation (10 items) and metacognitive sensitiveness (10)[1]. This catalogue is applied by parents every day, for two weeks, within three different temporal phases of the day, namely in the morning before going to school; in the afternoon, while children are playing both on their own and together with parents and/or siblings; at mealtime. Each unit of observation lasts thirty minutes and implies that parents record the behaviours, displayed by their children, according to the criterion of presence/absence of every behaviour listed in the catalogue.
- N. 1 "*task-based laboratory*" (Perricone Briulotta, 2011), which is aimed to determine the child's behavioural "repertoire", by including the different behavioural "inventories" got from the various observational units. This repertoire is made up of every skill and behaviour which, in parents' opinion, frequently characterises his/her child, and which could be a resource or, instead, an element of impairment for him/her (the child).
- The administration, to each parent, of the *Q-sort technique* (box 1) that is aimed to determine the profile of his/her own parental competence with respect to his/her child at risk of ADHD.
- N.2 *task-based laboratories*, one of which is aimed to get the parents to "build" a representative map which connect the child's dysfunctional behaviours with specific educational practices activated by them (the parents). The other laboratory is aimed to "build" a guide, a vade mecum of likely changes of the parental behaviours useful to also stimulate their child to change his/her disadaptive behaviours.
- *1stHomework*: it implies a stage of two-week practical training to be performed at home, where parents, according to some guidelines given by the trainer and suggested by the vade mecum, will try out the management of the new behavioural models, with his/her child. This is also a form of try-and-learn training path for parents, since they have the chance to activate new behavioural models and educational practices, in the attempt of modifying the relationship with their child; concurrently, they can determine a profile of their parental competence suitable for managing their child's problems.

[1]The catalogue is made up of a list of behaviours, detected according the criterion of coherence, and determined with relation to constructs of attention, self-regulation and metacognitive sensitiveness, by a group of experts of the field.

Box 1. The Q-Sort technique on parental competence

The Q-Sort scale, on parental competence, is a specific tool of observation, designed on purpose by the Research Unit of Pediatric Psychology of the Department of Psychology at the University of Studies of Palermo (Italy). It deals with a model of parental competence that refers to precise factors and indicators, retrieved by the literature of the field (Perricone, Morales, 2009). This scale is a descriptive technique (Cassiba, 1998; Stephenson, 1953; Block, 1961/1978; Perricone Briulotta, 2003) that, according to the self-observation mode with which parents of children are asked to describe his/her own behaviour, allows to activate a process of meta-observation, in terms of reflection on self and of the individual parental functions.

This tool, which is under validation, represents a specific contextualization of behaviours, concerning transversal factors of parental competence. It consists of a catalogue of 90 behaviours (Q-set), referring to the model of competence of the parents of children at risk of ADHD. Its indicators are the following

- *Emotional and cognitive coping,* where the *emotional* one is meant as parental self-regulation of emotions and stress reduction while facing disattention, hyperactivity and impulsivity displayed by children (e.g. "*when my son tends to be fidgety, I usually try to keep myself calm*". With respect to the *cognitive* coping, it deals with the changes in both representations and behaviours at risk of ADHD, as attitudes which can be modified by the child him/herself, in order to be not only a child with difficulties, but also with resources, (e.g.: "*I admit that, even though my child is easily distracted, s/he nevertheless succeed in carrying out the requested activities*"). It is a coping that refers to the ability of recognizing the specificity of the relation between parents and the difficulties displayed by their child (e.g.: "*It seems to me that when my child is fidgety, I can't succeed in staying with him/her*").
- *Cognitive and relational scaffolding,* which refers to parent's ability to control the impulsivity of his/her child, by proposing him/her rules, behavioural models, criteria to do something, etc. It is also related to the ability to ease his/her sustainment of attention by sharing focuses, providing him/her with practical strategies useful for selecting focuses and sustaining the concentration (e.g.: "*When my son is doing a task and s/he doesn't succeed in concentrating, I usually show him/her the steps to be observed to carry out the task*"). In respect of the relational level, the *scaffolding* refers to the abilities to provide models that rule the relationship with the others, in terms of observing and properly managing the conversational turn-taking ("*When my child and I talk each other, I usually invite him/her to observe his/her turn-taking*").
- *Caregiving,* in terms of parental responsivity as emotional tuning, whenever children display problem behaviour (e.g.: "*If my son cries because s/he doesn't want to carry out long-lasting tasks, I'll tell him/her that I understand how difficult concentrating is*"); in terms of cognitive responsivity, as parental support in managing the various everyday tasks of his/her child (e.g.: "*When my son carries out a task, I'll praise him/her*"); in terms of parental ability of adjusting his/her own educational model to the specific developmental needs of his/her child (e.g.: "*I try to reproach my son, whenever I realize s/he is misbehaving on purpose*").

The procedure of administration implies that parents grade the 90 behavioural examples of parental competence, written on cardboards, into 9 subgroups, according to a range of correspondence with their own behaviours (ibid.).

- N.1 *parole group,* with a group of parents of children at risk of ADHD, focusing on both the difficulties they have met during the homework, in order to find new management models for these difficulties.
- A *counselling setting*, involving each parental couple, whose purpose will be to find specific educational strategies useful for the proper development of their child.
- *2nd Homework*: each parental couple will experience again, in the every day relationship with their own child, the educational strategies identified during the counselling setting. They will be supervised, at distance, by the trainer, for one

month, through a "telephone counselling" (Polizzi, Morales, 2008). During this last phase, the parents will be administered a "*narrative interview*" (Atkinson, 2002), with which they are invited to report the changes of their child's behaviour, displayed as a consequence of the training. The data of the interview, when compared to those of the forum, could allow the trainer to identify a change of the representation that parents have about the disattention and hyperactivity problems of their child. Moreover, in order to evaluate the change promoted by the training, the parents will be administered again the tool utilised during the first phase of assessment (IPDAG).

Training for Preterm Children at Preschool Age

The training to be addressed to preterm children[2] at preschool age – recognized by the assessment path as children at risk of ADHD – is structured according to a *cognitive-behavioural* perspective (Kirby, Grimley, 1986), and it is aimed to develop or strengthen, in the child, early cognitive, metacognitive, emotional and social skills, whose absence makes children at risk of the syndrome.

In detail, the training promotes the processes that the above-mentioned research has detected as lacking in moderately preterm children:

- Selective attention processes, which allow to focus on activities without distraction, and processes of sustained or prolonged attention.
- Metacognition processes, concerning the child's ability of using strategies to understand better and keep on task, besides the ability of understanding what could be a source of distraction.
- Self-control processes, which are processes of behavioural self-regulation, modulation of activities depending on rules and external demands, and of expression of feelings.
- Problem solving, which is the skill of solving tasks and activities; as analysis of the characteristics of task; as research of alternatives useful for solutions.

The training implies, in respect of procedure and method, a path that comprises laboratory interventions to be performed over the course of six months. The interventions are performed according to two perspectives. The first one is the cognitive-behavioural perspective that utilise self-instructional procedures (Horn, Ialongo, Pascoe, Greenberg, Packard, Lopez, Wagner, and Puttler, 1991) aimed to activate self-talk strategies (internal dialogue, self-instruction) (Kendall & Braswell, 1985; Braswell & Bloomquist, 1991), self-monitoring (ib.), and problem solving in children. The second perspective is the metacognitive one (Cornoldi, De Beni and Gruppo MT, 2002) that deals with the development of metacognitive sensitiveness (ib.) and problem solving attitude of preschoolers. These skills are proved to be "calibrate"/sized according to the specific

[2] Parts and sequences of the training proposed within the research paths on the correlations between preterm birth and precursors of ADHD at preschool age, have been applied to measure both the efficacy and the impact of the choice of "rehabilitation" with respect to children's impairments. The model of rehabilitation is meant as psychological intervention, which allows to make the impaired processes function more properly, to be suitable for the health of the developmental trajectories.

cognitive functioning profile of preschoolers, who typically lack higher cognitive processes because of their age. Such missing cognitive processes are the abilities of thinking about his/her own cognitive modalities and the way of actively managing them (e.g. the comprehension of make-believe games, recognizing the difference between real objects and mental images), the skill of improving memory strategies and that of comprehending and ascribing mental states to themselves and to others.

In respect of the development of metacognitive attitudes, the goal of the training is also to foster a positive perception of self, i.e. a representation of self as a successful child in learning processes. The self-efficacy, in fact, besides the locus of control or the motivation, can ease the development of cognitive processes (ib.).

Moreover, as mentioned before, during the training, children will be involved in the monitoring of his/her likely change. Therefore, the training will be punctuated by segments of self-assessment, performed at the start of the path, and then at the end of every month of activities, through a worksheet for each child. The worksheet, consisting of six sketches, "asks" children to assess him/herself behaviour when at home and at school, with respect to attention, self-regulation and metacognitive attitude. To be more precise, two sketches are each related to a child who is attentive and inattentive; the other two are related to a child who is still and he is not; the last two show a child who is thinking and who is constantly speaking (see fig.1).

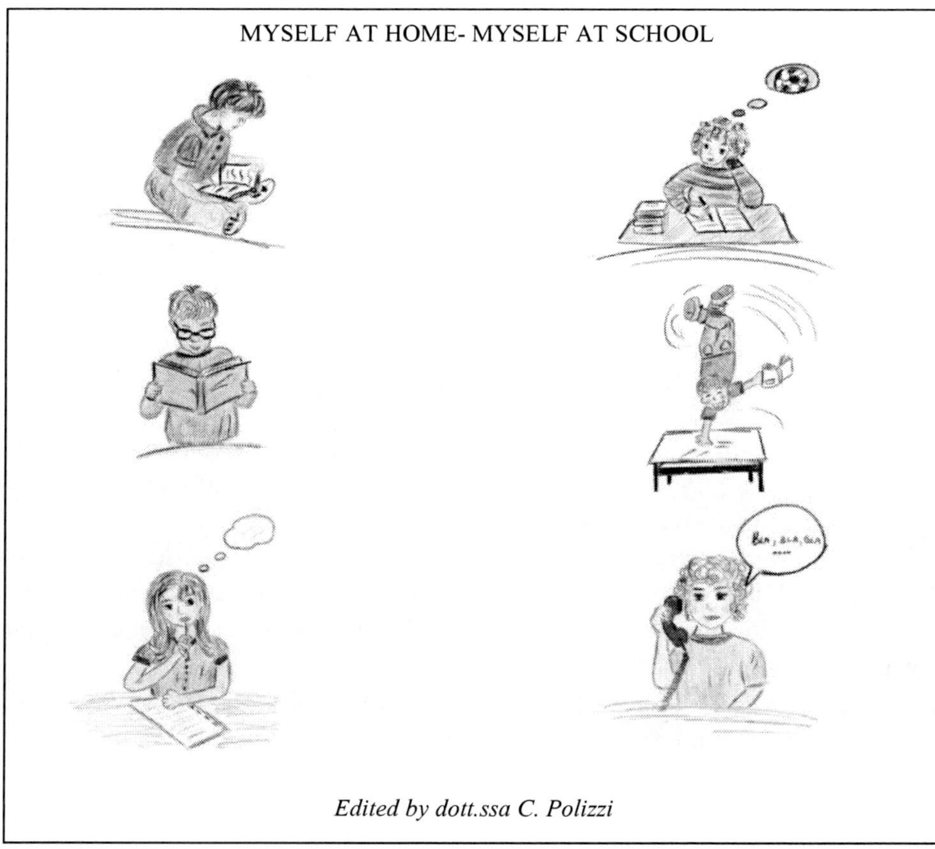

Figure 1. Sketches of self-assessment worksheet.

During the training, the trainer will monitor the likely changes in behaviour of each child, concerning the precursors of ADHD. At the end of every meeting with children, the trainer will apply a narrative technique, i.e. the technique of critical episodes (Perricone Briulotta, 2003), which allows to detect the presence of significant behaviours, with respect to the processes focalised by the treatment see (box 2). It will be possible, then, to verify the trend of change as a consequence of the treatment for each child.

To be more precise, the procedure of the training consists of two stages. The early phase, which lasts four weeks, is aimed to know the issues concerning the path and, at the same time, concerning the representation of self, with respect of the attention, self-regulation and metacognition skills; the phase of the real treatment, which lasts five months, is aimed to stimulate the change in absence of self-regulation, inattention and metacognition.

Box 2. Critical events technique

The technique implies the utilisation of a card, to detect critical episodes to be recorded together with contextual elements (time, situation, information about the episodes, etc.). It is also to be recorded the significant words that have been uttered, and/or the actions that have been displayed during the laboratory concerning the children undergoing the treatment.
DATE ....30/01/2012**................TIME...**9.30-11.30**.........**

SITUATION ...the trainer explains the part to be realized**....................................**

SHORT EPISODE .. While the trainer was explaining the task, the child X kept silent and listened to him/her without being distracted by what his/her peer was doing**...**

ANOTHER SIMILAR EPISODE.....the same behaviour has been also displayed during a later phase (in carrying out the task).......................................

ADDITIONAL INFORMATION ....

Early Stage

- N. 1 meeting with every child at risk of ADHD involved in the training. It is aimed to meet each other; to show the path they will be going to start; to explain and administer the worksheet for the self-assessment.
- N.1 *focus group* (Perricone Briulotta, 2005; 2011) on attention. It is aimed to build, together with them, a shared representation of the behaviours peculiar to an attentive child, about the value of the attention for child's wellbeing and about the outcomes to which the attention leads.
- N. 1 *focus group* (ibid.) on self-regulation. It is aimed to depict a shared idea about what self-regulating his/her own behaviour and emotions means for children, why it is so important and which benefits this action will bring to him/her.
- N. 1 *focus group* (ibid.) on metacognitive behaviour. It is aimed to build a negotiated model of how a child behaves when thinks.

It has to be remarked that all the three focus groups will be activated in every classroom where the children at risk of ADHD, involved in the training, are.

Treatment Phase

This stage implies the activation of specific fortnightly task-based laboratories (ibid.), addressed to small groups, consisting of up to a maximum of six children each, identified by the assessment path as at risk of ADHD. The explanation of these laboratories is attached (Attach. 1). The procedure applied by these laboratories allow to foster the activation of attention, self-regulation and metacognitive processes, through the planning and report of a task that implies a child's original production concerning the issues, as and when they will be tackled. Each month focuses the reference areas of the "experience field" fixed by the Italian Public Minister of Education (2007), according to infancy school (3-6 years old age). In detail

- 1st month – the laboratories will deal with the issues concerning the experience field "*knowing the world*", that is natural phenomena, space, time, measure, logical order, living organisms, technological contests and products;
- 2nd month –the laboratories will deal with the issues concerning the experience field "*the self and the other*", that is personal identity (competences, possible resources, needs, wishes, etc.), personal and family history, individual differences and civic coexistence;
- 3rd month – the laboratories will deal with the issues concerning the experience field "*body and motor control*" that isthe knowledge of body scheme, the representation of his/her own body, the control of body and its movements, the health of body and autonomy.
- 4th month – the laboratories will deal with the issues concerning the experience field "*dialogues and words*", that is communication, languages, cultures, values, building a story;
- 5th and last month – the laboratories will deal with the issues concerning the experience field "*languages, creativity and expression*", that is the different human forms of expression (music, drawing, painting, drama, etc.), multimedia language, artistic productions of cultural background.

Teacher Training

It is also planned the activation of an informative and formative path for the teachers of the reference school of the children involved in the training, to be performed during the six-month work with parents and children. The purpose of such training is to develop specific assessment competences on ADHD, in order to make teachers capable to recognize in his/her pupils, the presence of predictors of this disorder. It is also a training aimed to change the relationship between teacher and pupil at risk of ADHD, and to detect strategies, educational didactic methods, useful for developing the cognitive and metacognitive processes that are missing in such pupils.

With respect to procedure and method, the teacher's training implies

- n. 1 *Forum* on "preschoolers' attention difficulties and self-regulation", aimed to activate a debate on a narrative text concerning the case of a pupil who displays behaviours that could be precursors of ADHD. This intervention allows the trainer, together with the teachers, to "draw" a spectrum of not only every likely implication and problem connected to such difficulties, but also of the likely resources.
- N. 1 *task-based laboratory*, whose purpose is to set the guidelines for an educational didactic intervention of prevention of ADHD.
- N. 1 *task-based laboratory*, to design interventions to be performed in the classrooms where the children at risk of ADHD are.
- *Homework*: experimentation of the designed activities in classroom, as a support of the phase of the training addressed to children.
- *Supervision* with/through consulting setting
- As a conclusion, a *questionnaire with restitution*, to detect the perception the teachers have of the changes occurred as a consequence of the training, to the children at risk of ADHD, and the re-application of the assessment tools administered in the first phase (IPDA, IPDDAI).

Finally, the path implies the involvement of the ***family pediatricians***, referring to the children participant in the training, as further "actors" of the monitoring phase of attention, self-regulation and metacognition processes. Therefore, the trainer, together with the pediatrician, will apply a narrative interview on the changes in behaviours occurred to the children identified as at risk of ADHD, at the beginning, in the mid phase and at the end of the treatment.

Attachment 1. The Task-Based Laboratories in Child's Training

The task-based laboratory (Perricone Briulotta, 2011) is a method of working group designed from the perspective of social production and construction. It always implies, in fact, that the group of children is assigned a task concerning the realization of a real product according to the issue tackled by the laboratory.

The epistemological categories of this laboratory are related to

- *communication,* as the possibility to make the children's experiences and the issue of task-laboratory, "interact" with each other;
- *operativity*, as the condition of being able to do;
- *reasoning*, as the possibility of thinking about the path experienced in the laboratory, and about what has been made.

The laboratory consists of three sequential time-phases (i.e. dialogue between yesterday and today; reaction to task; metacognition) that would seem they activate the attention, self-regulation and metacognition processes considered by the training for children at risk of ADHD. To be more precise, it is reported one of the task-based laboratory performed during the second month of the training, and concerning the experience field "*the self and the other*". Such laboratory is focused on civic coexistence among children, and implies the task of making the Identity Cards of Little Red Cap's characters as good citizens of the world. The activities of the three phases are reported, and their connection with the processes, focalised by the training, is highlighted through the symbol (☼).

The trainer, in every phase of the laboratory, has utilised the *self-instruction* to guide children in utilising *self-talk* strategies, a sort of internal dialogue to divide the assigned task into different steps. The following guiding criteria are essential

- giving clear and concise rules, even through graphic exemplification;
- giving the rules with a positive approach rather than negative (e.g. "*you should stay seated while you're making this work*", rather than "*you shouldn't stand up while you are making this work*"), in order to highlight the planned behaviours;
- providing children with immediate feedback about what they are doing;
- praising children after every success of theirs;
- both praises and likely reproaches are to be made calling the child by his/her name, clarifying him/her to which behaviour is related.

Time-Phase 1 – Dialogue between Yesterday and Today (A)

During this time-phase, the connection between children's experiences with "civic coexistence" issue is fostered.

A1) The *Secret diary*: the trainer says: "*Now, let's try to pretend we open our own secret diaries; I'll start first and I'll show you how to do*(the trainer will close his/her eyes and put his/her hands at his/her head as if s/he is concentrating, then, still with his/her closed eyes, s/he will open his/her hands pretending to open a lined notebook and s/he will write with his/her fingers on it). "*Now, it's your turn. Try to do the same, please. After opening your diary, write what comes to your mind, thinking about a good citizen of the world, but don't forget! Don't tell anybody what you have written on your diary, it's a secret! When you finish, close your diary with your hands* (the trainer will show them how to do) *and save it wherever you like. For example, I want to hide mine in my pocket... please, watch how I'm doing it*".

☼ The activity of the Secret Diary, besides putting children in contact with the issue at emotional and affective levels, also involves processes of concentration, which imply a mental effort and the ability of self-regulating (e.g. keeping on staying seated or with their eyes closed for a time span decided by the trainer). Selective attention processes are also stimulated through the request of focusing on a specific issue, as well as memory processes that are useful for collecting information about the issue. Moreover, the utilization of mental images as a training of the mind, minimizes the tendency to impulsivity, and fosters the metacognitive sensitiveness.

A2) *Narration about the path*

In order to show the children the path they will follow and collect similar experiences, already made by other children before them, the trainer says: "*I'm sure, each of you have, at least once, tried to tell something new about a character of a fairy tale, adding details or removing others, beginning from physical characteristics and clothes, up to creating new actions, behaviours and stories, and adding characters. I'll show you how* (the trainer will go to the blackboard with a coloured chalk and draw Little Red Cap). *Look! I have drawn Little Red Cap, but if I cancelled the hood, like this, the girl could be her mother or another girl... What would you do? Do you remember a situation when you have done something similar?* (the trainer let the children speak and verbally underline what each child has said) *Today we're going to pretend to be the Delegates of the Mayor of a city of Fableland. As delegates we will have to sign the new Identity cards of the characters of the Little Red Cap fairy tale, who we are going to transform into good citizens of the world. This is our today's task".*

☼ This activity tells children in advance the path they are going to follow and recall to their mind personal experiences that could be related to. Their focus on the issue is constantly stimulated, and the selective attention is driven to the task, together with the motivation to accomplish it. Moreover, focusing on the task encourages concentration and self-regulation, in fact the children are invited to observe the times and steps proposed by the trainer.

A3) *Activation of the stimulus*

The trainer asks the children: "*Do you know who is the Mayor of a city, and what does he do? Raise your hand in turn to answer me, please*". After the children have answered, the trainer highlights that the Mayor is who guarantees the functioning of the city and all of its services; he gets the people to respect laws and rules; recognizes and guarantees the identity of each person by signing his/her Identity card where some personal information are fixed (name, residence, marital status, occupation, citizenship, etc.).

The trainer shows the children, as a stimulus, an A3 paper reproducing an Identity card, saying: " *Look at this Identity Card... it is just like the card you, as delegates of the Mayor, will have to create for each of the character of the Little Red Cap fairy tale. The likely behaviours, emotions, attitudes that can make each character a good citizen, will have to be written on this card*".

☼ This activity provides children with materials and information about both the issue and task. It tries further to motivate them to accomplish the task, producing the final product and guides them during the process of problem solving useful for making the product.

Time-Phase 2 – Task Response (B)

B1) Task motivation

The trainer shows to the children images as metaphors because they allow to say why it is important to make the new Identity cards of the characters of the fairy tale.

The images-metaphors are

- a magnifying glass: to watch closely/to fix aspects and determine new characteristics;
- a metre: to measure and compare/a measure to make clear how a good citizen has to behave;
- a compass: to understand how to rewrite the story of Little Red Cap in terms of citizenship.

The trainer says: "*Each of you, choose only one from these three images that helps you to say why the today's task is useful. I will choose the magnifying glass, for instance, because, in my opinion, an Identity Card allows me to know better every characteristics of a person. Now, before choosing, let's see what these images tell us, so you will choose better*".

Then, the trainer explains the meanings of the three metaphors, repeating them more times to get children to understand and memorize them.

Each child, after choosing, draws the image of the chosen metaphor on a paper. The trainer collects all the papers; he praises the children for what they have done and underlines the kind of choices of the group.

☼ This activity is aimed to encourage in the children a higher awareness about the utility of the task; it allows further to motivate the children to accomplish the task, producing the final product, and it guides them during the process of problem solving useful for making the product.

B2) *Task analysis*

The trainer says: "*Now we have to think about every important thing we need to do for making the Identity Card of the characters of Little Red Cap. For this reason I'll show you some important things that are in all Identity cards.*" Now, the children, in turn,

The trainer shows a board where an Identity Card is replicated, reading the contents (i.e. name, age, address, etc.) Now, the children in turn, detect other possible elements to be added in the Identity Card and written on the board. The silhouettes of the characters of Little Red Cap are shown to the children who, in turn, say what are the specific characteristics concerning age, sex, nationality, the actions that make them good citizens and the kind of signature, which will be added to the Identity cards. Every idea will be written on the board and, every time, the trainer will praise the child for his/her intervention. The children, who are not able to observe their turn, will be asked to do properly and will be also provided with further practical examples.

☼ This activity where the children hypothesise some criteria to accomplish the task, activates processes of problem solving and memory as the recalling of images, experiences concerning the issue of the task. It also activates processes of orientation, with respect to the realization of the product, which would foster the self-control in managing the task.

B3) Task planning

The trainer ask the children to choose, for each character, the characteristics that they think they are the most important among those they have said and written on the board. Therefore, he says: "*You have said a lot of things about what can be written on the Identity Card of Little Red Cap, concerning the actions that would make her a good citizen. Yet, some of these actions are more important than others, so let's choose which ones we think are the most important to be written on the Identity Card. Each of you, raise your hand before speaking and wait your turn, please*". The choices are made for each character and are written on the board. The trainer now tell the children that, to have a good product, they have to work first on the aesthetic aspect of the Identity Card, therefore he shows some possible materials (colours, coloured boards, fabrics, cardboards, etc.). The children decide, all together, which materials are to be utilised for each character.

☼ This activity encourages processes of problem solving in respect of the choices to be made, in order to accomplish the task. It also stimulates the metacognitive sensitiveness, since the children retrieve what they have already done in the early phase, and utilise such information to make assessment and make a selection. Moreover, this activity starts processes of foreseeing, in terms of mental imagination of the product and the ability of self-regulating with respect of the accomplishment of it.

B4) *Task accomplishment*

The children are divided in five subgroups. Each group is given the task to make the Identity Card of a specific character of the fairy tale. The children are divided in five subgroups to which is is given the task to make the Identity Card of a specific character of the fairy tale. To accomplish it, they are provided with some materials such as white paper, the specific silhouette of the character chosen, and other materials to embellish the silhouette (e.g. colours, glue, scissors, paper for collage, etc.). When the groups have realise their products, a gallery of all the Identity cards is organized after taking a photo of them.

☼ This activity, which implies the creation of a product by subgroups, activates processes of self-regulation and self-control, in terms of observation of rules and self-management in respect of the task given.

Time-Phase 3 – Metacognition (C)

C1 Metacognition of the product

The trainer says: "Today we pretended we were the delegates of the Mayor; we provided the characters of Little Red Cap with new Identity Cards as good citizens, but how difficult was it? Let's tell us by using a number from 1 up to 3 (1 little, 2 much, 3 very much). The trainer gives an example "It was much difficult for me, so I'll choose the number 2 and I'll write it on this sheet" then he says: "and how useful could be that? Let's tell us by using a number from 1 up to 3 (1 little, 2 much, 3 very much). Everything will be recorded on the board. Everything will be recorded on the board.

C2 Metacognition of the path

The children will record their work on their personal worksheet.

☼ This activity starts processes of analysis; assessment about difficulties and strong points of the task; metacognitive sensitiveness, in terms of considering about, and self-assessing their own behaviours during the experienced path.

REFERENCES

Allin, M., Henderson, M., and Suckling, J. (2004). Effects of very low birth weight on brain structure in adulthood. *Developmental Medicine & Child Neurology*, 46, 46–53.

Als, H., Gilkerson, L., Duffy, F.H., Mcanulty, G.B., Buehler, D.M., Vendenberg, K., Sweet, N., Sell, E., Parad, R.B., Ringer, S.A., Butler, S.C., Blickman, J.G., and Jones, K.J. (2003). A three-center, randomized, controlled trial of individualized developmental care for very low birth weight preterm infants: medical, neurodevelopmental, parenting, and caregiving effects. *Developmental and Behavioral Pediatrics*, 24, 399-408.

American Psychiatric Association. – A.P.A. (1994). *Diagnostic and Statistical Manual of Mental Disorders*, 4th edn, DSM IV. Washington: American Psychiatric Association.

Anderson, P. J., & Doyle, L. (2004). Executive functioning in school-aged children who were born very preterm or with extremely low birth weight. *Pediatrics*, 114, 50–57.

Atkinson, R. (2002). *Intervista narrativa, raccontare la storia di sé nella ricerca formativa, organizzativa e sociale.* Milano: Raffaello Cortina Editore.

Aylward, G.P. (2005). Neurodevelopmental outcomes of infants born prematurely. *Journal of Developmental and Behavioral Pediatrics*, 26, 427–440.

Baldini, L. (2009). Psicologia Pediatrica. Padova: Italia Piccin Nuova Libraria SPA.

Barkley, R.A. (1990). *Attention Deficit Hyperactivity Disorder: a Handbook for Diagnosis and Treatment*, New York: Guilford Press

Barkley, R.A. (1997). *Defiant Children: a Clinician's Manual for Assessment and Parent Training,* 2nd Edn. New York: Guilford Press

Befera, M. S., & Barkley, R. A. (1985). Hyperactive and normal girls and boys: mother–child interaction, parent psychiatric status and child psychopathology. *Journal of Child Psychology and Psychiatry,* 26, 439–452.

Bhutta, A.T., Cleves, M.A., Casey, P.H., Cradock, M.M., and Anand, K.J. (2002). Cognitive and behavioural outcomes of school-aged children who were born preterm: A meta-analysis. *JAMA,* 288, 728–737.

Block, J. (1978). *The Q-Sort method in personality assessment and Psychiatric Research*, Palo Alto. Consulting Psychological Press

Braswell, L., & Bloomquist, M.L. (1991). *Cognitive Behavioral Therapy with ADHD Children*. New York: Guilford Press.

Byrne, S.M., Bawden, H.N., Beattie, T.L., and De Wolfe, N.A. (2000). Preschoolers classified as having attention-deficit hyperactivity disorder (ADHD): DSM-IV symptom endorsement patterns. *Journal of Child Neurology*, 15 (8), 533-538.

Cherkes-Julkowski, M. (1998). Learning disability, attention deficit disorder and language impairment as outcomes of prematurity: A longitudinal descriptive study. *Journal of Learning Disabilities*, 31, 294–306.

Chiarenza, G.A., Bianchi, E., and Marzocchi, G.M. (2006). Le linee guida SINPIA per il trattamento cognitivo-comportamentale del DDAI. *Disturbi di attenzione e iperattività*, 1 (2), 177-194.

Chyi, L.J., Lee, H.C., Hintz, S.R., Gould, J.B., and Sutcliffe, T.L. (2008). School outcomes of late preterm infants: special needs and challenges for infants born at 32 to 36 weeks gestation. *J Pediatr.*, 153(1), 25–31.

Clark, C.A., Woodward, L.J., Horwood, L.J., and Moor, S. (2008). Development of Emotional and Behavioural Regulation in Children Born Extremely Preterm and Very Preterm: Biological and Social Influences. *Child Development*, 79, (5), 1444 – 1462.

Conners, C.K., Epstein, J.N., March, J.S., Angold, A., Wells, K.C., Klaric, J., Swanson, J.M., Abikoff, H.B., Arnold, L.E., Elliott, G.R., Greenhill, L.L., Hechtman, L., Hinshaw, S.P., Hoza, B., Jensen, P.S., Kraemer, H.C., Newcorn, J., Pelham, W.E., Severe, J.B., Vitiello, B., & Wigal, T. (2001). Multimodal treatment of ADHD in the MTA: an alternative analysis. *Journal of the American Academy of Child and Adolescent Psychiatry*, 40, 159-167.

Consensus Conference. (2003). *Indicazioni e strategie terapeutiche per i bambini e gli adolescenti con disturbo da deficit attentivo e iperattività*, Cagliari, 6-7 Marzo, Retrieved from http://www.aidaiassociazione.com/documents/consensusADHDita-pdf.

Cornoldi, C., De Beni, R., and Gruppo MT (2002). *Imparare a studiare – 2.* Trento: Erickson

Curatolo, P., D'Agati, E., and Moavero, R. (2010). The neurobiological basis of ADHD. *Italian Journal of Pediatrics*, 36:79. doi:10.1186/1824-7288-36-79

Daley, D. (2006). Attention deficit hyperactivity disorder: a review of the essential facts. *Child: Care, Health & Development*, 32 (2), 193–204.

Delobel-Ayoub, M., Arnaud, C., White-Koning, M., Casper, C., Pierrat, V., Garel, M., Burguet, A., Roze, J.C., Matis, J., Picaud, J.C., Kaminski, M., and Larroque, B. (2009). Behavioural problems and cognitive performance at 5 years of age after very preterm birth: the EPIPAGE Study. *Pediatrics*, 123(6), 1485-1492.

Egeland, B., Kalkoske, M., Gottesman, N. E., and Erickson, M.F. (1990). Preschool behaviour problems: Stability and factors accounting for change. *Journal of Child Psychology and Psychiatry,* 31 (6), 891-909.

Espy, K.A., Senn, T.E., Charack, D.A., Tyler, J., and Wieber, S. (2007). Perinatal pH and Neuropsychological Outcomes at Age 3 Years in Children Born Preterm: An Exploratory Study. *Developmental Neuropsychology*, 32(2), 669–682.

Foulder-Hughes, L.A., & Cooke, R.W. (2003). Motor, cognitive, and behavioural disorders in children born very preterm. *Dev Med Child Neurol.*, 45, 97–103.

Gillberg, C. (2003). Deficits in attention, motor control, and perception: a brief review. *Archives of Disease in Childhood*, 88, 904–910.

Hack, M., Taylor, H.G., Schluchter, M., Andreias, L., Drotar, D., and Klein, N. (2009). Behavioural outcomes of extremely low birth weight children at age 8 years. *J. Dev. Behav. Pediatr.*, 30, 122-130.

Heinonen, K., Räikkönen, K., Pesonen, Anu-K., Andersson, S., Kajantie, E., Eriksson, J.G., Wolke, D., and Lano, A. (2010). Behavioural symptoms of attention deficit/hyperactivity disorder in preterm and term children born small and appropriate for gestational age: A longitudinal study. *Pediatrics*, 10:91.

Hemgren, E., & Persson, K. (2006). Associations of motor co-ordination and attention with motor-perceptual development in 3-year-old preterm and full-term children who needed neonatal intensive care. *Child: care, health and development*, 33(1), 11–21.

Horn, W.F., Ialongo, N.S., Pascoe, J.M., Greenberg, G., Packard, T., Lopez, M., Wagner, M. and Puttler, L. (1991). Additive effects of psychostimulants, parent training and self-control therapy with ADHD children. *Journal of the American Academy of Child and Adolescent Psychiatry*, 30, 233-240.

Huddy, C.L.J., Johnson, A., and Hope, P.L. (2001). Educational and behavioral problems in babies of 32–35 weeks gestation. *Arch. Dis. Child. Fetal. Neonatal. Ed.*, 85(1): F23–F28.

Inder, T.E., Warfield, S.K., Wang, H., Huppi, P.S., and Volpe, J.J. (2005). Abnormal cerebral structure is present at term in premature infants. *Pediatrics*, 115, 286–294.

Kendall, P.C., & Braswell, L. (1985). *Cognitive-Behavioral Therapy for Impulsive Children.* New York: Guilford Press.

Kinney, H.C. (2006). The near-term (late preterm) human brain and risk for periventricular leukomalacia: a review. *Semin Perinatol.*, 30(2), 81– 88.

Kirby, E., & Grimley, L. (1986). *Understanding and treating attention deficit disorder,* USA: Pergamon Books. trad. It. (1989). *Disturbi dell'attenzione e iperattività.* Trento: Edizioni Erickson.

Krain, A.L., & Castellanos, F.X. (2006). Brain development and ADHD. *Clin Psychol Rev.,* 26, 433-444.

Lawson, K.R., & Ruff, H.A. (2004). Early focused attention predicts outcome for children born prematurely, *J Dev Behav Pediatr.*, 25(6), 399-406.

Marcotto, E., Paltenghi, B., and Cornoldi, C. (2002), La scala IPDDAI: contributo per la costruzione di uno strumento per l'identificazione precoce del disturbo da deficit di attenzione e/o iperattività. *Difficoltà di apprendimento*, 8 (2), 153-172.

McCormick, M., Gortmaker, S., and Sobol, A. (1990). Very low birth weight children: Behaviour problems and school difficulty in a national sample. *The Journal of Pediatrics*, 117, 688–693.

McGrath, M.M., & Sullivan, M.C. (2002). Neonatal morbidities and cumulative risk and school age outcomes. *Comprehensive Issues in Pediatric Nursing*, 45, 104–112.

McGrath, M.M., Sullivan, M., Devin, J., Fontes-Murphy, M., Barcelos, S., DePalma, J.L., and Faraone, S. (2005). Early precursors of low attention and hyperactivity in a preterm sample at age four. *Issues in Comprehensive Pediatric Nursing*, 28, 1–15.

Ministero della Pubblica Istruzione (2007). *Indicazioni per il curricolo per la scuola dell'infanzia e il primo ciclo d'istruzione*, Retrieved from: www.pubblica.istruzione.it.

National Institutes of Health (NIH) - Consensus Development Conference Statement. November 16-18. (1998). *Diagnosis and Treatment of Attention Deficit Hyperactivity Disorder.*16(2):1-37. Retrieved from http://consensus.nih.gov/1998/1998AttentionDeficit HyperactivityDisorder110html.

O'Keeffe, M.J., O'Callaghan, M., Williams, G.M., Najmanm J.M., and Bor, W. (2003). Learning, cognitive and attentional problems in adolescents born small for gestational age. *Pediatrics*, 112, 301-307.

Perricone Briulotta, G. (2003). *Agire l'osservazione. Modelli e percorsi.* Milano: McGraw Hill.

Perricone Briulotta, G. (2005). *Manuale di Psicologia dell'Educazione. Una prospettiva ecologica per lo studio e l'intervento sul processo educativo.* Milano: Mc Graw-Hill.

Perricone Briulotta, G. (2011). *Una giostra per la formazione. Modelli e metodologie nei Piani Operativi Nazionali della Scuola*, Milano: Franco Angeli

Perricone, G., Morales, M.R., (2009). *Madri in corsia. La competenza genitoriale nell'ospedalizzazione pediatrica.* Roma: Carocci.

Perricone, G., Scimeca, G. P., and Maugeri R. (2004). La nascita pretermine nell'ottica del "to care". *Età evolutiva*, 78, 85-92.

Peterson, B.S., Anderson, A.W., Ehrenkranz, R., Staib, L.H., Tageldin, M., Colson, E., Gore, J.C., Duncan, C.C., Makuch, R., and Ment, L.R. (2003). Regional brain volumes and their later neurodevelopmental correlates in term and preterm infants. *Pediatrics,* 111 (5), 939–948.

Polizzi, C., & Morales, M.R. (2008). *I costrutti di rappresentazione dei genitori nell'ospedalizzazione pediatrica*, in Perricone, G., Di Maio, M.T., and Nuccio, F.R. (a cura di), *Raccontando Aladino…Vincoli e possibilità del lavoro psico-socio-educativo in pediatria*, Milano: Franco Angeli (pp. 224-246).

Riello, M., Re, A.M., and Cornoldi, C. (2005). Costruzione di uno strumento rivolto alla famiglia per l'identificazione precoce del DDAI. *Disturbi di attenzione e iperattività,* 1 (1), 9-26.

Roberts, M.C., La Greca, A.M., and Harper, D.C. (1988). Journal of Pediatric Psychology: Another stage of development. *Journal of Pediatric Psychology*, 13, 1-5.

Saigal, S., den Ouden, L., and Wolke, D. (2003). School age outcomes in children who were extremely low birth weight from four international population-based cohorts. *Pediatrics*, 112, 943–950.

Sansavini, A., Guarini, A., Ruffilli, F., Alessandrini, R., Giovanelli, G., and Salvioli, G.P. (2004). Fattori di rischio associati alla nascita pretermine e prime competenze linguistiche rilevate con il MacArthur. *Psicologia Clinica dello Sviluppo*, 1, 47-67.

Shum, D., Neulinger, K., O'Callaghan, M., and Mohay, H., (2008). Attentional problems in children born very preterm or with extremely low birth weight at 7-9 years. *Arch Clin Neuropsychol.*, 23(1), 103-112.

Spirito, A., Brown, R., D'Angelo, E., Delameter, A., Rodrique, J., and Siegel, L. (2003). Society of Pediatric Psychology Task Force Report: Recommendations for the training of pediatric psychologists. *Journal of Pediatric Psychology*, 28, 85-98.

Stephenson, W. (1953). *The study of Behavior: Q-tecnique and its methodology.* Chicago: Chicago University Press.

Stoelhorst, G.M., Martens, S.E., Rijken, M., van Zwieten, PH., Zwinderman, A.H., Wit, J.M., Veen, S. and Leiden Follow-Up Project on Prematurity, (2003). Behaviour at 2 years of age in very preterm infants (gestational age < 32 weeks). *Acta Paediatr.*, 92, 595–601.

Strang-Karlsson, S., Raikkonen, K., Pesonen, A.K., Kajantie, E., Paavonen, E.J., Lahti, J., Hovi, P., Heinonen, K., Jarvenpaa, A.L., Eriksson, J.G., and Andersson, S., (2008). Very low birth weight and behavioral symptoms of attention deficit hyperactivity disorder in young adulthood: the Helsinki study of very-low-birth-weight adults. *Am J Psychiatry*, 165, 1345-1353.

Taylor, H., Klein, N., Munich, N., and Hack, M. (2000). Middle school-age outcomes in children with very low birth weight. *Child Development*, 71, 1495–1511.

Tenuta, F. (2007), *Il bambino prematuro: programmi di intervento e di sostegno psicologico.* Roma: Carocci Faber.

Terreni, A., Tretti, M.L., Corcella, P.R., Cornoldi, C., and Tressoldi, P.E. (2002). *IPDA. Questionario Osservativo per l'identificazione precoce delle difficoltà di apprendimento.* Trento: Erickson.

Theunissen, N.C.M., Veen, S., Fekkes, M., Koopman, H.M., Zwinderman, K.A.H., Brugman, E., and Wit, J. (2001). Quality of life in preschool children born preterm. *Developmental Medicine & Child Neurology*, 43, 460-465.

van Baar, A.L., Vermaas, J., Knots, E., de Kleine, M.J., and Soons, P. (2009). Functioning at school age of moderately preterm children born at 32 to 36 weeks' gestational age. *Pediatrics,* 124(1), 251-257.

INDEX

A

B

D

E

F

G

J

K

L

M

N

O

P

Q

R

S

T

U

V

W

Z